AF386343

Low-Dose Radiation Effects on Animals and Ecosystems II

Manabu Fukumoto
Editor

Low-Dose Radiation Effects on Animals and Ecosystems II

15 Years after the Fukushima Nuclear Accident

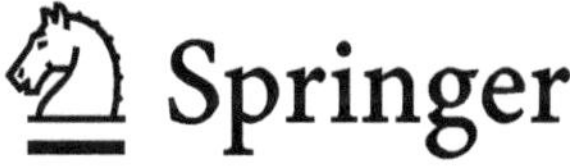 Springer

Editor
Manabu Fukumoto
International Research Institute of Disaster Science
Tohoku University
Sendai, Japan

ISBN 978-981-95-5558-1   ISBN 978-981-95-5559-8   (eBook)
https://doi.org/10.1007/978-981-95-5559-8

This book is an open access publication.

This Springer imprint is published by the registered company Springer Nature Singapore Pte Ltd.
The registered company address is: 152 Beach Road, #21-01/04 Gateway East, Singapore 189721, Singapore

If disposing of this product, please recycle the paper.

Foreword

An unprecedented crisis facing humanity is not something that occurs frequently, nor does it recur within a short period of time. Consequently, scientifically elucidating such a phenomenon and accurately assessing its impact is extremely difficult and requires careful and sustained consideration. The accident at the Fukushima Daiichi Nuclear Power Plant (FNPP) following the Great East Japan Earthquake in March 2011 stands as a paradigmatic example. As with the Chernobyl nuclear accident, this disaster had devastating effects not only on people living in radioactively contaminated areas but also on the animals and plants inhabiting those environments. Immediately after the accident, the authors of this book launched the Comprehensive dose evaluation project concerning animals affected by the FNPP accident (the Affected Animal Project). Through this initiative, they collected samples from contaminated livestock and euthanized wild Japanese macaques, establishing a systematic archive of radiation-related biological materials and contributing to the advancement of radiation protection research. Following the accident, residents within a 20-kilometer radius of the plant were evacuated. Although a significant increase in the incidence of pediatric thyroid cancer was reported during the first five years after the accident, the overall impact of contamination was later considered to have gradually diminished. Nevertheless, radioactive contamination of the environment and wildlife persists even today. Japanese macaques, which are phylogenetically close to humans, are particularly important subjects for comparison, as they have been continuously exposed to radioactive contamination. Based on my long-term research on the social ecology of Japanese macaques, I anticipate that the effects extend beyond internal physiological changes to encompass their ecology, social organization, and behavior. In 2020, the authors published a report documenting conditions up to seven years after the accident, entitled Low-Dose Radiation Effects on Animals and Ecosystems. The present volume is its sequel—a groundbreaking work that reveals the state of radioactive contamination in nonhuman animals 14 years after the accident. I encourage readers to engage with this book in order to deepen their understanding of what actually occurred in living organisms and ecosystems as a result of this unprecedented catastrophe, and how its effects are likely to continue unfolding. As the authors demonstrate, the biological effects of radioactive materials released during a nuclear reactor accident cannot be attributed solely to external radiation exposure; rather, they involve extremely complex processes. Long-term analyses based on continuous sampling of wildlife are indispensable for advancing our understanding of these phenomena. This book also highlights two important reasons for studying the effects of radioactive contamination on non-human animals. First, the ability to predict the biological consequences of radiation exposure will become increasingly crucial as humanity embarks on future space exploration. Second, it underscores a critical insight: while protecting nature from disasters ultimately helps protect people, protecting people does not necessarily ensure the protection of nature. This work offers a valuable opportunity to reflect deeply on how we should confront the future before us, including the large-scale, human-made disasters—such as the FNPP accident—that are likely to occur again. What concerns me is that in recent years, the perceived impact of the FNPP accident has diminished, resulting in reduced media attention and a tendency for research funding to be curtailed. Yet this research bears significance not only for Japan's future but for that of the entire planet. We sincerely hope that the authors' invaluable work will continue, and we look forward to the publication of a new report in the coming years, enriched by further discoveries.

Director, Research Institute for Humanity and Nature,   Juichi Yamagiwa
Former President, Kyoto University
Kyoto, Japan

Foreword

Fifteen years after the Fukushima Daiichi Nuclear Power Plant (FNPP) accident, ongoing evaluation of the impact of the accident is necessary since radiation effects are both instantaneous and also evolve over time. In the book *Low-Dose Radiation Effects on Animals and Ecosystems II*, Professor Fukumoto of Tohoku University presents updated research on biological and ecological impacts, including actual and predicted doses in heavily affected areas. Studies on wild macaques offer insight into potential human effects, while research on butterflies, fish, domestic animals, and cellular responses to ^{137}Cs microparticles expands understanding of ecosystem impacts. This book is relevant for the radiation accident community and the global radiation field, and serves as a resource for courses in radiation effects and ecology, as well as those in radiation protection.

As the world continues to grapple with the long-term consequences of nuclear accidents, the need for rigorous scientific inquiry has never been greater. This volume not only synthesizes cutting-edge data but also encourages interdisciplinary collaboration, fostering a deeper appreciation for both the complexity and resilience of affected ecosystems. Readers will find comprehensive analyses that illuminate the subtle yet significant ways in which low-dose radiation shapes biological processes, emphasizing the importance of vigilance in environmental monitoring and public health policy. The book stands as a testament to the dedication of researchers committed to advancing our understanding and guiding informed decisions for future generations.

The FNPP accident has served as a catalyst for renewed global focus on the effects of low-dose radiation, not just on immediate human populations but on entire ecosystems that form the backbone of environmental stability. Professor Fukumoto's research highlights the intricate connections between organisms and their surroundings, demonstrating how even minimal radiation exposures can ripple through food webs and alter species interactions over time. The inclusion of wild macaque studies is particularly compelling, as these animals share physiological similarities with humans, allowing researchers to extrapolate findings and anticipate possible health outcomes in human communities. By examining changes in blood chemistry, immune function, and reproductive success among affected macaque populations, the book paints a nuanced picture of biological adaptation and vulnerability in the face of contamination.

Furthermore, the exploration of radiation effects on butterflies and fish underscores the importance of biodiversity in ecosystem resilience. Butterflies, as sensitive bioindicators, reveal how radiation can impact genetic diversity and population dynamics, while studies of fish provide insight into aquatic ecosystem health and the movement of radioactive elements through water systems. The analysis of cellular responses to ^{137}Cs microparticles adds another layer of understanding, shedding light on sublethal effects that may accumulate over months or years, potentially influencing long-term survival and reproductive success across species.

This book is not merely a scientific compendium; it is a guide for policymakers, educators, and environmental stewards. By integrating findings from field observations, laboratory experiments, and predictive modeling, the volume equips readers with the knowledge needed to assess risk and implement effective radiation protection measures. Students and practitioners alike will benefit from its accessible yet comprehensive approach, making it a valuable addition to academic curricula and professional development in radiation safety and ecological management.

In summary, *Low-Dose Radiation Effects on Animals and Ecosystems II* offers a vital resource for understanding the subtle interplay between radiation and living systems. Through meticulous research and clear presentation, it advances the global conversation on nuclear safety, ecological integrity, and the collective responsibility to safeguard our planet for future generations. The insights presented in this book will inspire continued vigilance and innovation in responding to the ongoing challenges posed by nuclear accidents.

Professor, Northwestern University
Evanston, IL, USA

Gayle E. Woloschak

Preface

Nearly 15 years have passed since the Fukushima Daiichi Nuclear Power Plant (FNPP) accident. With approximately half of the 30-year half-life of cesium-137 (^{137}Cs) having elapsed, fieldwork research into the biological effects of the FNPP accident is thought to be at a major turning point. In Fukushima, decontamination and reconstruction efforts are progressing, and the areas contaminated with high levels of radioactive materials are steadily decreasing. However, ^{137}Cs remains present in the environment surrounding FNPP, continuing to contaminate flora and fauna. The previous book, *Low-Dose Radiation Effects on Animals and Ecosystems*, published 6 years ago, summarized the environmental contamination caused by radioactive materials and its impacts over the 8 years following the accident. This book is a sequel that adds new findings, including analysis results of wild Japanese macaques, primates with a genome structure very similar to humans. The FNPP accident is gradually fading from the memories of people around the world. However, with Russia's invasion of Ukraine and North Korea's nuclear missile program, concerns are growing about the future impact on the environment and human health from radioactive contamination caused by nuclear reactor attacks and atomic bombs. As a reflection of this social current, an illustrative example is the awarding of the Nobel Peace Prize for 2024 to Nihon Hidankyo (the Japan Confederation of A-and H-Bomb Sufferers Organizations). To achieve the extremely challenging goal of understanding the effects of sustained low-dose-rate radiation exposure on ecosystems and humans, we have been conducting ongoing study into the impact of the FNPP accident on animals. We believe that a scientifically accurate description of the ecological impacts of the accident, as we currently understand them, is essential for considering what steps should be taken to further our ongoing research, and will be beneficial for future generations.

We hope that this book will serve as a catalyst to rekindle people's interest in the biological effects of radioactive accidents.

<table>
<tr><td>Professor Emeritus, Tohoku University
Sendai and Tokyo, Japan</td><td>Manabu Fukumoto</td></tr>
</table>

Contents

Chapter 1
The Comprehensive Dose Evaluation Project Concerning Animals Affected by the Fukushima Daiichi Nuclear Power Plant Accident (Affected Animal Project): Fieldwork to Find Out What Happened and What Will Happen

Manabu Fukumoto

Abstract On April 22, 2011, 1 month and 11 days after the Fukushima Daiichi Nuclear Power Plant (FNPP) accident, the ex-evacuation zone was set within a 20-km radius of the plant. The livestock abandoned and wild animals in and around the ex-evacuation zone have been extremely valuable for analyzing the environmental pollution and the biological effects of internal and external exposure to radiation. We have launched "A comprehensive dose evaluation project concernining animals affected by the FNPP accident (Affected Animal Project)" to establish an archive system composed of samples and data from animals around FNPP to deepen our understanding of the biological effects of radiation and to improve protection against radiation. The ultimate goal of this project is to contribute to integrated radiation protection for ecosystems and humans through studies of animals affected by the FNPP accident.

In 2020, we published a book titled *"Low-Dose Radiation Effects on Animals and Ecosystems"* about the status of environmental contamination up to 7 years after the accident and the results obtained from the Affected Animal Project. This book is a sequel to that book and summarizes further findings 15 years after the accident.

Keywords Fukushima Daiichi Nuclear Power Plant (FNPP) accident · Evacuation zone · Animal · Fieldwork · Low-dose/low-dose-rate radiation · Long-term exposure · Thorotrast · Conversion factor

M. Fukumoto (✉)
International Research Institute of Disaster Science, Tohoku University, Sendai, Japan
e-mail: manabu.fukumoto.a8@tohoku.ac.jp

© The Author(s) 2026
M. Fukumoto (ed.), *Low-Dose Radiation Effects on Animals and Ecosystems II*,
https://doi.org/10.1007/978-981-95-5559-8_1

1.1 Introduction

The Fukushima Daiichi Nuclear Power Plant (FNPP) accident, which occurred on March 11, 2011, following the Great East Japan Earthquake, dispersed a large amount of radioactive materials into the environment. Even in Tsukuba, located 170 km southwest of FNPP, the peak amount of radioactive fallout was 100,000 times the usual background level [1, 2] (Fig. 1.1). Therefore, I thought that we would not be surprised if something were to happen in the future, even if not right now.

After the accident, farmers released their livestock from their barns when they were ordered to leave the evacuation zone set up within a 20-km radius of FNPP (ex-evacuation zone). As a result, herds of cattle and pigs flocked to the roads in the towns and villages where people had left, impeding safety there. There were also concerns about the distribution of contaminated meat in the market. Therefore, on May 12, the prime minister ordered the governor of Fukushima Prefecture to euthanize all livestock within the ex-evacuation zone. I thought that euthanizing livestock contaminated with radioactive materials solely for the purpose of disposal was unjustified, and that such livestock should serve to benefit future generations. Our laboratory took the lead in launching the "Comprehensive Dose Assessment Project Concerning Animals Affected by the Fukushima Daiichi Nuclear Power Plant Accident (Affected Animal Project)" [3]. After intense negotiations with the national, prefectural, and municipal governments, permission to enter the

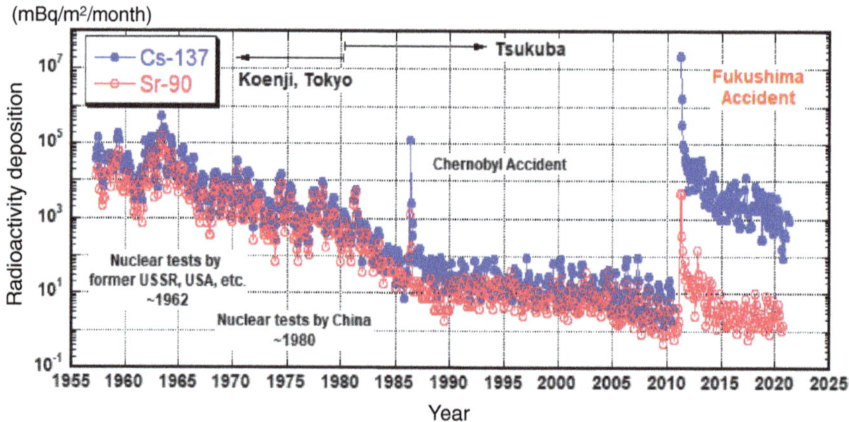

Fig. 1.1 Changes in monthly atmospheric radioactivity deposition at Meteorological Research Institute, Japan (1957-2021). The effect of atmospheric nuclear bomb tests conducted by the United States, the Soviet Union and the United Kingdom can be confirmed from 1957 when records began, until 1963 when the Partial Test Ban Treaty (PTBT) came into force. France and China continued atmospheric nuclear tests until 1974 and 1980, respectively. Since 1981, all nuclear bomb tests have been conducted underground, making additional contamination negligible. Chernobyl (Chornobyl) nuclear accident in 1986 and the FNPP accident in 2011 caused sharp increases and subsequent residual effects (Reproduced from Ref. [1]).

ex-evacuation zone was finally granted, and sampling became possible on August 26, more than 6 months after the accident. The euthanasia of livestock was completed in February 2014, when it was confirmed that no unleashed livestock had been found in the ex-evacuation zone. Accordingly, we have also finished collecting materials from livestock. However, we are still continuing the Affected Animal Project, focusing on compiling the results from the livestock organ archive we have built and collecting materials from euthanized wild Japanese macaques. We reported on the environmental contamination and its biological impacts during the first 7 years after the accident [4]. This book is a sequel to that report, presenting further findings 15 years after the accident.

1.2 The Significance and Characteristics of Fieldwork Revealed Through the Affected Animal Project

The purpose of science is to find the fundamental truth. While truth itself is singular, observed phenomena (facts) vary under different conditions. The scientific method is a framework for uncovering fundamental truths in previously unexplained objects from fragmented experimental and observational information by identifying and validating relationships and laws. The way of thinking must be logically and empirically supported, and systematic. Specifically, the term "scientific" implies that a phenomenon can be quantified and reproduced under identical conditions, and that the results are reliable and verifiable by others. Since biology deals with extremely complex living systems, a biological challenge can only be proven by comparing organisms in which exactly a single condition has been experimentally altered with those in which it has not. However, in many cases, controlled experiments are not feasible from an ethical and economic point of view to resolve issues that are crucial to clarify and understand. In particular, knowledge about the biological effects of radiation exposure can only be obtained from accidents and tragedies, since controlled experiments are not possible. Historically, it is an undeniable that the progress in research on radiation effects and protection has been driven by accumulating data obtained through fieldwork following major disasters including the Hiroshima–Nagasaki atomic bombs and the Chernobyl (Chornobyl) nuclear accident. Fieldwork refers to research activities to obtain objective scientific results through visiting sites where nature has already conducted experiments, directly observing the subject, and collecting data. Nature is fickle and never conducts experiments as we wish. Moreover, it never reproduces exactly the same experiment twice. Each field study is a once-in-a-lifetime experience. Consequently, the scientific value of fieldwork depends on the rigor of preparation, considering all possibilities without preconceptions, and on the ability to act promptly within the limited time available following an event of interest. Flexibility and motivation are especially crucial in the field.

1.3 Project Constituents

A high level of expertise, sustained enthusiasm, and stamina are essential for team members. Since a group of people with versatile expertise and strong scientific perspectives should work together efficiently and without omissions, the leader needs to always clarify the goals and establish a concise and qualified motto that describes the project. In addition, it is essential to hold debriefing meetings after each sampling round to identify problems encountered in the field and to implement necessary improvements.

1.4 Subject of Observation

A significant increase in the incidence of pediatric thyroid cancer began to be observed about 5 years after the Chernobyl (Chornobyl) nuclear accident, which is estimated to have scattered 10 times as much radioactive materials as the FNPP accident [5, 6]. More than 14 years have passed since the FNPP accident. No one is known to have been received extremely high radiation doses as a result of the accident. However, radioactive contamination of the environment and wildlife is still ongoing even in 2026. It remains to be seen whether the level of contamination around FNPP will affect any living organisms. Although some studies suggest that wildlife populations have declined dramatically within the Chornobyl exclusion zone (CEZ), recent evidence suggests that populations of several large mammal species increased within the CEZ during the first decade after the accident. Remote camera surveys conducted within the CEZ found no evidence of suppressed distributions for four mammal species with sufficiently high visitation rates to allow occupancy modeling [7, 8]. If the total radiation dose to animals is related to the effects of radiation, observation throughout the lifespan of medium-sized animals, which have relatively long lifespans of decades, is necessary. Radioactivity itself is a stable property from a physicochemical point of view, as demonstratd by its use in tracer studies. The biological effects of radioactive materials dispersed by a nuclear reactor accident cannot be attributed solely to temporary external exposure to radiation but involve extremely complex, temporally and spatially dynamic processes. Accordingly, careful analysis of each process is desirable (Fig. 1.2).

1.5 Dose Assessment

In analyzing effects of long-term exposure to low-dose-rate radiation, it is essential to identify which exposure condition best explains radiation effects as dependent varible. Independent variables can be combinations of external or internal exposure, or the combined exposure of both, and dose or dose rate. To achieve this, it is necessary to assess both dose rate and duration of exposure as accurately as possible, that is, to know how much radiation each organ was exposed to [9]. The International Commission on Radiological Protection (ICRP) recognized the need for a comprehensive and coherent

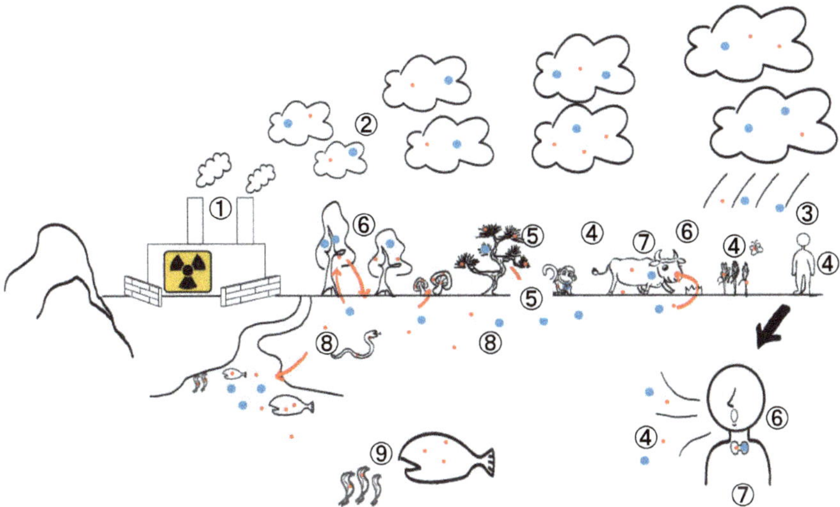

Fig. 1.2 Spread of contamination of the environment and human body due to a radioactive accident. The impact of contamination by radioactive materials from a nuclear accident involves very complex factors and pathways, including the passage of time, necessitating careful analysis at each stage. ① Differences in radiation quality and behavior due to the properties of radioactive materials that have been dispersed. ②The dynamics of the radioactive plume dependent on the particle size of the radioactive material and wind direction. ③ Differences in sedimentation from the plume due to weather. ④ Initial external and internal exposure due to the passage of the plume. ⑤ External exposure from radioactive materials deposited on trees and soil. ⑥ Recontamination due to the circulation of radioactive materials between soil and plants and persistent internal exposure of predators. ⑦ Differences in the distribution of radioactive materials in the body by organ. ⑧ Spread of contamination due to the movement of radioactive materials from the soil surface into the ground. ⑨ Contamination of aquatic organisms due to the transport of radioactive materials from land areas into water systems such as rivers and seawater.

radiological protection framework common to humans and environmental nonhuman organisms. Dosimetry of nonhuman biota exposed to environmental radiation sources is subject to variability in their ecology, morphology, biology, living conditions, and exposure situations. Therefore, the ICRP proposed a set of reference models for practical assessment tasks called Reference Animals and Plants (RAP) and developed dose conversion factors (DCs) to obtain dose per unit intake for internal exposure and dose per unit concentration in environment for external exposure [10, 11]. DC is expressed as (Gy/day)/(Bq/kg) to calculate a simplified dose to the organism under the assumption that radionuclides are uniformly distributed inside or outside the organism. Dose evaluation may further be significantly influenced by the spatial variation of radioactive contamination, the diversity of topography and landscape, and the behavior and vital activities of biota. Correspondingly, the International Atomic Energy Agency (IAEA) has launched a project, "Improving External Dosimetry for Terrestrial Animals and Plants" from 2022 to 2025. The project, in which we are participating, plans to develop a robust probabilistic framework for the assessment of external doses to terrestrial organisms by appropriately quantifying the inherent uncertainties arising from the spatial distribution of radioactivity in the environment, structure and water content of soil,

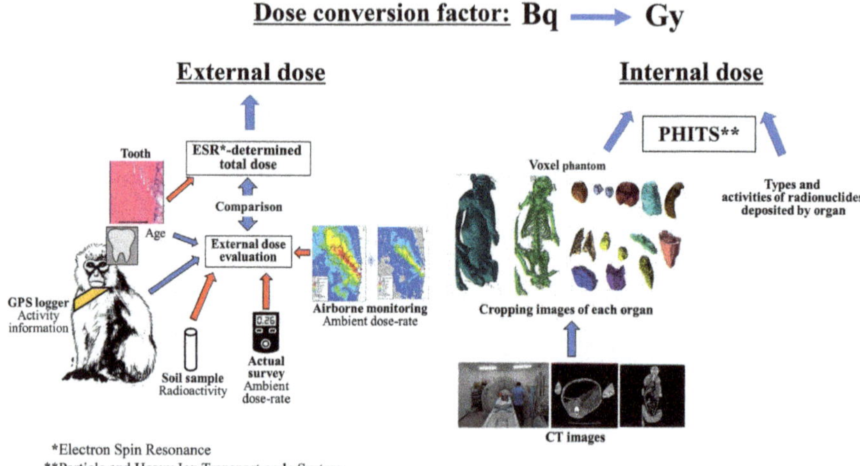

Fig. 1.3 How to standardize dose evaluation. External dose evaluation: Cumulative external dose of individual macaques is measured directly by electron spin resonance (ESR) using tooth enamel [18]. To determine the effective radioactive half-life in the environment, data on long-term changes in soil deposition of radioactive materials and air dose rate in a given area are collected. A glass dosimeter and a GPS logger are attached to a representative macaque from each group, and cumulative dose and behavior are analyzed over a certain period of time. Using the movement range obtained by analyzing the GPS data, radioactivity concentration in soil around the capture site is averaged. Cumulative external dose is calculated using the effective half-life of the ambient dose rate. These data are compared with the ESR dose to establish the optimal external dose evaluation method. Internal dose evaluation: Computed tomography (CT) imaging is performed, reconstructed into a 3D image, and each organ is segmented. The Digital Imaging and Communications in Medicine (DICOM) data of each organ are converted to voxel data. The organ weight is calculated by referring to the number and size of voxels and the tissue density. Dose coefficient for internal exposure of each organ is derived by Monte Carlo simulation using the Particle and Heavy Ion Transport System (PHITS) (Chapter 6 of this book).

vegetation type, terrain, and animal migration routes [12]. We therefore think the IAEA is merely looking at improving the accuracy of external exposure dose evaluation. However, since the Affected Animal Project suggests that dose rate rather than dose, and internal rather than external dose rate, is most relevant to biological effects, we believe that internal dose and dose-rate assessment needs to be refined as well (Fig. 1.3).

1.6   Pitfalls of Fieldwork: Time and Space

Living organisms are influenced by factors such as season, climate, and age. Furthermore, unlike plants, animals move around, making it difficult to standardize conditions for comparison. Several representative lessons learned through the activities of the Affected Animal Project are presented below. We conducted a behavioral study on unleashed cattle that were released after being fitted with Global Positioning System (GPS) devices. They moved within a 500-m radius, and the maximum and

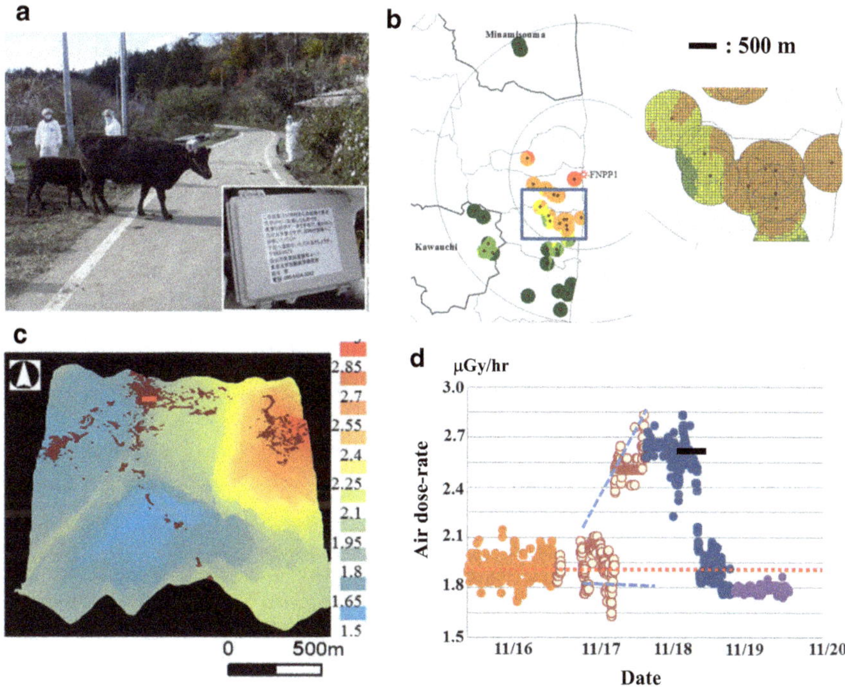

Fig. 1.4 Behavior survey of abandoned cattle and external exposure to radioactive Cs. (**a**) Installing a GPS logger system on the cattle nape (inset) (Kawauchi Village, between November 16 and 20, 2011). (**b**) Cattle moving around within a 500-m radius. (**c**) Overlaying behavioral area of cattle on the contamination map of radioactive Cs using a geographic information system. (**d**) Showing temporal change of external exposure dose rate obtained by cattle behavioral survey. Dose rate ranged from 1.63 to 2.85 μGy/h (mean: 2.21 μGy/h). External dose rate at the site where the cattle were captured was 1.9 μGy/h.

minimum air dose rates within this range differed by a factor of 2.5 (Fig. 1.4). To assess external radiation dose, the time spent at key points within the area must be taken into account. While fieldwork tells us what happened in the period between the time of the incident and that of the sample collection, we also have to consider the aging of the individuals. The count of γH2AX in peripheral lymphocytes of cattle, which reflects the number of DNA double-strand breaks, increases with age but decreases with long-term exposure [13]. At high altitudes, reduced oxygen concentration affects erythrocyte production. Therefore, when examining the effect of radiation on hematopoietic cells, it is preferable to investigate the relationship with radiation dose within the exposed group rather than comparing it to unexposed groups at different altitudes [14]. Animals in nature usually have reproductive (breeding) and nonreproductive (nonbreeding) seasons. It is known that not only testis size but also the expression of 2,000 genes related to various functions differ significantly between these two seasons, including those involved in spermatogenesis and supporting the reproductive system [15]. Therefore, comparisons between affected and unaffected control animals should be seasonally matched (Fig. 1.5).

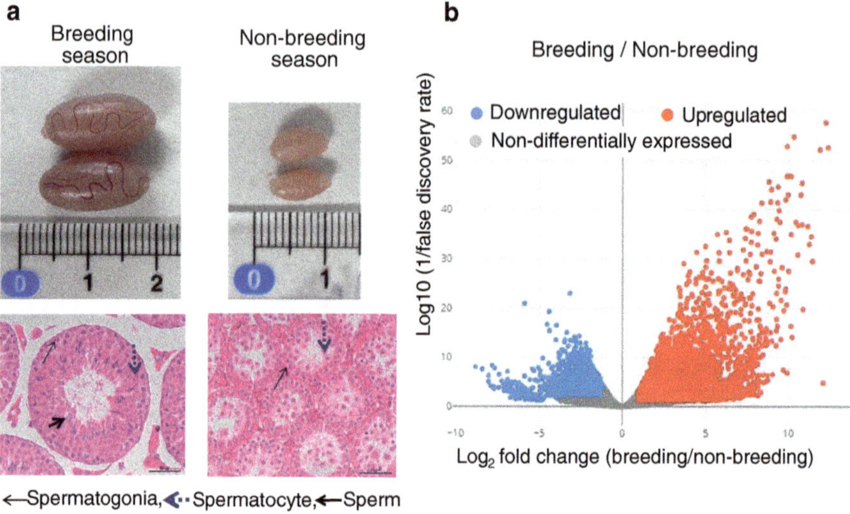

Fig. 1.5 Seasonal changes in Japanese wood mouse (*Apodemus speciosus*) testes. They have generally two breeding seasons per year, spring and autumn. (**a**) During the breeding season (*left*), spermatogenesis is observed, and the size and weight of the testes, and the diameter of the seminiferous tubules are significantly larger than those during the nonbreeding season (*right*) when spermatogenesis ceases. (**b**) The volcano plot shows that more genes are significantly upregulated than downregulated during the breeding season (Images are provided by courtesy of Prof. H Yamashiro and volcano plot reproduced from Ref. 15).

1.7 Future Prospects of the Affected Animal Project

With the aim of analyzing the human and biological effects of radiation in an ethically and economically rational and scientific manner, efforts are being made to consolidate information in databases and archives of epidemiology and animal experiments conducted to date [16]. Thorotrast, which is no longer in use, was a vascular contrast medium made of thorium dioxide that emits α-particles. After being administered to humans, most of Thorotrast accumulated in the liver, causing liver cancer decades later due to internal radiation exposure. When pathological specimens from Thorotrast cases were collected, their potential usefulness beyond diagnosis was not anticipated. However, steady and rapid advances in science and technology have since made it possible to perform genetic analysis even on poorly preserved specimens [17]. Based on this lesson, we are committed to archiving samples from the Affected Animal Project along with the accurate dose assessments and detailed information on the conditions at the time of collection, in a format accessible to any researcher. Such efforts will enable us to detect even subtle biological effects of long-term, low-dose-rate radiation exposure through comprehensive genetic, epigenetic, and omics analyses, including spatial transcriptomics. What would be the benefit to humans obtained from the Affected Animal Project? There are two possible answers. First, humans are expected to travel through space in the future, which will involve continuous exposure to radiation. Of course, a large proportion of exposure in space consits of particles, but it is impossible to know the effects of particle radiation without knowing the effects of photon radiation. Second, protecting disaster-stricken animals, that is, nature can help protect humans, whereas protecting humans does not always protect nature. These explain why this project is important for the future of humanity.

1.8   Outlook for Continuation of the Affected Animal Project

As discussed above, even though the Affected Animal Project is of critical importance, public memories of the FNPP accident have already begun to fade, and cooperation from the general public is becoming increasingly limited. It is therefore urgent that dedicated personnel and facilities be secured to continue storing and analyzing the invaluable samples. When the author retired from Tohoku University in 2016, the laboratory was closed, and only a small number of researchers have been continuing to collect and analyze samples of wild animals. From 2012 through the subsequent 4 years, a substantial national budget was allocated to the Affected Animal Project. Since the various pieces of research equipment purchased at that time belonged to the university, after the author retired, they were assigned to laboratories with purposes unrelated to this project. To maintain research activities, storage space is required for the minimum necessary samples and essential equipment. Above all, the most concerning aspect is the rapid decline in radiation levels resulting from decontamination efforts. Although beneficial for local residents, this decline hinders the implementation of this project, which aims to analyze the long-term biological effects of low-level radiation. It is necessary to continue steady research in mountainous areas where access is difficult and decontamination is not enforced. In light of recent global conflicts, including the Russian invasion of Ukraine and ongoing wars in the Middle East, the possibility of future accidents involving the release of radioactive material cannot be entirely ruled out, although such events are never desired. We hope that the experience of the Affected Animal Project will contribute to radiation protection and reasearch on the consequences of future radiation accidents.

References

1. Meteorological Res Inst (2022) Artificial radionuclides in the environment. (in Japanese) https://www.mri-jma.go.jp/Dep/ap/ap4lab/recent/ge_report/2021Artifi_Radio_report/2021Artifi_Radio_report.pdf
2. Kinase T, Adachi K, Sekiyama TT et al (2020) Temporal variations of Sr and Cs in atmospheric depositions after the Fukushima Daiichi Nuclear Power Plant accident with long-term observations. Sci Rep 10:21627. https://doi.org/10.1038/s41598-020-78312-3
3. Takahashi S, Inoue K, Suzuki M et al (2015) A comprehensive dose evaluation project concerning animals affected by the Fukushima Daiichi Nuclear Power Plant accident: its set-up and progress. J Radiat Res (Suppl 1):i36–i41. https://doi.org/10.1093/jrr/rrv069

4. Fukumoto M (ed) (2019) Low-dose radiation effects on animals: long-term study on the Fukushima nuclear accident. Springer Open. https://link.springer.com/book/10.1007/978-981-13-8218-5

5. Ron E (2007) Thyroid cancer incidence among people living in areas contaminated by radiation from the Chernobyl accident. Health Phys 93(5):502–511. https://doi.org/10.1097/01.HP.0000279018.93081.29

6. Imanaka T (2019) Comparison of radioactivity release and contamination from the Fukushima and Chernobyl Nuclear Power Plant accidents. In: Fukumoto M (ed) Low-dose radiation effects on animals and ecosystems. Springer, Singapore. https://doi.org/10.1007/978-981-13-8218-5_20

7. United Nations Scientific Committee on the Effects of Atomic Radiation (2020/2021) Sources, effects and risks of ionizing radiation. UNSCEAR 2020/2021 Report Volume II, Scientific Annex B. (https://www.unscear.org/unscear/uploads/documents/publications/UNSCEAR_2020_21_Annex-B-CORR.pdf)

8. Webster SC, Byrne ME, Lance SL et al (2016) Where the wild things are: influence of radiation on the distribution of four mammalian species within the Chernobyl exclusion zone. Front Ecol Environ 14:185–190. https://doi.org/10.1002/fee.1227

9. Urayama T, Takamura Y, Yamada K et al (2025) Evaluation of organ doses to Japanese macaques for internal dose using voxel phantom. In: Low-dose radiation effects on animals: long-term study on the Fukushima nuclear accident II. Springer Open

10. International Commission on Radiological Protection (ICRP) (2008) Environmental protection – the concept and use of reference animals and plants. ICRP Publication 108 Ann. ICRP 38 (4–6). https://www.icrp.org/publication.asp?id=icrp%20publication%20108

11. ICRP (2017) Dose coefficients for nonhuman biota environmentally exposed to radiation. ICRP Publication 136 Ann ICRP 46(2). https://icrp.org/publication.asp?id=ICRP%20Publication%20136

12. International Atomic Energy Agency (IAEA) (2022) Improving external dosimetry for terrestrial animals and plants. https://www.iaea.org/projects/crp/k41023

13. Nakamura AJ, Suzuki M, Redon CE et al (2017) The causal relation between DNA damage induction in bovine lymphocytes and the Fukushima nuclear power plant accident. Radiat Res 187(5):630–636. https://doi.org/10.1667/RR14630.1

14. Urushihara Y, Suzuki T, Shimizu Y et al (2018) Haematological analysis of Japanese macaques (Macaca fuscata) in the area affected by the Fukushima Daiichi Nuclear Power Plant accident. Sci Rep 8(1):16748. https://doi.org/10.1038/s41598-018-35104-0

15. Annaka K, Tokita S, Jin Shibata J et al (2026) Seasonal switches in testicular gene programs underlie spermatogenic plasticity in the large Japanese field mouse (Apodemus speciosus). Theriogenology Wild 8:100147. https://doi.org/10.1016/j.therwi.2026.100147

16. Zander A, Paunesku T, Gayle E Woloschak GE (2019) Radiation databases and archives – examples and comparisons. Int J Radiat Biol 95:1378–1389. https://doi.org/10.1080/09553002.2019.1572249

17. Fukumoto M (2014) Radiation pathology: from thorotrast to the future beyond radioresistance. Pathol Int 64:251–262. https://doi.org/10.1111/pin.12170

18. Mitsuyasu Y, Oka T, Takahashi A et al (2023) Estimation of external dose for wild Japanese macaques captured in Fukushima prefecture: decomposition of electron spin resonance spectrum. Radiat Prot Dosim 199:1620–1625. https://doi.org/10.1093/rpd/ncad146

Part I
Evaluation of Environmental Contamination and Radiation Dose from Radionuclides Released by FNPP

Chapter 2
Verification of the Initial Impact Assessments Made by the Worldwide Experts on the Fukushima Daiichi Nuclear Plant Accident

Hiroshi Yasuda

Abstract Since the Fukushima Daiichi Nuclear Power Plant accident (hereinafter referred to as the "FNPP accident") occurred in March 2011, many experts around the world have conducted assessments of radiation doses and health effects attributed to the FNPP accident. During the several weeks after the accident, while the state of the nuclear reactor was not accurately grasped, the radiation exposures of the local residents were estimated based on the anticipated environmental behavior of various radionuclides. However, notable differences were observed in the doses and risks assessed by different researchers and research institutes. As 13 years have passed, research on the causes and progress of the FNPP accident has advanced significantly, and we now have a better understanding of the situation and consequences of the accident. In this article, the author briefly reviews the contents of relevant scientific articles published during the initial 3 years (2011–2014) after the FNPP accident and tries to evaluate how correct or incorrect the early assessments were through a comparison with more recent publications.

Keywords Fukushima Daiichi Nuclear Power Plant (FNPP) · Nuclear accident · Dose assessment · Health risk · Uncertainty · UNSCEAR

2.1 Introduction

Owing to the large-scale earthquake that occurred off the coast of Miyagi Prefecture on March 11, 2011, and the subsequent tsunami that hit the Pacific coast of Fukushima Prefecture approximately 1 h later, the Tokyo Electric Power Company's Fukushima Daiichi Nuclear Power Plant (hereinafter referred to as "FNPP") lost its electric power supply and made it impossible to cool the reactors, which led to core

H. Yasuda (✉)
Research Institute for Radiation Biology and Medicine, Hiroshima University, Hiroshima, Japan
e-mail: hyasuda@hiroshima-u.ac.jp

© The Author(s) 2026

M. Fukumoto (ed.), *Low-Dose Radiation Effects on Animals and Ecosystems II*,
https://doi.org/10.1007/978-981-95-5559-8_2

meltdowns at three reactors (Units 1–3). This accident was later ranked as Level 7, the highest level of severity, on the International Nuclear and Radiological Event Scale (INES) [1].

First, at 15:36 on March 12, approximately 1 day after the earthquake and tsunami, a hydrogen explosion occurred at Unit 1, where the cooling water level had dropped, and the building structure was severely damaged. While the water supply at Unit 3 was able to continue using batteries until March 13, it was eventually interrupted, and at 11:01 on March 14, a hydrogen explosion occurred at Unit 3 also, and the upper part of the building was broken. At Unit 2, a hydrogen explosion did not occur, and the building structure remained ~intact, it was later found that the containment vessel of Unit 2 had been seriously damaged by high pressure. At Unit 4, an explosion occurred in the early morning hours of March 15 due to hydrogen leakage from Unit 3, and the building was destroyed. As a result of these explosions and damages, as well as artificial vent operations to prevent further damage to the pressure vessels, large amounts of radionuclides, such as iodine-131 (^{131}I) and cesium-137 (^{137}Cs), were released into the atmosphere. Additionally, because of the core meltdowns, part of the nuclear fuel penetrated the containment vessel and spread underground, reached the groundwater, and consequently released various radionuclides including strontium-90 (^{90}Sr) and plutonium-239 (^{239}Pu) into the ocean. The release of radionuclides into the aqueous environment continues (as of March 2026), albeit most of the underground tainted water has been collected and processed.

On the other hand, amidst the difficult situation caused by the natural disasters and ongoing nuclear accident, such as large-scale power outages, infrastructural damage, termination of public services, and sheltering or evacuation of local residents, there were limited data regarding the release and dispersion of radioactive materials into the environment, including the monitoring data of radiation levels within the FNPP site as well as residential areas where electric power supply was interrupted due to the earthquake and tsunami. Consequently, crucial data for approximately 4 days after the occurrence of the accident (March 11–15, 2011) were missing in the critically affected area near FNPP. As a result, estimations of dispersion, deposition, and public doses caused by released radioactive materials, particularly short-lived radionuclides such as ^{131}I, Tellurium-132 (^{132}Te), and ^{133}I, were accompanied by large uncertainties.

In this article, the author reviews the early dose and health risk assessments conducted during the initial 3 years (2011–2014) after the FNPP accident and discusses how accurate these estimates were through a comparison with more recent publications.

2.2 Early Assessments Conducted by Scientists

In the days to months after the accident, many scientists in related fields conducted research on the impact of the FNPP accident based on limited monitoring data and presumed reactor conditions (temperature, pressure, effects of venting, etc.). They attempted to clarify the source term, that is, what kind of radionuclides were released at what timing and in what quantities from the damaged nuclear facilities. However, owing to the lack of critical information, large gaps were observed among the results of evaluations performed by different researchers and research institutions. For example, on March 22, 2011, 10 days after the accident, the French Institute for Radiation Protection and Nuclear Safety (IRSN) reported on their website that the estimated amount of ^{131}I released into the atmosphere was 90 PBq and that of ^{137}Cs was 10 PBq [2], while Austria's Central Institution for Meteorology and Geodynamics (ZAMG) reported on the same day that the estimated atmospheric releases of ^{131}I and ^{137}Cs were 400 PBq and 33 PBq, respectively [3].

The most representative early publication on the scientific impact assessment of the FNPP accident is considered to be the 2013 Report of the United Nations Scientific Committee on the Effects of Atomic Radiation (UNSCEAR) [4]. UNSCEAR announced a plan for documenting the 2013 Report in May 2011, 2 months after the accident, which stated the overall work to collect and analyze a large amount of information related to the FNPP accident and then to present scientifically sound perspectives on the health effects on affected people within 2 years. According to this document plan, UNSCEAR established an expert group that brought together approximately 80 scientists in relevant fields from the United Nations member states and began writing the report in late 2011. The group worked together with experts from the United Nations specialized agencies such as the International Atomic Energy Agency (IAEA), World Health Organization (WHO), World Meteorological Organization (WMO), Food and Agriculture Organization of the United Nations (FAO), and Preparatory Committee for the Comprehensive Nuclear-Test-Ban Treaty Organization (CTBTO).

UNSCEAR collected and analyzed information such as papers in academic peer-reviewed journals and official reports from government agencies published within approximately 2 years after the accident, until the first half of 2013. From the vast amount of information collected, UNSCEAR scientists carefully identified the most reliable information and used it for further analysis. For example, regarding the source term, they presented a probable range of the total atmospheric release of ^{131}I as 100–500 PBq and that of ^{137}Cs as 6–20 PBq, selected the source term reported by Terada et al. (120 PBq for ^{131}I and 9 PBq for ^{137}Cs) [5] as it was judged to be the most reasonable in light of the observations, and used this source term for model simulations of atmospheric diffusion and deposition with the cooperation of WMO.

Based on limited observations and model calculations of radionuclides released into the atmosphere, UNSCEAR assessed the radiation doses of Japanese residents for three exposure routes: external exposure, respiratory inhalation, and oral ingestion. The residents were classified into three age groups (0–5 years old represented by 1-year-old infant, 6–15 years old by 10-year-old children, and 16 years old and older by 20-year-old adults). For each group, the effective dose and the doses to several critical organs (thyroid, bone marrow, and female breasts) were estimated. District- or prefecture-average doses were calculated for non-evacuees, and group (settlement) average doses for evacuees. These calculations were performed for three periods (within the first year, for 10 years after the accident, and for the period up to age 80).

Some of the short-lived radionuclides, such as ^{132}I (half-life: 2.28 h), ^{132}Te (half-life: 3.20 d), and ^{133}I (half-life: 20.8 h), were presumed to have caused considerable exposure of the local residents for several days after the FNPP accident. However, their monitoring data were lacking, and the levels of these radionuclides were required to be estimated from the data of other radionuclides having relatively long half-lives measured 3 months or later after the accident. For this purpose, measurements of ground surface depositions of ^{134}Cs (half-life: 2.06 y) and ^{137}Cs (half-life: 30.0 year) were commonly used. Comprehensive data on atmospheric radionuclide concentrations were provided by the CTBTO monitoring station outside Fukushima Prefecture. Based on these observations, the atmospheric dispersions and depositions of major radionuclides, such as ^{131}I (half-life: 8.06 day) and ^{137}Cs, were estimated by a combination of model simulations. Other important inputs used to assess public exposure for several weeks after the accident included air dose rates estimated through the above process, evacuation records managed by the local governments, population size of districts and settlements, local food intake patterns, and radioactivity in representative local foodstuffs measured with germanium semiconductor detectors.

Figure 2.1 shows the distribution of the estimated effective doses received by residents of each municipality during the first year in Fukushima Prefecture and neighboring prefectures, excluding evacuation zones [4], which are color-coded by dose level. The highest dose (around 4 mSv) as a municipality average was found in Fukushima City and Nihonmatsu City located to the west of the FNPP, followed by Souma City, Date City, Koriyama City, and Iwaki City. While the dose level in Fukushima Prefecture was clearly higher than in other prefectures overall, some areas, such as southern Miyagi Prefecture and northern Tochigi Prefecture, showed relatively high dose levels.

The geological distribution of thyroid doses of infants (1 year old) estimated by UNSCEAR for the first year after the accident is shown in Fig. 2.2 [4]. Unlike the effective dose (Fig. 2.1), Iwaki City located to the south of FNPP presented the highest dose exceeding 50 mGy. Overall, the thyroid dose levels in Fukushima Prefecture were higher than those in other surrounding prefectures, whereas the levels in some areas in the prefectures located to the south (Ibaraki, Tochigi, Gunma, etc.) were estimated to have been considerably higher.

UNSCEAR estimated the doses of evacuated local residents for each settlement/group who evacuated with different patterns (routes, methods, and timings) from two areas: the precautionary evacuation area within a 20-km radius zone from the FNPP site and the deliberate evacuation area extending northwestward beyond the 20-km zone where high radiation levels were observed. As a result, the estimated effective dose of some groups reached approximately 10 mSv, which exceeded the highest level of district-average doses of non-evacuated residents (Fig. 2.1). Regarding the thyroid doses, the infants in some evacuation groups received 80 mGy or higher, which significantly exceeded the dose levels of any non-evacuees. Based on these estimates, UNSCEAR stated that the inferred risks of developing thyroid

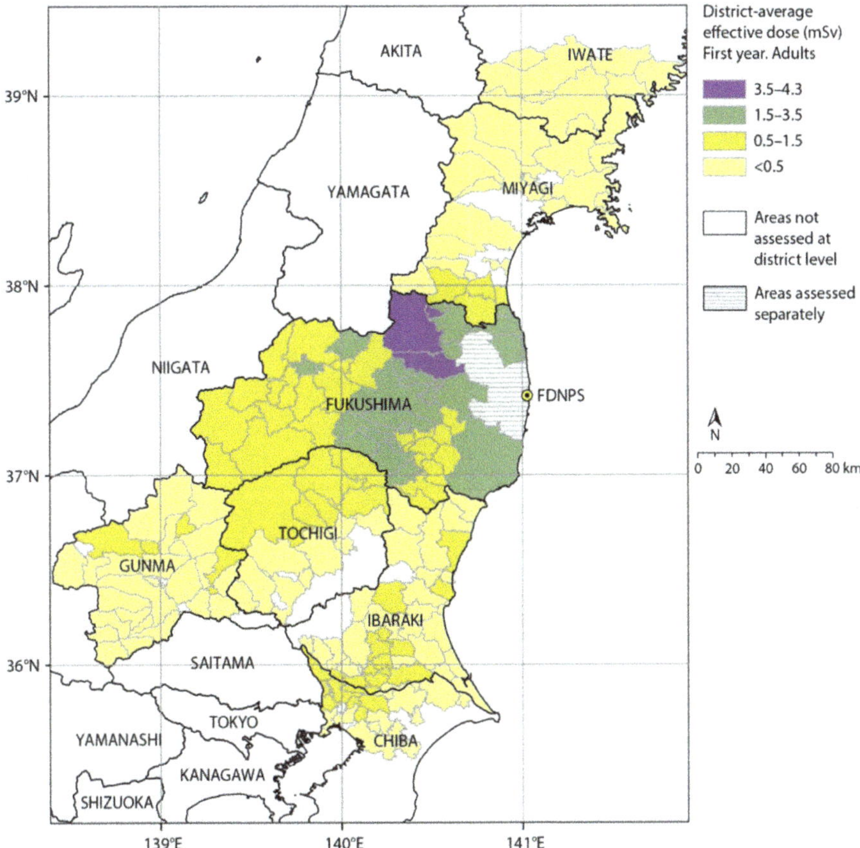

Fig. 2.1 The district-average effective doses in the first year following the accident for adults living in and near Fukushima Prefecture [4] (Reproduced by permission of UNSCEAR).

cancer were relatively small compared to that of spontaneous thyroid cancer and thus would be indiscernible.

UNSCEAR also made long-term dose projections for residents in the 2013 Report for 10 years after the accident and also until they reach the age of 80. The projection indicated that most of the cumulative dose after the second year (2012~) could be attributed to external exposure to the gamma rays from radioactive cesium ([134]Cs and ^{137}Cs) deposited onto the ground. Based on these predicted dose levels, UNSCEAR stated the following conclusions regarding the impact of the FNPP accident on public health.

- The doses received by the Japanese population due to the accident were generally low.
- In the highest-dose case, the lifetime risk increase would be ~0.1%. Therefore, no discernible changes in future cancer rates and hereditary diseases are expected to appear due to radiation exposure as a result of the FNPP accident.

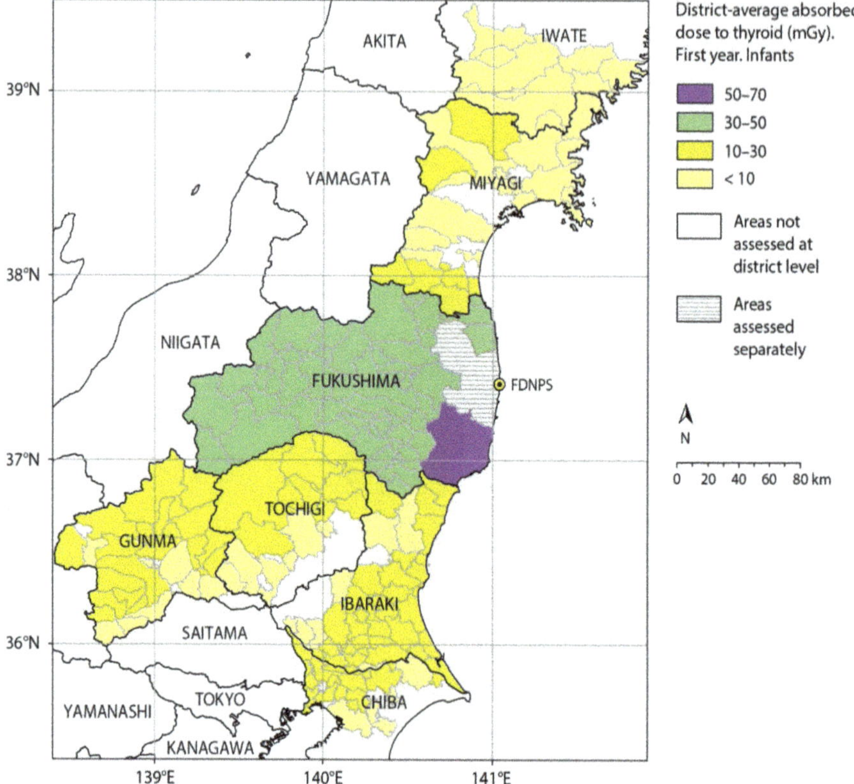

Fig. 2.2 The district-average absorbed doses to the thyroid in the first year following the accident for 1-year-old infants living in and near Fukushima Prefecture [4] (Reproduced by permission of UNSCEAR).

- In addition, no increases in the rates of birth defects are expected to appear.
- Nevertheless, there is a theoretical possibility that the risk of thyroid cancer among the group of children most exposed to radiation could increase.
- The situation needs to be closely followed and further assessed in the future.

2.3 Were the Early Assessments Correct?

This section discusses the accuracy of the early assessments made by scientists during the first 3 years on the doses and health effects of the FNPP accident. Although it is undeniable that there are still large uncertainties that make it difficult to obtain correct answers owing to the lack of initial-phase monitoring data, the author has attempted to evaluate the reliability of early assessments regarding the dose and risk of the FNPP accident by comparing recent data published in peer-reviewed articles since 2014.

Regarding the source term, that is, the estimated amounts of radionuclides released into the atmosphere, these have been constantly reported for the past decade. Selected source-term estimates of the atmospheric releases of ^{131}I and ^{137}Cs are shown in Table 2.1 [5–13].

In comparison with the recently presented values, the source term of ^{137}Cs (9 PBq) [5] adopted in the UNSCEAR 2013 Report is considered to be reasonable, as the variation is within a factor of approximately 2. The validity of this estimate has been verified by Kadowaki et al. [14] through comprehensive analyses. On the other hand, it is implied that the UNSCEAR's source term of ^{131}I (120 PBq), which affects the thyroid dose estimates, is still accompanied by a larger uncertainty with a factor of approximately 4.

The validity of the estimated doses of local residents can be judged through comparison with the data of the Fukushima Health Management Survey (called the "Survey" hereafter), which began 3 months after the FNPP accident [15, 16]. In this Survey, the external exposure doses of the residents in Fukushima Prefecture were estimated based on the monitored or presumed air dose rates in the affected area and the behavioral records of each resident obtained through a questionnaire survey. According to the survey results as of March 2020 [16], nearly 100% of people received less than 5 mSv in effective dose from external radiation (Table 2.2), with the highest dose of approximately 25 mSv. These dose levels were in good agreement with the estimates in the UNSCEAR 2013 Report (Fig. 2.1). In addition, from the geographical dose distribution obtained in this Survey, the highest doses were seen in Fukushima City and Nihonmatsu City, as shown by UNSCEAR in the 2013 Report (Fig. 2.1).

As for the thyroid doses of the local residents mainly due to ^{131}I and other short-lived radionuclides (^{132}I, ^{132}Te, etc.), there are still large uncertainties owing to the lack of monitoring data, as in the source term. Here, we attempt to verify the early

Table 2.1 Selected source-term estimates of the total amounts of ^{131}I and ^{137}Cs released into the atmosphere during the FNPP accident.

Author	Year of publication	Total release [PBq]	
		^{131}I	^{137}Cs
Chino et al. [6]	2011	150	12
Terada et al. [5] (employed in the UNSCEAR 2013 Report)	2012	120	9
Kobayashi et al. [7]	2013	200	13
Achim et al. [8]	2014	400	11
Winiarek et al. [9]	2014	–	12–19
Katata et al. [10]	2015	151	15
Yumimoto et al. [11]	2016	–	8
Kim et al. [12]	2017	754	29
Terada et al. [13]	2020	120	10

Table 2.2 Estimated external dose levels of the residents in Fukushima Prefecture due to the FNPP accident for the initial 4 months (as of March 31, 2020) [16].

Dose level	Percentage
External exposure (n = 475,190)	
<1 mSv	62.2%
<2 mSv	93.8%
<5 mSv	99.8%
5–25 mSv	0.2%
Internal exposure (n = 344,565)	
<1 mSv	99.9%

risk estimation of radiation-induced thyroid cancer through a comparison with the regional data of thyroid cancer incidence rates obtained from the Fukushima Health Management Survey [16]. Regarding this issue, Ohira et al. [17] classified municipalities in Fukushima Prefecture into five groups (A to E) according to the estimated external exposure doses, as shown in Fig. 2.3, and analyzed the incidence of thyroid cancer in each group. According to the results of their analyses (Table 2.3), thyroid cancers appeared to be slightly more common in Groups A to C, where higher external dose levels were observed, while the number of cancer cases was not enough to detect a statistically significant difference. This finding agrees well with the predictive statement in the UNSCEAR 2013 Report, that is, "no discernible changes in future cancer rates and hereditary diseases are expected. Nevertheless, there is a theoretical possibility that the risk of thyroid cancer among the group of children most exposed to radiation could increase."

It should be noted that UNSCEAR published the 2020/2021 Report [18] which presented lower estimated doses for residents in Japan than those in the 2013 Report. However, these updated estimates have confronted severe criticisms from many scientists, particularly in Japan [19, 20]. Thus, in the current situation, in which UNSCEAR is requested to resolve some critical questions raised by these scientists, it is considered to be inappropriate to discuss the accuracy of the early assessment of the FNPP accident (i.e., the contents of the UNSCEAR 2013 Report) by using the information presented in the UNSCEAR 2020/2021 Report.

As one of the important findings obtained from the Survey [16], the age distribution of children who developed thyroid cancer after the FNPP accident is clearly different from that after the Chernobyl accident, which occurred in 1986 [21]. In the Chernobyl accident, the incidence rate of thyroid cancer was significantly higher in small children (1–6 years old) whose thyroid tissues are considered to be highly sensitive to radiation exposure. In contrast, few cases of thyroid cancer have been found in small children in Fukushima, and the highest incidence rate was observed among high school students (16–18 years old). Based on these data, most of the postaccident thyroid cancers reported in Fukushima Prefecture are attributed to the highly sensitive diagnostic technology employed in the Survey to detect early-stage thyroid cancers that were originally present in some local children.

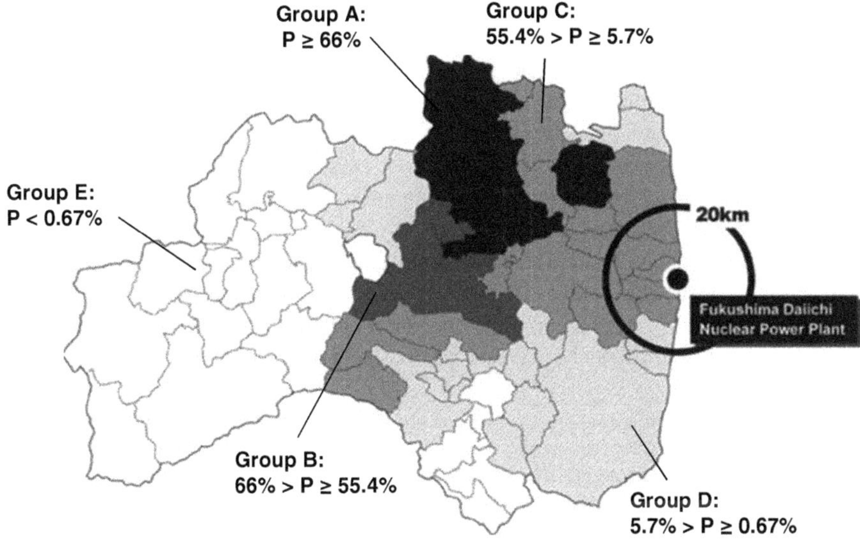

Fig. 2.3 Geographic details of the highest-dose (Group A), high-middle-dose (B), middle-dose (C), low-middle-dose (D), and lowest-dose (E) areas, according to the first 4-month external radiation doses estimated by the Fukushima Health Management Survey [16, 17].

Table 2.3 Characteristics of the subjects investigated and adjusted relative risks (RRs) with 95% confidence intervals (CIs) regarding thyroid cancers of children in Fukushima Prefecture [17].

Variable	Group (illustrated in Fig. 2.3)				
	A	B	C	D	E
Number of subjects, n	52,693	44,743	44,875	67,893	31,628
Age at the accident [y], mean	8.3	8.0	8.2	7.9	7.6
Number of cancer cases, n	15	18	18	13	5
Cancer incidence rate [n per 100,000]	13.5	19.2	17.3	9	8.3
Age- and sex-adjusted RR (95% CI)	1.62 (0.59–4.46)	2.32 (0.86–6.24)	2.20 (0.82–5.93)	1.02 (0.36–2.86)	- (ref.)
Multivariable-adjusted RR including obesity (95% CI)	1.68 (0.61–4.62)	2.40 (0.89–6.48)	2.16 (0.80–5.82)	1.05 (0.37–2.95)	- (ref.)

2.4   Conclusion

It was attempted here to verify the accuracy of early assessments conducted during the initial 3 years (2011–2014) by world-class scientists on the doses of the residents affected by the FNPP accident, focusing mainly on the contents of the UNSCEAR 2013 Report [4]. According to comparisons with recent data including the health status of local residents, no critical contradiction was found in the major findings (radionuclide dispersions and depositions, public doses, and health implications) in the early assessment. More specifically, no significant increase in adverse health effects such as leukemia, solid cancers, or birth defects directly attributed to radiation exposure would be discernible, although there is still a large uncertainty in the thyroid doses and risks of individual children. In addition, regarding worker exposure and the effects on the ecosystem, the assessment results and perspectives presented in the 2013 Report are considered reasonable, although descriptions about these issues have been omitted here.

Finally, it should be noted that there remain some questions difficult to answer in regard to the doses and health effects of the FNPP accident, as raised in the recent UNSCEAR report [18]. It is strongly hoped that scientists in the relevant field will continue working to solve these issues and build a higher level of credibility.

Acknowledgments Sincere appreciation is expressed to Prof. Manabu Fukumoto (Tohoku University) for offering the opportunity to write this article. The author also acknowledges the efforts of all scientists and administrative staff who have made great contributions to the assessments of doses and health effects of the FNPP accident.

References

1. International Atomic Energy Agency (IAEA) (2015) The Fukushima Daiichi accident, Report by the Director General. IAEA, Vienna. https://www-pub.iaea.org/mtcd/publications/pdf/pub1710-reportbythedg-web.pdf
2. Institut de Radioprotection et de Sûreté Nucléaire (2011) L'IRSN publie une évaluation de la radioactivité rejetée par la centrale de Fukushima Daiichi (Fukushima I) jusqu'au 22 mars 2011 (in French). https://www.irsn.fr/fr/actualites_presse/actualites/pages/20110322_evaluation-radioactivite-rejets-fukushima-terme-source.aspx#.YNv5d-j7S-Y. Accessed on 30 June 2021
3. Zentralanstalt für Meteorologie und Geodynamik (2011) Accident in the Japanese NPP Fukushima: Spread of radioactivity/first source estimates from CTBTO data show large source terms at the beginning of the accident/weather currently not favourable/low level radioactivity meanwhile observed over U.S. East Coast and Hawaii (Update: 22 March 2011 15:00). http://www.zamg.ac.at/docs/aktuell/Japan2011-03-22_1500_E.pdf. Accessed on 30 June 2021
4. United Nations Scientific Committee on the Effects of Atomic Radiation (2014) UNSCEAR 2013 report to the general assembly with scientific annexes, annex A: levels and effects of radiation exposure due to the nuclear accident after the 2011 great East-Japan earthquake and tsunami. New York, United Nations. https://www.unscear.org/unscear/en/publications/2013_1.html. Accessed on 1 May 2024
5. Terada H, Katata G, Chino M et al (2012) Atmospheric discharge and dispersion of radionuclides during the Fukushima Dai-ichi Nuclear Power Plant accident. Part II: verification of the source term and analysis of regional-scale atmospheric dispersion. J Environ Radioact 112:141–154. https://doi.org/10.1016/j.jenvrad.2012.05.023
6. Chino M, Nakayama H, Nagai H et al (2011) Preliminary estimation of release amounts of ^{131}I and ^{137}Cs accidentally discharged from the Fukushima Daiichi Nuclear Power Plant into the atmosphere. J Nucl Sci Technol 48:1129–1134. https://doi.org/10.1080/18811248.2011.9711799
7. Kobayashi T, Nagai H, Chino M et al (2013) Source term estimation of atmospheric release due to the Fukushima Dai-ichi Nuclear Power Plant accident by atmospheric and oceanic dispersion simulations: Fukushima NPP accident related. J Nucl Sci Technol 50(3):255–264. https://doi.org/10.1080/00223131.2013.772449

8. Achim P, Monfort M, Le Petit G et al (2014) Analysis of radionuclide releases from the Fukushima Dai-ichi Nuclear Power Plant accident part II. Pure Appl Geophys 171:645–667. https://doi.org/10.1007/s00024-012-0578-1

9. Winiarek V, Bocquet M, Duhanyan N et al (2014) Estimation of the caesium-137 source term from the Fukushima Daiichi Nuclear Power Plant using a consistent joint assimilation of air concentration and deposition observations. Atmos Environ 82:268–279. https://doi.org/10.1016/j.atmosenv.2013.10.017

10. Katata G, Chino M, Kobayashi T et al (2015) Detailed source term estimation of the atmospheric release for the Fukushima Daiichi Nuclear Power Station accident by coupling simulations of an atmospheric dispersion model with an improved deposition scheme and oceanic dispersion model. Atmos Chem Phys 15:1029–1070. https://doi.org/10.5194/acp-15-1029-2015

11. Yumimoto K, Morino Y, Ohara T et al (2016) Inverse modeling of the ^{137}Cs source term of the Fukushima Dai-ichi Nuclear Power Plant accident constrained by a deposition map monitored by aircraft. J Environ Radioact 164:1–12. https://doi.org/10.1016/j.jenvrad.2016.06.018

12. Kim T-W, Rhee B-W, Song J-H et al (2017) Estimation of in-plant source term release behaviors from Fukushima Daiichi reactor cores by forward method and comparison with reverse method. J Radiat Prot Res 42:114–129. https://doi.org/10.14407/jrpr.2017.42.2.114

13. Terada H, Nagai H, Tsuduki K et al (2020) Refinement of source term and atmospheric dispersion simulations of radionuclides during the Fukushima Daiichi Nuclear Power Station accident. J Environ Radioact 213:106104. https://doi.org/10.1016/j.jenvrad.2019.106104

14. Kadowaki M, Furuno A, Nagai H et al (2021) Validity of the source term for the Fukushima Dai-ichi Nuclear Power Station accident estimated using local-scale atmospheric dispersion simulations to reproduce the large-scale atmospheric dispersion of ^{137}Cs. J Environ Radioact 237:106704. https://doi.org/10.1016/j.jenvrad.2021.106704

15. Yasumura S, Hosoya M, Yamashita S et al (2012) Study protocol for the Fukushima health management survey. J Epidemiol 22:375–383. https://doi.org/10.2188/jea.JE20120105

16. Fukushima Prefectural Government. Fukushima Revitalization Station: Health of residents of the prefecture. https://www.pref.fukushima.lg.jp/site/portal-english/en03-03.html. Accessed on 1 May 2024

17. Ohira T, Ohtsuru A, Midorikawa S et al (2019) External radiation dose, obesity, and risk of childhood thyroid cancer after the Fukushima Daiichi Nuclear Power Plant accident: the Fukushima health management survey. Epidemiology 30:853–860. https://doi.org/10.1097/EDE.0000000000001058

18. United Nations Scientific Committee on the Effects of Atomic Radiation (2021) UNSCEAR 2020/2021 report to the general assembly with scientific annexes, annex B: levels and effects of radiation exposure due to the accident at the Fukushima Daiichi Nuclear Power Station: implications of information published since the UNSCEAR 2013 report. United Nations, New York. https://www.unscear.org/unscear/publications/2020_2021_2.html. Accessed on 1 May 2024

19. Kato T, Yamada K, Hongyo T (2023) Area dose–response and radiation origin of childhood thyroid cancer in Fukushima based on thyroid dose in UNSCEAR 2020/2021: high 131I exposure comparable to Chernobyl. Cancer 15:4583. https://doi.org/10.3390/cancers15184583

20. Hamaoka Y (2023) The novel terminology 'discernible' undiscerned conclusions:: a critical review of UNSCEAR 2020/21 Fukushima Report. https://doi.org/10.51094/jxiv.286

21. Takamura N, Orita M, Saenko V, Yamashita S, Nagataki S, Demidchik Y (2016) Radiation and risk of thyroid cancer: Fukushima and Chernobyl. Lancet Diabetes Endocrinol 4:P647. https://doi.org/10.1016/S2213-8587(16)30112-7

Chapter 3
Radioactive Contamination by the Fukushima Daiichi Nuclear Power Plant Accident: Radiation Survey in Iitate Village and Future Perspectives of Cesium-137 Contamination

Tetsuji Imanaka

Abstract Iitate Village is located 30–45 km northwest of Fukushima Dai-ichi Nuclear Power Plant (FNPP) and suffered serious radioactive contamination by the FNPP accident in March 2011. Our team has been conducting car-borne radiation surveys on main roads in Iitate Village since the end of March 2011. The average ambient radiation dose rate of 0.31μSv/h was obtained by the last car-borne survey on April 1, 2023, which was 1/35 of the initial value of 10.8μSv/h on March 29, 2011.

Meanwhile, the aerial monitoring data taken by the Nuclear Regulatory Authority Japan (NRA) in October 2022 using helicopters at 300 m above ground indicated an average ambient dose rate of 0.82μSv/h in Iitate Village. The difference between our car-borne survey and the aerial monitoring reflects heavy contamination of the forest occupying 75% of Iitate Village without decontamination.

Future perspectives of areas contaminated by the FNPP accident are given based on NRA's aerial monitoring data in October 2022. In 2122, that is, 100 years later, the area size of significant cesium-137 (^{137}Cs) contamination more than 40 kBq/m^2 will remain 350 km^2, while the serious contamination more than 500 kBq/m^2 will almost disappear.

Keywords Iitate Village · Radioactive contamination · Cesium-137 (^{137}Cs) · Car-borne survey · Aerial monitoring

T. Imanaka (✉)
Institute for Integrated Radiation and Nuclear Sciences, Kyoto University, Kumatori-cho, Sennan-gun, Osaka, Japan
e-mail: imanaka@rri.kyoto-u.ac.jp

M. Fukumoto (ed.), *Low-Dose Radiation Effects on Animals and Ecosystems II*,
https://doi.org/10.1007/978-981-95-5559-8_3

3.1   Introduction

The Fukushima Daiichi Nuclear Power Plant (FNPP) accident began on March 11, 2011, triggered by the earthquake and tsunami. At the time of earthquake, three units (Unit 1, Unit 2, and Unit 3) out of six units of FNPP were in operation at full power. These three units were successfully shutdown by automatically inserting emergency control rods into reactor cores. Approximately an hour later, a large tsunami hit FNPP, which led to a blackout of electric power to remove the decay heat of reactor cores after shutdown. The meltdown process of Unit 1 began in the evening of March 11, Unit 3 in the morning of March 13, and Unit 2 in the evening of March 14 [1–4].

A large amount of radioactivity leakage into the environment began in the morning of March 12 and continued until the end of March. During this period, approximately 300 PBq of iodine-131 (^{131}I), 15 PBq of cesium-134 (^{134}Cs), 15 PBq of cesium-137 (^{137}Cs), and other radionuclides were released. The released amounts of ^{131}I and radioactive cesium (^{134}Cs + ^{137}Cs) corresponded to 5% and 2.1%, respectively, of the total accumulated in the reactor cores of Units 1–3. Because of the prevailing westerlies above the Japanese islands, approximately 80% of radionuclides flowed toward the direction over the Pacific Ocean, while the remaining 20% were directed toward land and deposited there [4, 5].

Ambient dose rates recorded during March 2011 at five points in Fukushima Prefecture [6] and Shinjuku, Tokyo [7], are shown in Fig. 3.1. The first peak at Minamisoma City on March 12 was caused by a hydrogen explosion at the reactor building of Unit 1. From the early morning of March 15, radioactive plumes from Unit 2 flowed toward the south, which moved over Iwaki City, forming a radiation peak at 4:00 a.m., passing over Ibaragi Prefecture and Chiba Prefecture, arriving at

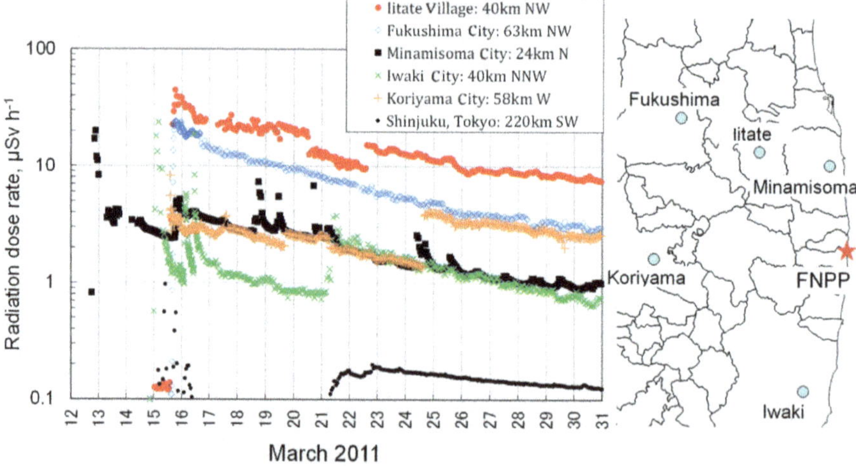

Fig. 3.1 Radiation dose rate in March 2011 at five points in Fukushima Prefecture (light blue circles on the right-hand map), and Shinjuku, Tokyo.

Shinjuku, Tokyo, at around 10:00 a.m. In the afternoon of March 15, as the wind direction changed to west and to northwest, heavy deposition of radionuclides occurred in Namie Town, Iitate Village, and Fukushima City where arrival of radioactive plumes coincided with rain or snow.

Our group, a radiation survey team of Iitate Society for Radioecology (IISORA) [8], has been periodically conducting car-borne radiation surveys in Iitate Village since the end of March 2011. In this chapter, the results of our survey activities are described as well as the results of recent aerial radiation monitoring by Nuclear Regulatory Authority Japan (NRA) using helicopters. Future perspectives of the ground contamination level for the entire contaminated area and Iitate Village are also shown, assuming that ^{137}Cs is the only remaining contaminant due to the FNPP accident from now to the future.

3.2 Radiation Survey in Iitate Village

Iitate Village, with population of approximately 6000, is located in the Abukuma Moutains, at 30–45 km northwest of the FNPP site on the Pacific coast. When the FNPP accident occurred in March 2011, there was no preparedness for a radiological emergency in Iitate Village. A portable radiation MP (monitoring post) was set next to the Iitate Village Office on March 13. A sharp increase in ambient dose rate began in the afternoon of March 15 when radioactive plumes from FNPP arrived. The MP recorded a maximum value of 44.7μSv/h at 18:20 on March 15 [6].

Because of the unexpected scale of the FNPP accident, the emergency headquarters did not function as planned. Little information was available through the mass media about radioactive contamination around FNPP. Therefore, to investigate the situation around the contaminated areas by ourselves, we decided to organize a small survey team and visited Iitate Village at the end of March. On March 29, our first car-borne survey was conducted, and we measured ambient dose rate at 130 points on main roads within Iitate Village to assess the situation of the village [9, 10]. The radiation dose rate inside the car was measured using two CsI scintillation survey meters (PDR-101, ALOKA Ltd, Japan). Measured values inside the car were converted to ambient dose rates on the road by dividing the shielding factor obtained from the ratio of dose rate inside and outside the car. The ambient dose-rate map based on the measurements taken on March 29, 2011, is shown in Fig. 3.2. The average ambient radiation dose rate on March 29, 2011, was 10.8μSv/h. A maximum of 30μSv/h was measured in the rice field of Nagadoro, south district of Iitate Village. We took soil core samples and analyzed radionuclide composition in our laboratory, from which we estimated radiation dose rate on the night of March 15 to be approximately 200μSv/h [9].

After the first visit in March 2011, our team repeated the radiation survey within Iitate Village at least once a year, excluding the period of the COVID-19 pandemic from 2020 to 2022. The last survey was conducted on April 1, 2023 [11]. The results of our car-borne survey are summarized in Table 3.1. The temporal change of the

Fig. 3.2 The result of our first car-borne survey in Iitate Village on March 29, 2011.

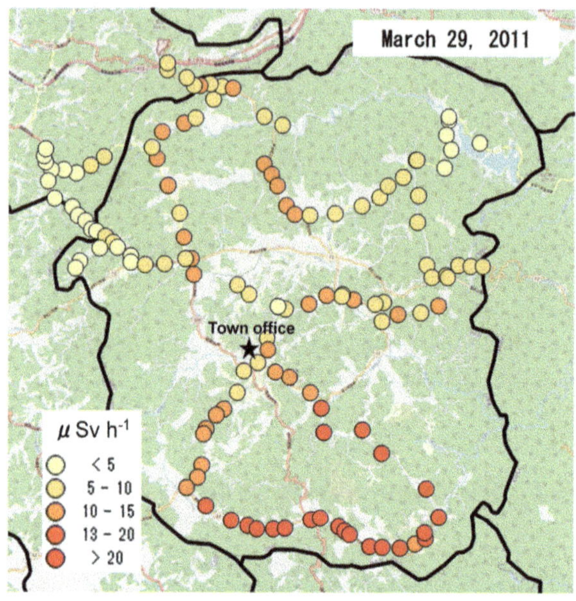

Table 3.1 Summary of car-borne survey in Iitate Village.

Date	Number of measurements	Average ± SD	Median	Min	Max
Mar 29, 2011	130	10.8 ± 7.2	9.2	2.4	24
Oct 5, 2011	122	2.8 ± 1.4	2.6	0.65	7.6
Mar 27, 2012	139	2.6 ± 1.6	2.3	0.42	8.0
Mar 17, 2013	170	2.2 ± 1.3	2.0	0.44	7.6
Apr 26, 2014	238	1.7 ± 1.1	1.5	0.31	7.2
Mar 26, 2015	257	1.2 ± 0.89	1.0	0.21	5.9
Mar 26, 2016	236	0.82 ± 0.61	0.65	0.14	4.4
Apr 1, 2017	249	0.59 ± 0.47	0.43	0.13	3.2
Mar 31, 2018	261	0.55 ± 0.41	0.44	0.12	3.1
Mar 30, 2019	264	0.49 ± 0.41	0.35	0.07	2.9
Apr 1, 2023	276	0.31 ± 0.25	0.23	0.04	2.1

Unit: μSv/h

average dose rate measured in Iitate Village is plotted in Fig. 3.3. Currently, the average dose rate decreased to 1/35 of our first visit in March 2011. The solid black line indicates the theoretical curve calculated considering only the physical decay of the initially deposited radionuclides. The rapid decrease observed after our first visit reflects the decay out of short half-lived nuclides of tellurium-132/iodine-132 (^{132}Te/^{132}I) and ^{131}I. The measured average agreed well with the theoretical decay curve up to 2014. Then, the measured average values became lower than the theoretical values, which can be attributed to the large-scale decontamination in Iitate Village.

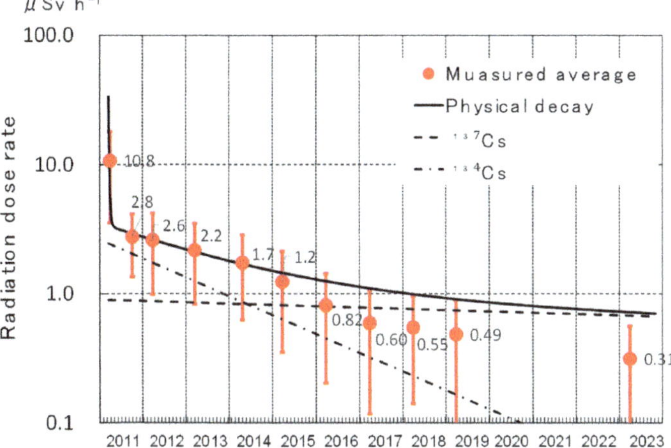

Fig. 3.3 Temporal change in the average dose rate of our car-borne survey in Iitate Village. Solid line indicates theoretical reduction only considering the physical decay of radionuclides of ^{132}Te/^{132}I, ^{131}I, ^{134}Cs, and ^{137}Cs with a composition fitting to 10.8 μSv/h on March 29, 2011.

3.3   Current Situation and Future Prediction of ^{137}Cs Contamination

Ambient radiation dose-rate distribution map of the left panel in Fig. 3.4 is drawn by plotting our car-borne suvey data measured at 276 points on April 1, 2023. The right panel is also the ambient dose-rate distribution map created from aerial heli-copter monitoring data for 3623 meshes in Iitate Village measured by NRA in October 2022 [12]. All our survey data were measured on main roads around which decontamination was completed. On the other hand, aerial monitoring data were taken at 300 m above the ground, which strongly reflects the state of contamination of the forest occupying 75% of Iitate Village, where decontamination has not been carried out. The difference in the average dose rate between the two maps (0.31μSv/h from the car-borne and 0.83μSv/h from the arial monitoring) indicates that high levels of contamination still remain in forest, especially in the southern part of Iitate Village.

As 12 years have passed since the FNPP accident occurred, it is clear that ^{137}Cs with a half-life of 30 year is the primary radionuclide of contamination. It is also known that atoms of radioactive cesium are firmly fixed within the clay minerals of Japanese soil[13, 14]. Therefore, we can assume that ^{137}Cs will hardly migrate from its current position. Considering only the physical attenuation of ^{137}Cs with an assumption of a natural background of 0.05 μSv/h, the future decreasing trend of radiation dose for both car-borne survey and for arial monitoring is shown in Fig. 3.5.

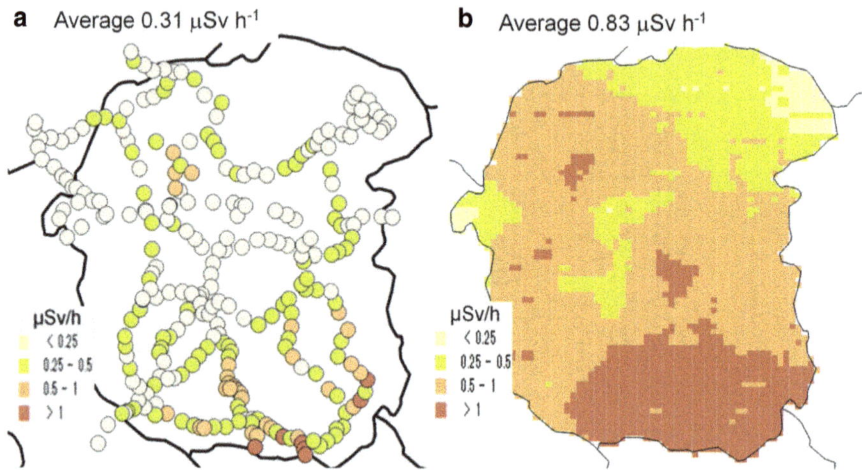

Fig. 3.4 Current distribution of radiation levels in Iitate Village. (**a**) Our car-borne survey at 276 points on April 1, 2023. (**b**) Aerial helicopter monitoring data by NRA assigned to 3623 meshes within Iitate Village on October 21, 2022.

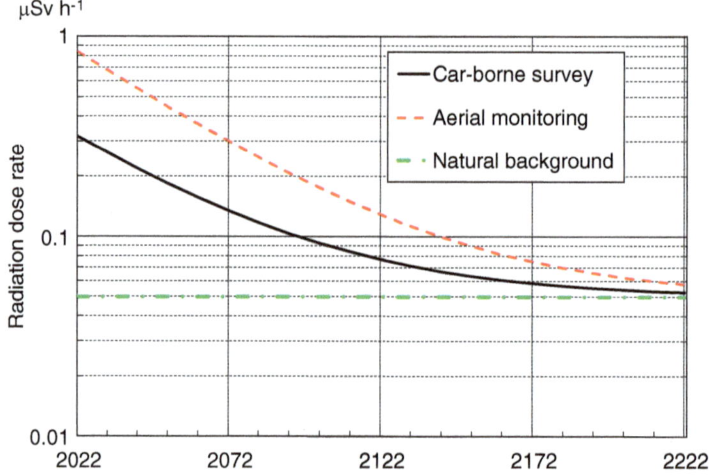

Fig. 3.5 Future decreasing tendency of radiation dose rate in Iitate Village considering the physical decay of ^{137}Cs and natural background of 0.05 µSv/h. The solid line starts at our car-borne of 0.31 µSv/h on April 1, 2023 and the red broken line at 0.82 µSv/h of the NRA aerial survey in October 2022.

From the author's personal experience as a researcher investigating radioactive contamination in the environment, radiation doses up to 0.1µSv/h in Japan can be regarded as levels within the range of natural background variations. If the ambient dose rate exceeds 0.2µSv/h, some artificial radiation sources should be suspected.

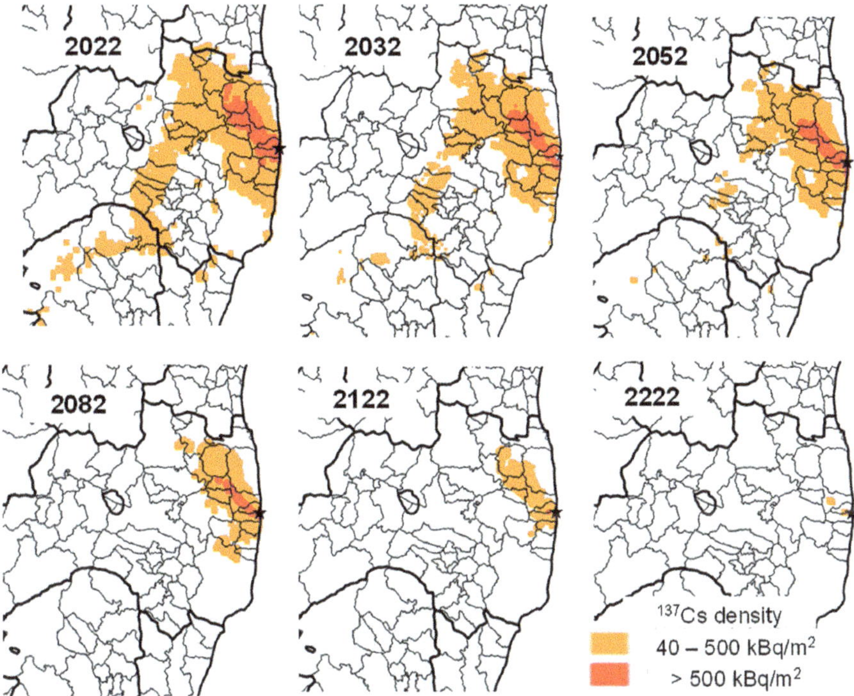

Fig. 3.6 Future density maps of ^{137}Cs contamination: current (2022), 10 years (2032), 30 years (2052), 60 years (2082), 100 years (2122), and 200 years (2222) later.

From Fig. 3.5 we can say that it will take 70 years in residential areas and 120 years in forested areas for radiation levels in Iitate Village to decrease within the range of natural background in Japan.

Maps of the future ^{137}Cs contamination density up to 200 years later, calculated based on the October 2022 aerial monitoring data by NRA [15], are shown in Fig. 3.6..

The ^{137}Cs contamination density of 40 kBq/m^2 corresponds to the level above which the radiation control area should be set in facilities dealing with radioisotopes according to Japanese radiation regulations. The density of 500 kBq/m^2 was chosen as close to 550 kBq/m^2, above which residents around Chernobyl must relocte. Areas of contamination are summarized in Table 3.2 by dividing in the whole area related to the FNPP accident and Iitate Village. It is noted that the current 3200 km^2 area more than 40 kBq/m^2 is equivalent to 1.5 times the Tokyo Metropolitan of 2200 km^2, and the 277 km^2 area more than 500 kBq/m^2 is 4.4 times the area within the Yamanote loop line in central Tokyo.

Table 3.2 Perspective of ^{137}Cs contaminated area by the FNPP accident up to 2222: total area and Iitate Village.

Year	Total area		Iitate Village	
	40–500 kBq/m^2	>500 kBq/m^2	40–500 kBq/m^2	>500 kBq/m^2
2022	2873 km^2	277 km^2	189 km^2	42 km^2
2032	2298 km^2	230 km^2	204 km^2	26 km^2
2052	1402 km^2	143 km^2	222 km^2	4.1 km^2
2082	811 km^2	48 km^2	202 km^2	0 km^2
2122	349 km^2	0.1 km^2	74 km^2	0 km^2
2222	2 km^2	0 km^2	0 km^2	0 km^2

3.4 Conclusion

The average ambient dose rate of 0.31μSv/h was obtained by our most recent carborne survey in Iitate Village on April 1, 2023, which decreased to 1/35 of 10.8μSv/h on March 29, 2011. Meanwhile, the average dose rate in Iitate Village of 0.83μSv/h was deduced from the aerial monitoring data by NRA in October 2022. The difference between the two averages indicates that strong ^{137}Cs contamination remains in the forest part of Iitate Village for more than 12 years. Currently, the total areas of ^{137}Cs contamination density of 40–500 kBq/m^2 and above 500 kBq/m^2 are 2,900 km^2 and 277 km^2, respectively. Considering the half-life of 30 years of ^{137}Cs, it should be recognized that significant ^{137}Cs contamination will continue for 50–100 years more.

References

1. The National Diet of Japan Fukushima Nuclear Accident Independent Investigation Commission (2012) The official report of The Fukushima Nuclear Accident Independent Investigation Commission. http://warp.da.ndl.go.jp/info:ndljp/pid/3856371/naiic.go.jp/en/report/. Accessed 5 July 2024
2. TEPCO (2011) Fukushima Nuclear Accident Analysis Report, June 20, 2012. https://www.tepco.co.jp/en/press/corp-com/release/betu12_e/images/120620e0104.pdf. Accessed 5 July 2024
3. Imanaka T, Hayashi G, Endo S (2015) Comparison of the accident process, radioactivity release and ground contamination between Chernobyl and Fukushima-1. J Radiat Res 56(suppl):i56–i61. https://academic.oup.com/jrr/article/56/suppl_1/i56/2580293. Accessed 5 July 2024
4. Imanaka T (2020) Comparison of radioactivity release and contamination from the Fukushima and Chernobyl nuclear power plant accidents. In: Fukumoto M (ed) Low-dose radiation effects on animals and ecosystems: long-term study on the Fukushima Nuclear Accident. Springer, pp 249–259
5. Aoyama M, Kajino M, Tanaka T et al (2016) ^{134}Cs and ^{137}Cs in the north Pacific Ocean derived from the March 2011 TEPCO Fukushima dai-ichi nuclear power plant accident, Japan. Part two: estimation of ^{134}Cs and ^{137}Cs inventories in the north Pacific Ocean. J Oceanogr 72:67–76. https://doi.org/10.1007/s10872-015-0332-2
6. Fukushima prefecture HP, Results of past radiation monitoring. (in Japanese). https://www.pref.fukushima.lg.jp/sec/16025d/kako-monitoring.html. Accessed 5 July 2024

7. Tokyo Metropolitan Institute of Public Health Home Page. (in Japanese) https://monitoring.tmiph.metro.tokyo.lg.jp/mp_shinjuku_air_week_list.html. Accessed 5 July 2024
8. Iitate-mura Society for Radioecology HP. https://www.iitate-sora.net/. Accessed 5 July 2024
9. Imanaka T, Endo S, Shizuma K et al (2011) Interim Report on Radiation Survey in Iitate Village area conducted on March 28th and 29th. http://www.rri.kyoto-u.ac.jp/NSRG/seminar/No110/Iitate-interim-report110404.pdf. Accessed 5 July 2024
10. Imanaka T, Endo S, Sugai M et al (2012) Early radiation survey of Iitate village, which was heavily contaminated by the Fukushima Daiichi accident, conducted on 28 and 29 March 2011. Health Physics 102:680–686
11. IISORA Radiation Survey Team (2023) Report of radiation survey in Iitate village after 12 years from the FNPP accident. (in Japanese) http://www.rri.kyoto-u.ac.jp/NSRG/temp/2023/Iitate23-4-16.pdf. Accessed 5 July 2024
12. Nuclear Regulation Authority Home Page, Airborne Monitoring Survey Results. March 10, 2023 (in Japanese). https://radioactivity.nra.go.jp/ja/results/airborne/air-dose. Accessed 5 July 2024
13. Kato H, Onda Y, Hisadome K et al (2017) Temporal changes in radiocesium deposition in various forest stands following the Fukushima Dai-ichi Nuclear Power Plant accident. J Environ Radioact 166:449–457
14. Ito E, Miura S, Aoyama M et al (2020) Global ^{137}Cs fallout inventories of forest soil across Japan and their consequences half a century later. J Environ Radioact 225:106421
15. Japan Atomic Energy Agency Home Page, Database for Radioactive Substance Monitoring Data (in Japanese). https://emdb.jaea.go.jp/emdb/contents/12/. Accessed 5 July 2024

Part II
Contamination and Dosimetry of Individual Animals

Chapter 4
Radioactive Cesium Concentrations in Raw Milk and Beef of Cattle Fed Contaminated Feed

Takashi Numabe, Hidehiko Suzuki, Masatoshi Suzuki, Hideaki Yamashiro, and Manabu Fukumoto

Abstract After the Fukushima Daiichi Nuclear Power Plant (FNPP) accident, maintaining the safety of agricultural products in the event of radiation accidents has become a major social concern. In order to predict the transfer of radioactive materials to dairy products and minimize the spread of contamination to food, we conducted tests in which cattle were fed feed containing relatively low levels of radioactive cesium (^{134}Cs + ^{137}Cs) derived from the FNPP accident. This study consists of two parts: (1) determination of the transfer of radioactive Cs to milk, and (2) measurement of radioactive Cs contamination in tissues corresponding to edible beef in cattle prior to slaughter. Radioactive Cs concentration in milk rose within 1 day after feeding contaminated feed and began to decrease witin 1 day after switching to uncontaminated feed, but it took 4–8 weeks to fall below detection limits. Fecal excretion showed changes similar to those in milk. After even 1 week of continuous feeding of contaminated food, accumulation of radioactive Cs was observed in organs and muscles. We have established a method to estimate radioactive Cs concentration in skeletal muscles using radioactivity values measured by placing the probe of a sodium iodide (NaI) survey meter in close contact with the body surface of live cattle (external measurement). A strong positive correlation between the external measurement (cps) and radioactive Cs concentration (Bq/kg) in slaughtered beef was verified even below 50 Bq/kg.

T. Numabe
Miyagi Agricultural Department Corporation, Sendai, Japan

H. Suzuki
Agriculture Department, Miyagi Prefectural Government, Sendai, Japan

M. Suzuki · M. Fukumoto (✉)
International Research Institute of Disaster Science, Tohoku University, Sendai, Japan
e-mail: manabu.fukumoto.a8@tohoku.ac.jp

H. Yamashiro
Faculty of Agriculture, Niigata University, Niigata, Japan

M. Fukumoto (ed.), *Low-Dose Radiation Effects on Animals and Ecosystems II*,
https://doi.org/10.1007/978-981-95-5559-8_4

Keywords Fukushima Daiichi Nuclear Power Plant (FNPP) accident ·
Radioactive cesium (Cs) · Contaminated feed · Transfer coefficient · Milk · Beef ·
External measurement

4.1 Introduction

In Japan, cattle are often fed homegrown forage such as grass, rice straw, and live-stock corn harvested by farmers themselves. The Fukushima Daiichi Nuclear Power Plant (FNPP) accident occurred in March 2011 released large amounts of radioactive material, particularly radioactive cesium, into the environment. In this chapter, unless otherwise specified, the total amount of cesium-134 (^{134}Cs) and cesium-137 (^{137}Cs) is referred to as the amount of radioactive Cs. A survey conducted by the Tokyo Metropolitan Government on July 8 and 9, 2011, detected radioactive Cs in beef shipped from a fattening farm in Minamisoma City, Fukushima Prefecture, exceeding the provisional regulatory value for food products (500 Bq/kg), which was attributed to feeding homemade forage containing contaminated rice straw [1]. The detection of radioactive Cs exceeding the provisional regulatory value in rice straw for livestock feed (300 Bq/kg) produced in Miyagi Prefecture, adjacent to northern Fukushima Prefecture, prompted a request for voluntary restraint on the use of grass produced in Miyagi Prefecture, which had a significant negative impact on the livestock industry. Therefore, we began developing a system to ensure that milk and beef containing detectable levels of radioactive Cs would not enter the market. Our goals were: (1) to separate contaminated milk at the time of milking, thereby preventing its mixing with uncontaminated milk during raw milk process-ing, and (2) to avoid unnecessary slaughter by making it possible to accurately measure radioactive Cs concentration in the edible parts of cattle (i.e., beef) prior to slaughter. In order to obtain criteria for determining the safety of homemade forage, we carried out radioactivity inspection tests in which dairy cows were fed silage (lactic acid-fermented pasture grass) contaminated with radioactive materials, and studied the transfer of radionuclides into milk, fecal excretion, and organ distribu-tion. Fm, the transfer coefficient of radionuclides from feed to milk, has been widely employed to quantify radionuclide transfer to milk as the equilibrium ratio of the radioactivity concentration in milk to the daily dietary radionuclide intake. Fm has been reported to show less variation among individuals within an experimental herd than the percentage of ingested radionuclides excreted in milk [2]. The Fm value was calculated to evaluate the validity of the results of this study. We further estab-lished a method for estimating radioactive Cs concentration in the edible parts based on the measurement of radioactivity on the body surface of live cattle.

4.2 Tests to Study Transfer of Radioactive Cesium from Feed to Milk

4.2.1 Cattle and Mixed Feed

Three independent tests were conducted, and similar results were obtained. Therefore, we present representative results in this chapter. An individually housed lactating Holstein cow (mid-lactation, second calving, body weight 500 kg) was used. We designed the mixed feed to meet 16% crude protein and 73% total digestible nutrients in accordance with the Japanese Feeding Standards for dairy cattle. The mixed feed ingredients such as compound feed, corn silage, hay cubes, crushed corn, vitamins, and other ingredients were purchased and confirmed to be free of detectable radioactivity. Feeding and milking were carried out twice a day, and the cow had free access to silage, water, and mineral blocks. Raw milk yield was 12 kg/day, with a composition of 4.1% milk fat, 3.1% milk protein, and 8.5% nonfat solids.

4.2.2 Feeding Test with Radiocontaminated Silage

The silage contaminated with radioactive material due to the FNPP accident was collected and molded in Miyagi Prefecture in June 2011. The only radioactive material detected was radioactive Cs, with radioactivity concentration of 817 Bq/kg (235 Bq/fresh grass equivalent, 80% moisture). In the radioactive feeding test, mixed feed and contaminated silage were fed for 9 days. From the 10th day onward, feeding was continued after switching to uncontaminated silage. Raw milk was collected periodically, and 2 L each was used as sample milk for radioactivity measurement. Feces were collected rectally or immediately after defecation and stored frozen until measurement. At the end of the radioactive feeding period, the cow was dissected, and the organ concentrations of radioactive materials were measured.

4.2.3 Radioactivity Measurement

Samples were thoroughly stirred and mixed, then packed in Marinelli beakers, and radioactivity was measured. The measurement was performed in a high-purity germanium semiconductor detector (ORTEC Co., Oak Ridge, TN) for 2000–5400 s.

4.2.4   Transfer Coefficient to Milk

The transfer coefficient to milk (Fm) is defined as the fraction of a radionuclide transferred to one liter of milk relative to the amount ingested by the animal per day at equilibrium, and is calculated using the following equation.

$$\mathrm{Fm}\left(\mathrm{day}\,/\,\mathrm{L}\right) = \text{radionuclide in milk}\left(\mathrm{Bq}\,/\,\mathrm{L}\right)/\text{intake of radionuclide in feed}\left(\mathrm{Bq}\,/\,\mathrm{day}\right)$$

4.3   Feeding Contaminated Silage and Transfer of Radioactive Cesium to Milk and Distribution in Organs

We fed dairy cows silage contaminated by the FNPP accident and examined the transition of radioactivity transferred to their bodies and livestock products. Since radioactive Cs was the only radioactive substance significantly detected in the contaminated silage, studies on radioactive Cs were subsequently conducted (Fig. 4.1).

Radioactive Cs levels in milk clearly increased the day after the start of feeding contaminated silage, and an increase was observed 12 h after feeding in the earliest

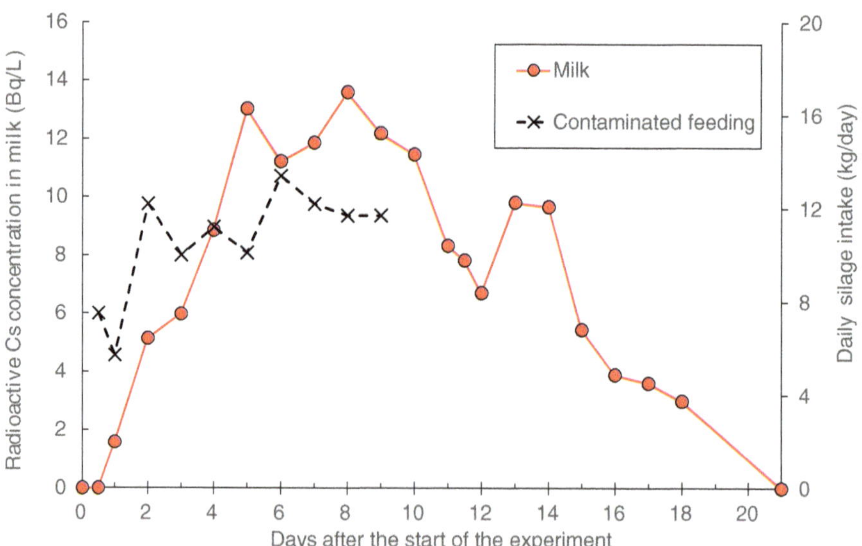

Fig. 4.1 A representative case showing radioactive Cs transfer into and clearance from milk via dietary intake. Radioactive Cs concentration in milk reached near saturation levels 5 days after the start of feeding contaminated silage, and began decreasing the day after switching to uncontaminated silage. Feeding intake verification was conducted once a day. Solid circles: radioactive Cs concentration in milk; crosses: daily intake of radioactive Cs contaminated silage.

individual. However, even after continuing to feed contaminated silage for more than10 days, the concentration saturated after about 5 days and then leveled off. Next, we examined the time until radioactive Cs became undetectable after switching to uncontaminated feed. Radioactive Cs in milk began to decrease the day after cessation of contaminated intake. The time required to decrease to undetectable levels was approximately twice the time required to reach saturation following the start of contaminated intake, amounting to 12 days in the dairy cow shown in Fig. 4.1. The day after we started feeding contaminated silage, radioactive Cs was also detected in feces. The excretion pattern of radioactive Cs in feces was similar to that in milk, including the decrease after cessation of contaminated feed. (data not shown)

Assuming that the intake of silage was approximately 10 kg/day, the transfer coefficient to milk (Fm) on the day of switching was 3.2×10^{-3} day/L. Two other feeding tests were conducted using silage with radioactive Cs concentrations of 2,100 Bq/kg and 604 Bq/kg, which yealded similar Fm values of 3.2×10^{-3} and 2.5×10^{-3} day/L, respectively. According to data provided by the International Atomic Energy Agency (IAEA), the Fm value ranges from 6.0×10^{-4} to 6.8×10^{-2} (mean 4.6×10^{-3}) [3]. Fm varies according to maintenance management and feed composition, and characteristics such as dry matter digestibility. The Fm value in this study is consistent with the report of IAEA, indicating that our results can be applied to agricultural strategies around the world. The cow fed contaminated silage for 8 days was dissected, and the highest radioactive Cs concentration was found in the kidneys, followed by the liver, digestive organs, and skeletal muscles.

4.4 Measuring Radioactivity from the Body Surface of Live Cattle to Determine the Amount of Radioactivity in the Muscle [4]

4.4.1 Establishment of a System to Predict Radioactive Cesium Concentration in Cattle Prior to Slaughter

Radioactivity measurements from the body surface of live cattle (external measurements) were performed by determining the radioactivity count rate (cps) on the body surface of live cattle using a 2-inch or a 3-inch NaI survey meter (SAM940; Berkeley Nucleonics Co., San Rafael, CA). Two challenges arose in accurately measuring the radioactivity of live cattle muscle, that is, edible parts prior to slaughter: (1) How could we mitigate the effect of environmental background radiation, such as natural radiation or radiation emitted from radioactive materials floating in the atmosphere or deposited on soil due to the FNPP accident? (2) What part of the body and what measurement time should be used to obtain stable data? In order to minimize background count, it was ultimately necessary to wrap a 1-cm-thick lead shield (Fig. 4.2a) around the NaI detector of the survey meter (Fig. 4.2b). Since the environmental

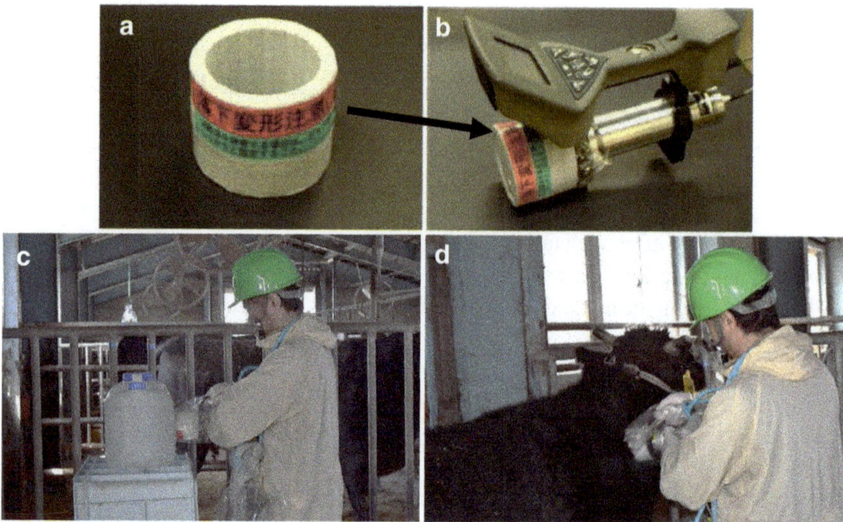

Fig. 4.2 External measurements to estimate radioactive Cs concentration in beef prior to slaughter. Emvironmental background radiation was blocked by tightly attaching a handmade heavy lead shield, weighting ca 5 kg (**a**), to the probe of the NaI scintillation survey meter (**b**). Baseline radioactivity was measured using a polyethylene tank filled with uncontaminated water as a phantom for cattle (**c**). External measurements were taken on the neck or buttocks of cattle fed contaminated feed (**d**). The body part of the cattle to be measured, the location where the cattle was held, and the direction in which the survey meter was applied were kept constant.

background count rate varied depending on the measurement location, the external measurement was conducted at a fixed location within the barn (Fig. 4.2c).

Radioactivity in the cattle muscle was calculated by subtracting baseline radioactivity from the external measurement. Measuring baseline radioactivity using a polyethylene tank filled with uncontaminated water as a phantom (Fig. 4.2c), we found that the value was affected by weather conditions. If it rained or snowed on the day of the measurement, naturally existing radionuclides such as bismuth-214 and lead-214 fell together, causing the measured values to increase. When snowfall exceeded 5 cm, radiation from soil was blocked, resulting in lower measured values. As the snow melted, the measured values gradually increased, and when the depth decreased to about 1 cm, the values became the same on sunny and cloudy days. Simultaneously, ambient count rate was measured without the water phantom. Measurements on the surface of the polyethylene tank were about 20% lower than the ambient count rate, indicating that background radiation from the ground was shielded by the cattle body. For the external measurement, the neck and buttock muscles (rump) were selected so that organs were not included in the measurement range (Fig. 4.2d). The detector was pressed onto the skin just above the muscle. Measurements were taken twice for 30 s each, and the average value was taken as the measured value. Each time, the external measurement was performed after the cattle was fixed in position and orientation. The cattle became accustomed to maintaining a certain standing posture during the external measurement work at the pretest stage. It was necessary to keep the measurement range and direction of the survey meter constant.

4.4.2   Conclusions and Discussion

Over a 2-month period from September to October 2011, external measurements were performed in the neck of 169 beef cattle delivered to slaughterhouses in Miyagi Prefecture using the NaI survey meter equipped with the lead shield. After slaughter, radioactive Cs concentration in beef was measured by Υ-ray spectral analysis using a germanium semiconductor detector. As a result, it was found that the correlation coefficient between external measurement values (cps) and radioactive Cs concentrations in beef (Bq/kg) was greater than 0.9, and that the external measurement could detect radioactive Cs concentrations of 21 Bq/kg or higher in beef (Fig. 4.3).

Therefore, we drew a calibration curve by applying data correlation, enabling accurate estimation of radioactivity concentrations in beef even below 50 Bq/kg. Based on the results of this study, an inspection system has been established whereby cattle are shipped only if they pass the non-invasive external meausrement. Cattle determined through the external measurement to have edible parts exceeding regulatory limits are returned to their respective farms Accurate measurement of radioactivity in live animals prior to slaughter has made it possible to ensure safe and secure production, distribution, and consumption of meat without wasting valuable

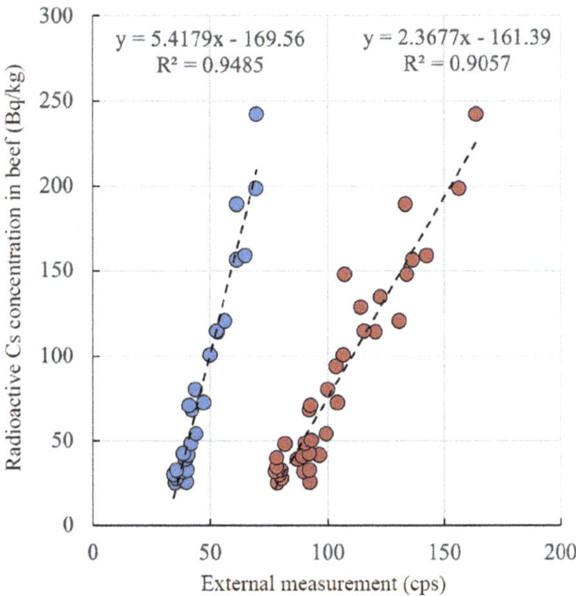

Fig. 4.3 Correlation between external measurements and radioactivity concentrations in beef. The larger the diameter of the probe, the higher the measured value and the gentler the slope of the regression line, resulting in higher sensitivity. External measurements were carried out using a 2-inch (blue circles) or a 3-inch (red circles) NaI survey meter.

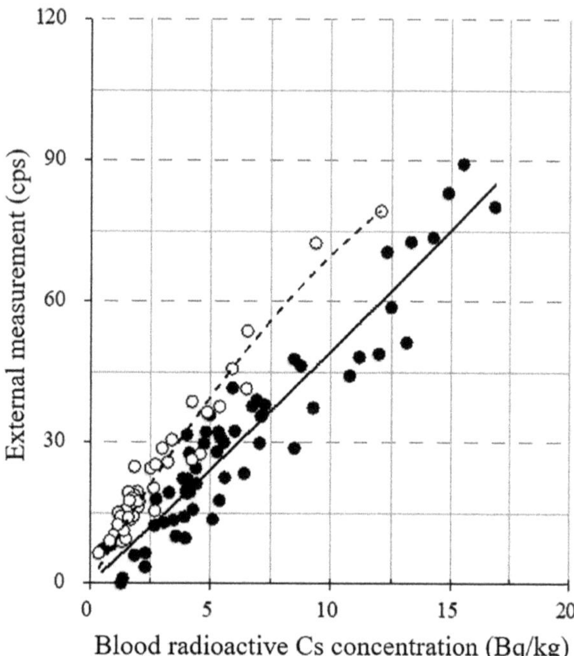

Fig. 4.4 Correlation between radioactive Cs concentrations in regularly collected blood samples and corresponding external measurements of the skeletal muscle (neck). Solid circles: cattle continuously fed radioactive Cs contaminated feed; open circles: cattle switched to uncontaminated feed after continuously fed radioactive Cs contaminated feed. The data sets were each fitted with a linear model (solid line) and a quadratic model (dashed line) (Adapted from Ref. 4).

livestock. According to public data released by Miyagi Prefecture, as of March 2020, 110,600 cattle passed the external measurement and were slaughtered, and none of them exceeded the provisional regulatory limit for radioactive Cs. Furthermore, it became clear that the external measurement (cps)/blood radioactivity concentration (Bq/kg) ratio was consistently higher after switching to uncontaminated feed compared with the period during which contaminated feed continued to be fed (Fig. 4.4).

By calculating the ratio of externally measured radioactivity to blood radioactive Cs concentration, we can determine whether the feed consumed by cattle is contaminated, that is, whether radioactive Cs is continuing to accumulate in the body or is being excreted.

References

1. https://www.mofa.go.jp/j_info/visit/incidents/pdfs/press/20110725/foreign-press-briefing-20110725-kantei.pdf (in Japanese)
2. Ward GM, Johnson JE, Sasser LB (1967) Transfer coefficients of fallout cesium-137 to milk of dairy cattle fed pasture, green-cut alfalfa, or stored feed. J Dairy Sci 50(7):1092–1096
3. International Atomic Energy Agency (IAEA) (2020) Handbook of parameter values for the prediction of radionuclide transfer in terrestrial and freshwater environments. IAEA-TRS 472. https://www-pub.iaea.org/MTCD/Publications/PDF/trs472_web.pdf
4. Suzuki M, Suzuki H, Ishiguro H et al (2019) Correlation of radiocesium activity between muscle and peripheral blood of live cattle depending on presence or absence of radiocontamination in feed. Radiat Res 192(6):589–601

Chapter 5
Radiation Monitoring and Detection System for Soil/Waste and Cattle Model

Emiko Isogai, Jun Saito, Hisahi Shinoda, Tsutomu Sekine, and Yoshiyuki Higuchi

Abstract We used a radiation monitoring and detection system (RMDS) with split-aram technology to measure the radioactivity of soil/waste and a cattle phantom. The system was designed to distinguish between the background and samples contaminated with cesium-137 (^{137}Cs).

Before the RMDS trial, the radioactivity levels measured using an NaI (Tl) scintillation counter were 3000 Bq/kg for soil (gross $\pm$1.9%, net $\pm$5%) and 130,000 Bq/kg for waste (gross $\pm$5.7%, net $\pm$5.6%). The RMDS provides stable results by performing self-shielding measurements based on passing vehicles after installation.

The phantom used for the test was based on a cattle weight of 620 kg. The ^{137}Cs concentration of the phantom assumed a uniform 100 Bq/kg using soil contaminated with ^{134}Cs and ^{137}Cs after the Fukushima Daiichi Nuclear Power Plant accident. Experimental data confirmed the presence of radioactive Cs in the soil. The 620 kg phantom produced measurements of 108.4 $\pm$ 12.5 Bq/kg (1st run) and 104.9 $\pm$ 8.0 Bq/kg (2nd run). When a 520 kg phantom was used, the result was 97.4 $\pm$ 8.7 Bq/kg, and the difference was not significant between the two phantom weights. Should a nuclear disaster recur, the first screening should involve a whole-body counter for livestock, and clean feeding management can reduce the uptake of contaminating radionuclides. Using RMSD measurements of radioactive cesium and a phantom for calibration could contribute to food safety in livestock production.

E. Isogai (✉)
Graduate School of Agricultural Science, Tohoku University, Sendai, Aoba-ku, Japan
e-mail: isogai.a7@tohoku.ac.jp

J. Saito
Niki Glass Co. Ltd, Tokyo, Shinagawa-ku, Japan

H. Shinoda
Graduate School of Dentistry, Tohoku University, Sendai, Aoba-ku, Japan

T. Sekine
Institute for Excellence in Higher Education, Tohoku University, Sendai, Aoba-ku, Japan

Y. Higuchi
Faculty of Symbiotic Systems Science, Fukushima University,
Fukushima, Kanayagawa, Japan

M. Fukumoto (ed.), *Low-Dose Radiation Effects on Animals and Ecosystems II*,
https://doi.org/10.1007/978-981-95-5559-8_5

Keywords Radioactive cesium (Cs) · Radioactivity monitoring · Soil · Waste · Whole-body · Cattle

5.1　Introduction

The Fukushima Daiichi Nuclear Power Plant (FNPP) accident in March 2011 released large amounts of artificial radioactive substances into the environment [1]. Radioactive materials were removed from local inhabited areas using methods such as decontamination, and a wastewater disposal plan was released for the region on June 11, 2012. The soil and waste are expected to be disposed of both inside and outside of the Fukushima Prefecture by 2045. Currently, the large amount of generated waste is stored in distinct areas of the prefecture. The volume of soil and waste must be sorted and reduced, its radioactive concentration measured, and then moved to interim storage facilities for reconstruction to proceed.

On April 22, 2011, the evacuation zone consisted of a 20-km radius surrounding the FNPP, and approximately 3,400 cattle, 31,500 pigs, and 630,000 chickens were stranded in this area. On May 12, 2011, the Japanese government ordered Fukushima Prefecture to euthanize the cattle that inhabited the evacuation zone.

Prior to the FNPP accident, the radiation limit for contaminated meat as determined by the International Atomic Energy Agency (IAEA) was 1,000 Bq/kg. Since that time, more conservative limits of 500 Bq/kg and, subsequently, 100 Bq/kg have been established in Japan. We previously reported that radioactive cesium (^{134}Cs + ^{137}Cs) easily accumulates in the muscle and is associated with blood [2]. The amount of radioactive cesium in the blood is a useful marker for estimating the levels in muscle, even in areas with low radioactivity [3, 4]. Although this technique could detect high-risk cattle before they enter the market, the time and costs involved are prohibitive. In addition, an NaI (Tl) scintillation counter can be used to estimate radioactive Cs levels through direct contact with the skin of live cattle [5]; however, measurements from outside the body introduce issues such as high background interference. Furthermore, an NaI (Tl) scintillation counter is extremely heavy and difficult to handle. Screening methods that are simple, fast, and absent of background noise are critical when dealing with live cattle.

We developed a passage-type radiation monitoring and detection system (RMDS) for soil/waste and livestock phantoms. The system can distinguish between the background and contaminated samples and operates in a rapid and easy-to-handle manner.

5.2 Materials and Methods

5.2.1 Soil/Waste

Soil and waste (weeding sheet or litter layer) were obtained from the area of Date City (Reizan-cho) between November 18 and 22, 2013 (air dose: 0.33–040 μSv/h). The samples were then placed in flexible 1-t container bags.

5.2.2 Radiation Monitoring and Detection System (RMDS) for Soil/Waste

We used an RMDS with split-aram technology (Nucsafe, Inc. [now Rapiscan Co. Ltd.], Tennessee, USA) on the soil/waste in Reizan-cho [6, 7]. The device allowed for nondestructive inspection. Each panel had a gamma-ray detector with photomultiplier tubes at both ends of a polyvinyl toluene (PVT) crystal, as shown in Fig. 5.1. The equipment continued to operate while the soil or waste was loaded onto the truck or crane. The radioactivity was measured at a speed of approximately 5 km/h. Before the RMDS trial, the samples were measured using an NaI (Tl) scintillation counter (EMF211, EMF Japan Co. Ltd.), and the radioactivity was 3,000 Bq/kg for soil and 130,000 Bq/kg for waste. The trial was performed three times for soil and four times for waste.

5.2.3 Phantom Cattle

We prepared a cattle-type phantom using tough tenor containers (square bag-in-box, 10 L and 20 L; AS One Co., Ltd., Japan) as shown in Fig. 5.2. Soil contaminated with radioactive Cs released from the FNPP was uniformly mixed with a superabsorbent polymer and diluted with tap water in the tenor container. The soil particles were then uniformly dispersed in gel. The radioactivity of the soil samples was determined using gamma-ray spectrometry with three high-purity germanium (HPGe) detectors (Ortec Co., USA). The final concentration of radioactive Cs in the square bag was adjusted to 100 Bq/kg. The livestock phantom was created with 36 storage units representing the main body parts (20 kg × 24 and 10 kg × 12) and two units representing the neck parts (10 kg × 2). Hata reported that muscle tissue accounts for approximately 60% of the total mass of cattle [8], and the muscle content was estimated by the Statistics Department of the Ministry of Agriculture, Forestry and Fisheries (http://www.toukei.maff.go.jp/dijest/tikusan/tiku03/tiku03. html) as 311 kg/cow. A muscle mass of 311 kg corresponds to an estimated weight of 690 kg. The phantom used weighed 620 kg excluding the head, legs, or tail. We

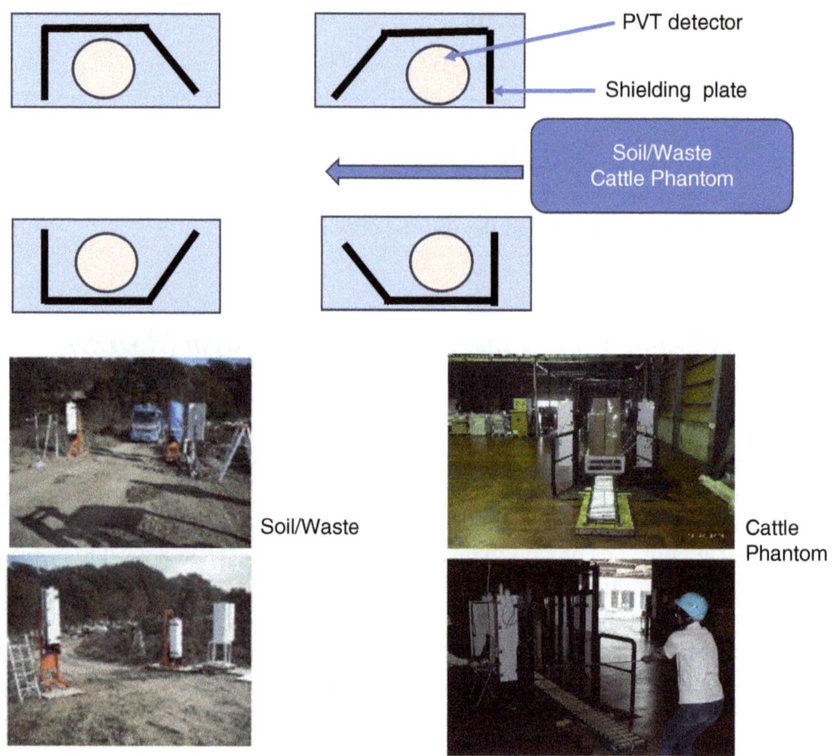

Fig. 5.1 Monitoring system and test run. Left photographs: The radioactivity was measured at a speed of about 5 km/h by loading onto the truck or crane. Trial was performed three times for the soil and four times for the waste. Right photographs: The test was performed by pulling the phantom livestock past the detector arrays at approximately 2 m/s. A total of 40 runs was performed consecutively. The test runs were recorded using a data collection tool and stored in a database for retrieval.

also prepared a 520-kg phantom consisting of 26 storage units for the main body parts (20 kg × 24 and 10 kg × 2) by removing 10 kg × 10.

5.2.4   Monitoring System for Cattle Model

The RMDS test was performed by pulling the phantom at approximately 2 m/s, as shown in Fig. 5.1. Forty runs for the 620-kg phantom (eliminating malfunctions such as derailment) were conducted at Sendai (air dose: 0.04–0.05 μSv/h) in June 2013, while 14 runs were performed for the 520-kg phantom. Test runs were recorded using a data collection tool and stored in a database for retrieval. Data were expressed as means ± standard deviations.

5.3   Results and Discussion

We used an RMDS to monitor the soil/waste in Reizan-cho, Fukushima (air dose: 0.33–0.40 µSv/h) [8], after determining the radioactivity using an NaI (Tl) scintillation counter. The radiation doses of the soil and waste were 3,000 Bq/kg and 130,000 Bq/kg, respectively. The measurement data were gross $\pm1.9\%$ (net $\pm5\%$) in the soil and gross $\pm5.7\%$ (net $\pm5.6\%$) in the waste. The RMDS provided stable results by performing self-shielding measurements based on passing vehicles after installation, sampling in advance, and calculating conversion factors. The monitoring system consisted of four cylindrical PVT detectors encased in a three-sided stainless-steel shield, as shown in Fig. 5.2. This system can be used to determine contamination levels of soil and waste.

A separate phantom was prepared as a positive control for the cattle model. The control contained radioactive material that was uniformly distributed as the soil particles. Furthermore, the size and shape of the phantom could be freely adjusted.

The RMDS detectors are configured in a "split detection" scheme, which allows for the differentiation of individually contaminated cows within a contiguous line of animals. Two pairs of detectors were set up in an entry/exit configuration. The screening time for each test was approximately 1 min. The background spectrum from the PVT detector exhibited a different waveform when radioactive Cs was

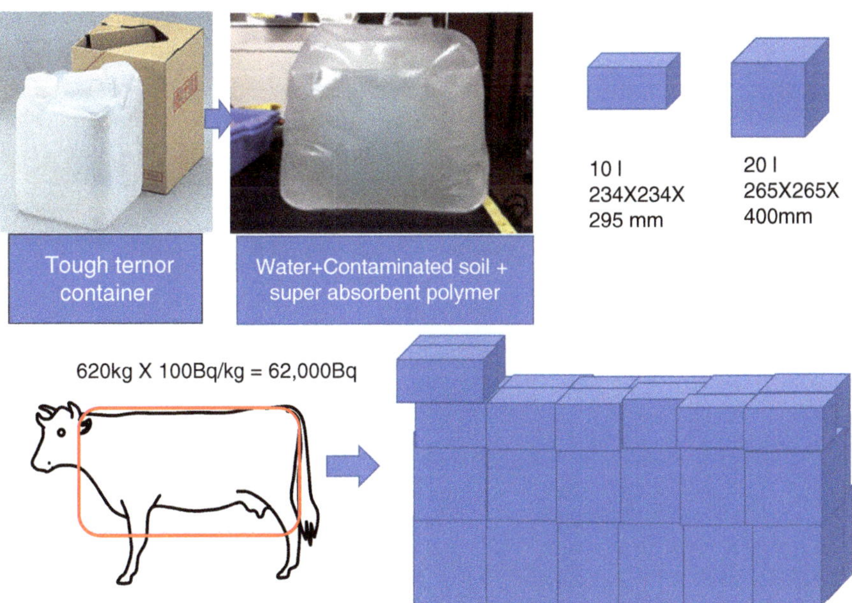

Fig. 5.2 Phantom (cattle type). As radiation sources, contaminated soil with radioactive Cs released from the FNPP was used. The sample was uniformly mixed with superabsorbent polymer and diluted with tap water in the tough tenor container. A livestock phantom was created with 36 storage units.

present, which reflects the difference in Compton scattering of the radioactive Cs. The RMDS analyzes the sample based on Compton scattering. Clear photoelectric peaks (region of interest [ROI]) were observed for the phantom (100 Bq/kg), whereas no peaks were observed for the control (Fig. 5.3). The measurements for the 620-kg phantom were 108.4 ± 12.5 Bq/kg (1st run) and 104.9 ± 8.0 Bq/kg (2nd

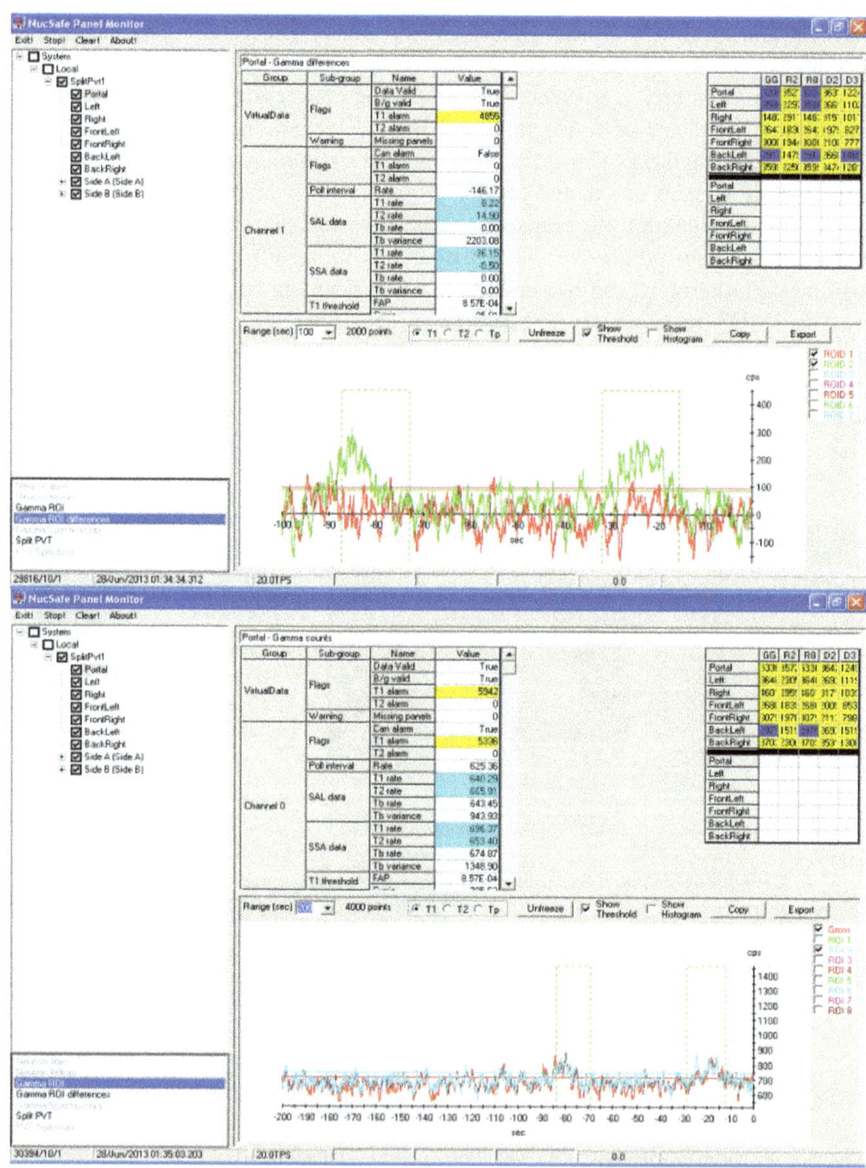

Fig. 5.3 Results of RMSD. Upper: Clear photoelectric peaks (ROI) are observed in the phantom (100 Bq/kg). Lower: Control—no peaks observed.

Table 5.1 RMSD measurement for livestock phantom.

Phantom weight (kg)	Trial run	RMSD measurement (mean ± SD)		
620	40	108.4 ± 12.5	⎱ NS*	
620	20	104.9 ± 8.0	⎰ ⎱ NS	⎱ NS
520	20	97.4 ± 8.7	⎰	⎰

*not significant (unpaired t test)

run) (Table 5.1). The 520-kg phantom returned a value of 97.4 ± 8.7 Bq/kg. The difference was not significant between the 620-kg and 520-kg phantoms. The RMDS measurement of radioactive cesium could contribute to food safety in livestock production.

*Not significant (unpaired t test)

When we tested the RMDS with humans (Sendai citizens, 5 runs, approximately 4 km/h), no peaks were observed. An estimation of a whole-body counter for the residents of Korosten City, Ukraine, had been performed, which showed that the median body burden of ^{137}Cs decreased from 1996 to 2008 [9]. After 2003, more than half of the participants had internal exposure doses below the detectable level [9]. After the FNPP accident, the results obtained from the Namie residents (approximately 5 Bq for ^{134}Cs and 20 Bq for ^{137}Cs) were much lower than those from Korosten City [10]. In Iwaki City, most of the participants registered below 300 Bq/body in the first (October 2012 to February 2013) and second screening (May to November 2013) [11]. Similarly, Bernhardsson et al. reported the internal and external exposure of inhabitants living in the Bryansk region of Russia between 1990 and 2008 [12]. Thus, the whole-body counter can be useful for temporal and spatial comparisons between people.

In vivo whole-body counters are calibrated using phantoms such as the bottle manikin absorption phantom [13]. These phantoms contain point sources, rod sources, uniform sources, or radionuclides distributed in soft tissues. Point sources have been previously used with RMDSs [6]. Muscle tissues show the highest deposition of ^{137}Cs, and no statistical difference in ^{137}Cs activity concentration was observed among the three representative positions of cattle muscle (longissimus, biceps femoris, and masseter muscle) [2]. Therefore, a phantom was created with radioactive material evenly distributed throughout. For small livestock such as calves and pigs, standard samples can be easily created by rearranging the blocks. Since each detector in the RMDS is an independent panel, measurements can be adjusted to the size of the particular animal.

When a nuclear disaster such as the FNPP accident occurs, livestock and animals around the facility continuously ingest low levels of radioactive material [14]. The correlation of radiocesium activity concentration of radioactive Cs between the muscle and peripheral blood of live cattle can vary depending on the presence or absence of ^{137}Cs contamination in the feed, and it is possible to protect food safety without the need to slaughter cattle after a nuclear disaster [5]. If contamination can be easily detected, the livestock can be isolated and fed uncontaminated feed for several months. A whole-body counter may be useful in these situations, similar to that for humans. The biological half-life for living animals is significantly shorter than the physical half-life, thereby allowing the radioactive activity to be removed from the animals more quickly. Faster excretion of radioactive Cs means that livestock can be returned to the meat or dairy market within a reasonable time frame. Clean feeding management can reduce the uptake of contaminating radionuclides [15]. This method has been used with cattle in the former USSR and Western Europe after the Chernobyl accident (5000 and 20,000 cattle, respectively). If a nuclear disaster recurs, a whole-body counter should be used for the first screening of livestock.

5.4 Conclusion

Passage-type RMDSs can distinguish between the background and contamination in soil/waste and livestock phantoms. These systems are easy to handle and require only a short measurement time. The separate phantom consists of uniformly distributed radioactive material in the soil, which is useful for measuring a variety of systems because of the ability to freely manipulate its size and shape.

References

1. Kinoshita N, Sueki K, Sasa K et al (2011) Assessment of individual radionuclide distributions from the Fukushima nuclear accident covering central-east Japan. Proc Natl Acad Sci USA 108:19526–19529. https://doi.org/10.1073/pnas.1111724108
2. Fukuda T, Kino Y, Abe Y et al (2013) Distribution of artificial radionuclides in abandoned cattle in the evacuation zone of the Fukushima Daiichi nuclear power plant. PLoS One 8:e54312. https://doi.org/10.1371/journal.pone.0054312
3. Fukuda T, Hiji M, Kino Y et al (2016) Software development for estimating the cesium radioactivity in skeletal muscle from that in blood of cattle. Anim Sci J 87:842–847. https://doi.org/10.1111/asj.12490
4. Fukuda T, Kino Y, Abe Y et al (2015) Cesium radioactivity in peripheral blood is linearly correlated to that in skeletal muscle. Anim Sci J 86:120–124. https://doi.org/10.1111/asj.12301
5. Suzuki M, Suzuki H, Ishiguro H et al (2019) Correlation of radiocesium activity between muscle and peripheral blood of live cattle depending on presence or absence of radiocontamination in feed. Radiat Res 192:589–601. https://doi.org/10.1667/RR15418.1
6. Niki Glass Co. Ltd (2012) Demonstration of the Nucsafe livestock monitoring system Yokohama, Japan, Report for Nucsafe livestock monitoring system-September 2012
7. Higuchi Y, Hamada H, Itakura S et al (2013) Demonstration of pass-through decontamination waste – radiation measuring device using PVT detector (Japanese). https://kensetsu.ipros.jp/news/detail/24145/attachFile/. Accessed 21 Oct 2023
8. Hata H (2000) Nutritional and physiological aspects in production of cattle fed roughage, Research bulletin of the livestock farm, Faculty of agriculture, Hokkaido University (Japanese) 17:29–38. http://hdl.handle.net/2115/48956. Accessed 29 Sept 2023
9. Hayashida N, Sekitani Y, Kozlovsky A et al (2011) Screening for 137Cs body burden due to the chernobyl accident in Korosten City, Zhitomir, Ukraine: 1996–2008. J Radiat Res 52:629–633. https://doi.org/10.1269/jrr.11017

10. Hosokawa Y, Nomura K, Tsushima E et al (2017) Whole-body counter (WBC) and food radi-ocesium contamination survey in Namie, Fukushima Prefecture. PLoS ONE 12:e0174549. https://doi.org/10.1371/journal.pone.0174549
11. Orita M, Hayashida N, Nukui H et al (2014) Internal radiation exposure dose in Iwaki city, Fukushima prefecture after the accident at Fukushima Dai-ichi Nuclear Power Plant. PLoS One 9:e114407. https://doi.org/10.1371/journal.pone
12. Bernhardsson C, Zvonova I, Rääf C et al (2011) Measurements of long-term external and internal radiation exposure of inhabitants of some villages of the Bryansk region of Russia after the Chernobyl accident. Sci Total Environ 409:4811–4817. https://doi.org/10.1016/j.scitotenv.2011.07.066
13. Manohari M, Sugumar P, Deepu R et al (2022) Comparison of Indian BOMAB and ICRP voxel phantom for calibration of shadow shield whole body counter. Appl Radia Isot 180:110020. https://doi.org/10.1016/j.apradiso.2021.110020
14. Takahashi S, Inoue K, Suzuki M et al (2015) A comprehensive dose evaluation project con-cerning animals affected by the Fukushima Daiichi Nuclear Power Plant accident: its set-up and progress. J Radiat Res 56:i36–i41. https://doi.org/10.1093/jrr/rrv069
15. Chernobyl forum expert group Environment (2006) Environmental consequences of the Chernobyl accident and their remediation: twenty years of experience. https://www-pub.iaea.org/MTCD/Publications/PDF/Pub1239_web.pdf. Accessed 29 Sept 2023

Chapter 6
Evaluation of Organ Doses to Japanese Macaques for Internal Dose Using Voxel Phantom

Takumi Urayama, Yuta Takamura, Kosei Yamada, Tsuyoshi Kajimoto, Kenichi Tanaka, Masatoshi Suzuki, Yohei Inaba, Koichi Chida, Manabu Fukumoto, and Satoru Endo

Abstract The purpose of this study is to calculate organ doses for Japanese macaques. Voxel phantoms of six macaques with different body weights were fabricated, and internal dose-rate conversion coefficients for cesium-134 (^{134}Cs), ^{137}Cs, iodine-129 (^{129}I), and ^{131}I were estimated. As a result, it was found that there is a correlation between body weight and dose-rate conversion coefficients. A function of conversion coefficients to body weights was derived for each organ. Organ doses for ^{134}Cs and ^{137}Cs were estimated from the measured ^{134}Cs and ^{137}Cs concentration data of 246 Japanese macaques affected by the Fukushima Daiichi Nuclear Power Point accident. Each mean of the internal organ dose was generally less than 191 mGy for absorbed dose. The effective dose for macaques was estimated using the tissue weighting factors for humans to be 158 mSv, which is quite higher than the effective dose for humans, reported to be less than 1 mSv.

T. Urayama · Y. Takamura · K. Yamada · T. Kajimoto · S. Endo (✉)
Quantum Energy Applications, Graduate School of Advanced Science and Engineering, Hiroshima University, Higashi-Hiroshima, Japan
e-mail: endos@hiroshima-u.ac.jp

K. Tanaka
Division of Liberal Arts Sciences, Kyoto Pharmaceutical University, Kyoto-shi, Kyoto, Japan

M. Suzuki · Y. Inaba · K. Chida
International Research Institute of Disaster Science, Tohoku University, Sendai, Miyagi, Japan

Course of Radiological Technology, Health Sciences, Tohoku University Graduate School of Medicine, Sendai, Miyagi, Japan

M. Fukumoto
International Research Institute of Disaster Science, Tohoku University, Sendai, Miyagi, Japan

Pathology Informatics Team, RIKEN Center for Advanced Intelligence Project, Chuo-ku, Tokyo, Japan

M. Fukumoto (ed.), *Low-Dose Radiation Effects on Animals and Ecosystems II*,
https://doi.org/10.1007/978-981-95-5559-8_6

Keywords Japanese macaque · Japanese macaque phantom · Voxel phantom ·
Dose-rate conversion coefficients · Internal organ dose · Fukushima Daiichi
Nuclear Power Plant (FNPP) accident

6.1 Introduction

In the wake of the Fukushima Daiichi Nuclear Power Plant (FNPP) accident in 2011,
the effects of long-term exposure to low-dose and low-dose-rate radiation have
attracted public interest. Therefore, a study has been conducted to clarify the effects
of continuous exposure to radioactive materials emitted from FNPP. A survey of various organisms such as cattle, snakes, and wild boars inhabiting land within a 20-km
radius of the Fukushima ex-evacuation zone has been conducted [1, 2].

In this study, Japanese macaques inhabiting the ex-evacuation zone are the focus
because they are the closest primate species to humans and have an average lifespan
of more than 20 years. Therefore, they are expected to be continuously exposed to
low-dose, low-dose-rate radiation since the FNPP accident occurred. In animals
affected by the FNPP accident, both external and internal exposure persists over-
time, making it necessary to accurately estimate the radiation doses to organs [3].
The whole-body internal and external doses have been calculated using conversion
factors for a phantom that assumes the Japanese macaque is an ellipsoid [6]. The
internal organ dose-rate conversion coefficient is a value used to calculate the organ
dose rate by multiplying the actually measured organ-specific radioactivity concentration. In our previous study, a voxel phantom for 15 body parts (brain, eyeball,
thyroid, lung, heart, stomach, liver, spleen, kidney, intestine, bladder, testis, bone,
bone marrow, and other component—mainly skeletal muscles and soft tissues) was
created from computed tomography (CT) images of a macaque weighing 11 kg
(hereafter referred to as the 11-kg phantom) to calculate internal radiation dose by
organ [4]. However, since organ doses are highly dependent on the mass of the
organs, accurate estimation of organ doses requires consideration of the size of the
macaque. Therefore, in this study, voxel phantoms with body weights of approximately 1 kg, 3.5 kg, 5.5 kg, 7.5 kg, 11 kg, and 22 kg were created based on the 11-kg
phantom [4]. Internal organ dose-rate conversion coefficients for cesium-134
(^{134}Cs), ^{137}Cs, iodine-129 (^{129}I), and ^{131}I were then estimated. A Monte Carlo simulation code of the Particle and Heavy Ion Transport System (PHITS) [5] was used to
estimate conversion coefficients for each of the six voxel phantoms. By using conversion coefficients for the voxel phantoms created in this study, it is possible to
calculate doses that take body weight into account. We calculated internal dose from
^{134}Cs and ^{137}Cs concentrations in each organ using the conversion coefficients
derived in this study.

6.2 Materials and Methods

6.2.1 *Japanese Macaque Voxel Phantom*

Six voxel phantoms weighing from 1 to 22 kg were created using that of the 11-kg phantom [4]. Figure 6.1 shows an example of a voxel phantom. We used 3D Slicer to modify the voxel size of the 11-kg phantom and created voxel phantoms adapted to different body weights using DICOM2PHITS [7, 8]. The voxel size was changed for five different weights while keeping the side-length ratio the same. The voxel size for each phantom is listed in Table 6.1.

6.2.2 *Organ Radioactivity Concentration*

For dose estimation, we used data from 246 Japanese macaques collected from 2013 to 2021 as part of the FNPP accident Affected Animal Project. The data include the capture date and location, weight of the macaque, age, and ^{134}Cs and ^{137}Cs concentrations in each organ. Capture sites were divided into five main districts: Namie Town, Fukushima Prefecture (22 animals); Haramachi (95 animals), Kashima (106 animals), and Odaka (18 animals) Wards of Minamisoma City, Fukushima Prefecture; and Miyagi Prefecture (5 animals) for nonaffected control.

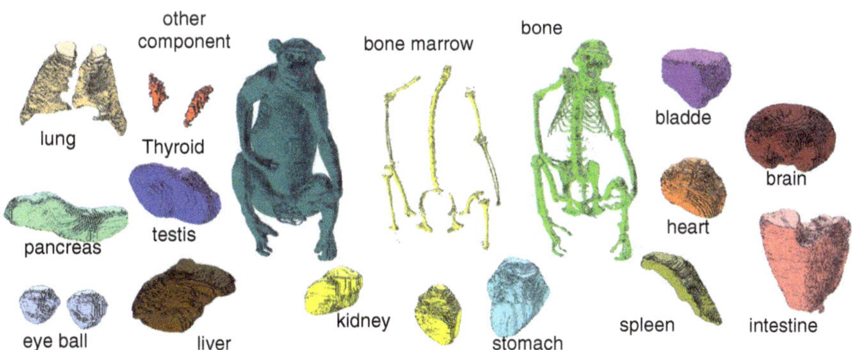

Fig. 6.1 Created voxel phantom of a Japanese macaque.

Table 6.1 Weight and voxel size for each phantom.

Body weight (kg)	Voxel size (mm × mm × mm)
0.99	0.00608 × 0.00608 × 0.00445
3.45	0.00923 × 0.00923 × 0.00676
5.60	0.01085 × 0.01085 × 0.00794
7.39	0.01190 × 0.01190 × 0.00871
11.09	0.01366 × 0.01366 × 0.01000
22.37	0.01721 × 0.01721 × 0.01260

Radioactivity was measured in the following organs: brain, eyeball, thyroid, lung, heart, stomach, liver, kidney, spleen, pancreas, bladder, testis, and femoral muscle. Due to collection conditions, ^{134}Cs and ^{137}Cs concentrations could not be measured in some organs, which varied from individual to individuals. However, since the radioactivity concentration in femoral muscle was measurable for all individuals, for organs in which ^{134}Cs and ^{137}Cs concentrations could not be measured, the radioactivity concentration was estimated using the correlation from the regression line created for individuals in which ^{134}Cs and ^{137}Cs concentrations could be measured in both femoral muscle and organs.

6.2.3 PHITS Simulation

As shown in previous papers, a geometry was defined with a 10 m × 10 m × 10 m volume of air on a 0.5 m × 10 m × 10 m volume of soil. The voxel phantom of the Japanese macaque was placed in the center of the soil surface. Sixteen organs and other component, each with deposited radionuclides, were designated as radiation source organs. The organs for which internal exposure dose is considered were defined as target organs. The β-particles and γ-rays from ^{134}Cs, ^{137}Cs, ^{129}I, and ^{131}I were generated in the source organ, and the energy deposition in each target organ was calculated using PHITS. The energy and emission probability of β-particles were referred to the website of the National Nuclear Data Center (NNDC) [9], and the β-particle energy distribution including internal conversion electrons was obtained from previous papers [10–12].

6.2.4 Calculation of Internal Organ Dose-Rate Conversion Coefficients

The internal dose-rate conversion coefficient for each organ was estimated, as before, from the energy deposition calculated by PHITS as follows [14]:

$$n_{ij} = A \frac{m_i}{m_j} \left(\varepsilon_{ij}^{\gamma} I_{\gamma} + \varepsilon_{ij}^{\beta} I_{\beta} \right) \tag{6.1}$$

where n_{ij} is the internal organ dose-rate conversion coefficient [(μGy/d)/(Bq/kg)] for the i-th source organ (mass m_i [kg]) to the j-th target organ (mass m_j [kg]); A is the unit conversion coefficient $1.60218 \times 10^{-7} \times 3600 \times 24$ [(μJ/d)/(MeV/s)]; $\varepsilon_{ij}^{\gamma}$ and ε_{ij}^{β} are the calculated energy deposition in MeV from γ-ray and β-particles, respectively; and I_{γ} and I_{β} are the γ-ray and β-particle emission rates, respectively [13].

6.2.5 Dose Calculations for ^{134}Cs and ^{137}Cs

The internal dose from ^{134}Cs and ^{137}Cs was calculated with reference to the fact that the contribution of ^{134}Cs and ^{137}Cs occupies 90% of the total body dose for external dose [6]. The internal dose for each organ was estimated from the calculated internal organ dose-rate conversion coefficients and the measured radioactive concentration as follows:

$$D_j = \sum_i B_i n_{ij} \int_d^o e^{\left(-\frac{\ln2}{T}t\right)} dt \tag{6.2}$$

where D_j is the internal dose in organ j (μGy), B_i is ^{134}Cs or ^{137}Cs concentration in organ i (Bq/kg); n_{ij} is the organ dose-rate conversion coefficient [(μGy/d)/(Bq/kg)] in organ j when the source organ is i; d is the number of days since the accident (March 15, 2011); o is the date of collection of macaque samples; and T is the half-life.

6.3 Results

6.3.1 Internal Organ Dose-Rate Conversion Coefficients

Figure 6.2 shows the relationship between the body weight of Japanese macaque and the internal organ dose-rate conversion coefficients in four organs and other component for ^{134}Cs, when the source and target organs are the same. Conversion coefficients were dependent on body weight, which was observed even when the source and target organs were different. When the source and target organs are the same, weight-dependent conversion coefficients could be fitted by a quadratic equation of $\ln(M)$. The function is shown as follows:

$$n_{ij} = a_1 + a_2 \times \ln(M) + a_3 \times \{\ln(M)\}^2 \tag{6.3}$$

where n_{ij} is the internal organ dose-rate conversion coefficient, and a_1, a_2, and a_3 are the fitting parameters. The parameters are summarized in Table 6.2. The difference between the conversion coefficients calculated by PHITS and fitted curve was less than 1%, which is a good agreement. Even when the source and target organs were different from each other, the difference was within less than 10%, except for the eyeball and the testis, which were small in volume. This difference was considered to be due to the statistical fluctuation of the energy deposition in the PHITS calculation. To obtain the coefficient of the macaque with any weight, the coefficient, n_{ij}, was fitted using a function of the body weight, M.

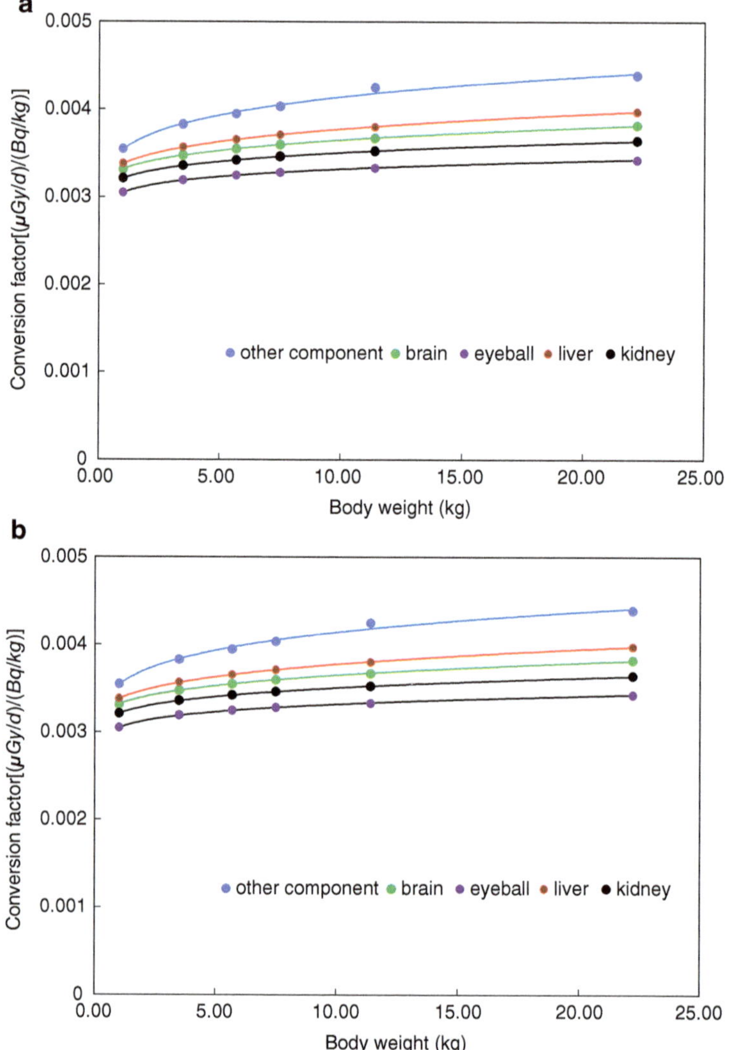

Fig. 6.2 Relation between internal organ dose-rate conversion coefficients and body weight for brain, eyeball, liver, kidney, and other component when the source and target organs are the same for (**a**) ^{134}Cs and (**b**) ^{137}Cs.

We compared conversion coefficients to determine the contribution of radioactive cesium from each target organ to internal dose of the liver as a source organ (Fig. 6.3). It was shown that the contribution of radiation dose from the target organ itself to internal dose is obviously larger than that from other source organs. For these, we concluded that it is sufficient to consider internal dose of a certain target organ only if the target organ itself and other component are source organs.

Table 6.2 presents the fitting parameters (a_1, a_2, a_3) for each radionuclide in Eq. (6.3).

Table 6.2 Coefficient of $n_{ij} = a_1 + a_2 \cdot \ln(M) + a_3 \cdot \{\ln(M)\}^2$ when (a) source i and target organ j are the same and (b) tissue is the source organ.

(a) Source organ

		Tissue	Bone	Bone marrow	Brain	Eyeball	Heart	Lung	Liver	Stomach	Spleen	Kidney	Pancreas	Intestine	Bladder	Testis	Thyroid
^{134}Cs	a_1	3.87×10^3	2.72×10^3	2.24×10^3	3.06×10^3	2.61×10^3	2.98×10^3	2.21×10^3	3.23×10^3	3.29×10^3	2.78×10^3	2.86×10^3	2.69×10^3	3.88×10^3	2.93×10^3	2.85×10^3	1.85×10^3
	a_2	1.07×10^3	5.53×10^4	3.50×10^4	5.17×10^4	3.35×10^4	4.98×10^4	3.50×10^4	6.32×10^4	6.55×10^4	4.14×10^4	4.33×10^4	3.58×10^4	1.06×10^3	4.26×10^4	4.43×10^4	4.08×10^4
	a_3	4.71×10^4	1.97×10^4	4.44×10^5	3.37×10^4	1.56×10^4	2.99×10^4	4.44×10^5	4.00×10^4	4.33×10^4	2.13×10^4	2.43×10^4	1.84×10^4	5.85×10^4	2.85×10^4	2.35×10^4	-2.48×10^5
^{137}Cs	a_1	3.56×10^3	2.98×10^3	3.32×10^3	3.32×10^3	3.05×10^3	3.28×10^3	2.64×10^3	3.38×10^3	3.41×10^3	3.16×10^3	3.21×10^3	3.11×10^3	3.63×10^3	3.25×10^3	3.21×10^3	2.23×10^3
	a_2	4.20×10^4	3.67×10^4	2.35×10^4	2.35×10^4	2.41×10^4	2.43×10^4	4.15×10^4	2.78×10^4	2.81×10^4	2.26×10^4	2.36×10^4	2.41×10^4	3.94×10^4	2.40×10^4	2.36×10^4	5.42×10^4
	a_3	1.53×10^4	3.99×10^5	9.94×10^5	9.94×10^5	2.88×10^5	8.20×10^5	-5.60×10^5	1.22×10^4	1.31×10^4	6.21×10^5	5.95×10^5	2.88×10^5	1.90×10^4	6.87×10^5	5.95×10^5	-8.48×10^5
^{129}I	a_1	8.51×10^4	9.16×10^4	7.93×10^4	8.31×10^4	8.05×10^4	8.28×10^4	7.95×10^4	8.42×10^4	8.44×10^4	8.18×10^4	8.21×10^4	8.11×10^4	8.71×10^4	8.26×10^4	8.15×10^4	7.87×10^4
	a_2	3.47×10^5	5.42×10^5	8.38×10^6	3.54×10^5	1.52×10^5	3.06×10^5	1.09×10^5	4.37×10^5	4.33×10^5	2.50×10^5	2.62×10^5	1.99×10^5	5.65×10^5	3.04×10^5	1.08×10^4	6.54×10^6
	a_3	5.03×10^6	-4.52×10^6	3.63×10^6	9.25×10^6	7.70×10^6	1.25×10^5	4.50×10^6	7.56×10^6	9.63×10^6	9.57×10^6	1.17×10^5	9.92×10^6	3.25×10^6	1.15×10^5	-8.38×10^5	2.28×10^6
^{131}I	a_1	3.21×10^3	2.76×10^3	2.55×10^3	3.00×10^3	2.80×10^3	2.97×10^3	2.52×10^3	3.06×10^3	3.08×10^3	2.88×10^3	2.92×10^3	2.84×10^3	3.26×10^3	2.95×10^3	2.92×10^3	2.21×10^3
	a_2	3.65×10^4	2.90×10^4	2.44×10^4	1.75×10^4	1.89×10^4	1.80×10^4	2.65×10^4	2.05×10^4	2.28×10^4	1.68×10^4	1.76×10^4	1.72×10^4	3.32×10^4	1.65×10^4	1.77×10^4	4.00×10^4
	a_3	1.23×10^4	3.60×10^5	-5.71×10^6	1.05×10^4	1.85×10^5	8.43×10^5	-1.63×10^5	1.22×10^4	1.21×10^4	6.28×10^5	6.14×10^5	4.21×10^5	1.80×10^4	8.39×10^5	6.11×10^5	-6.22×10^5

(b) Target organ

		Tissue	Bone	Bone marrow	Brain	Eyeball	Heart	Lung	Liver	Stomach	Spleen	Kidney	Pancreas	Intestine	Bladder	Testis	Thyroid
^{134}Cs	a_1	3.87×10^3	1.62×10^3	1.46×10^3	7.51×10^4	8.67×10^4	1.34×10^3	1.66×10^3	1.05×10^3	9.76×10^4	1.27×10^3	1.11×10^3	1.17×10^3	1.07×10^3	1.70×10^3	1.14×10^3	2.65×10^3
	a_2	1.07×10^3	7.62×10^4	8.63×10^4	4.38×10^4	4.54×10^4	8.21×10^4	7.40×10^4	6.57×10^4	6.06×10^4	7.42×10^4	6.32×10^4	6.77×10^4	6.49×10^4	1.04×10^3	6.94×10^4	9.14×10^4
	a_3	4.71×10^4	4.63×10^4	3.73×10^4	1.57×10^4	1.75×10^4	3.61×10^4	4.71×10^4	1.98×10^4	1.73×10^4	3.04×10^4	2.05×10^4	2.47×10^4	2.06×10^4	4.97×10^4	2.57×10^4	7.66×10^4
^{137}Cs	a_1	3.56×10^3	8.43×10^4	5.67×10^4	2.76×10^4	3.98×10^4	5.17×10^4	9.13×10^4	4.07×10^4	3.65×10^4	5.34×10^4	4.65×10^4	4.89×10^4	4.07×10^4	6.53×10^4	4.68×10^4	1.66×10^3
	a_2	4.20×10^4	1.04×10^4	2.53×10^4	1.37×10^4	1.01×10^4	2.44×10^4	6.91×10^5	1.84×10^4	1.84×10^4	1.86×10^4	1.59×10^4	1.75×10^4	1.90×10^4	3.07×10^4	1.76×10^4	-1.30×10^4
	a_3	1.53×10^4	1.84×10^4	1.26×10^4	5.11×10^5	6.79×10^5	1.23×10^4	1.88×10^4	7.63×10^5	6.03×10^5	1.16×10^4	7.84×10^5	9.19×10^5	7.22×10^5	1.72×10^4	1.01×10^4	3.57×10^4
^{129}I	a_1	8.51×10^4	2.85×10^4	4.02×10^5	2.10×10^5	2.30×10^5	5.97×10^5	6.85×10^5	4.24×10^5	3.69×10^5	5.54×10^5	4.31×10^5	4.65×10^5	3.97×10^5	3.97×10^5	5.12×10^5	1.08×10^4
	a_2	3.47×10^5	7.43×10^5	1.07×10^5	3.17×10^6	6.35×10^6	2.79×10^5	3.33×10^5	1.46×10^5	1.09×10^5	2.46×10^5	1.64×10^5	1.80×10^5	1.28×10^5	1.28×10^5	2.40×10^5	6.15×10^5
	a_3	5.03×10^5	-3.64×10^5	-7.49×10^6	-3.68×10^6	-1.93×10^6	-1.04×10^5	-3.47×10^6	-7.39×10^6	-7.58×10^6	-6.79×10^6	-4.09×10^6	-6.67×10^6	-6.48×10^6	-6.48×10^6	-6.63×10^6	2.28×10^6
^{131}I	a_1	3.21×10^3	6.46×10^4	4.74×10^4	2.31×10^4	3.21×10^4	4.30×10^4	7.05×10^4	3.38×10^4	3.07×10^4	4.34×10^4	3.76×10^4	4.02×10^4	3.38×10^4	5.45×10^4	3.82×10^4	1.25×10^3
	a_2	3.65×10^4	1.26×10^4	2.26×10^4	1.17×10^4	9.49×10^5	2.18×10^4	9.73×10^5	1.65×10^4	1.62×10^4	1.78×10^4	1.49×10^4	1.61×10^4	1.74×10^4	2.72×10^4	1.62×10^4	-4.96×10^6
	a_3	1.23×10^4	1.83×10^4	1.13×10^4	4.68×10^5	5.55×10^5	1.18×10^4	1.67×10^4	6.95×10^5	5.50×10^5	1.00×10^4	6.63×10^5	8.36×10^5	6.28×10^5	1.68×10^4	8.76×10^5	2.97×10^4

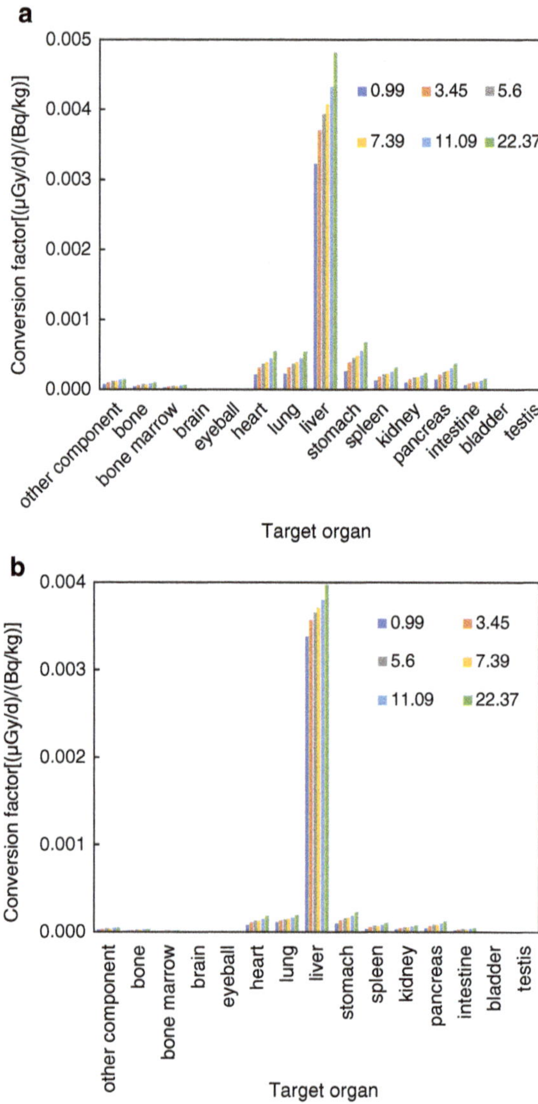

Fig. 6.3 Conversion coefficients for (**a**) ^{134}Cs and (**b**) ^{137}Cs when the source organ is the liver.

6.3.2 ^{134}Cs and ^{137}Cs Concentrations

Figure 6.4 shows the correlation between ^{134}Cs and ^{137}Cs concentrations in femoral muscle and brain, and Fig. 6.5 shows the correlation between femoral muscle and thyroid. The mean difference from the regression line was almost the same for both ^{134}Cs and ^{137}Cs: 16% for the brain and 23% for the femoral muscle.

Fig. 6.4 Correlation of radioactive Cs concentrations in femoral muscle and brain for (**a**) ^{134}Cs and (**b**) ^{137}Cs.

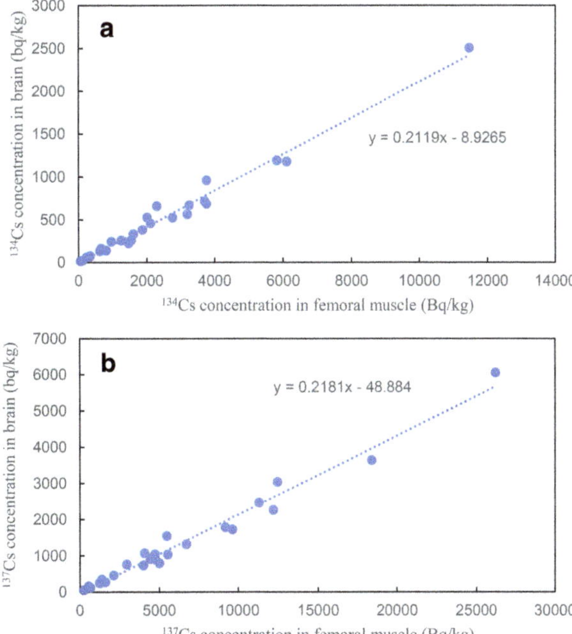

Fig. 6.5 Relation of radioactive Cs concentrations in femoral muscle and liver for (**a**) ^{134}Cs and (**b**) ^{137}Cs.

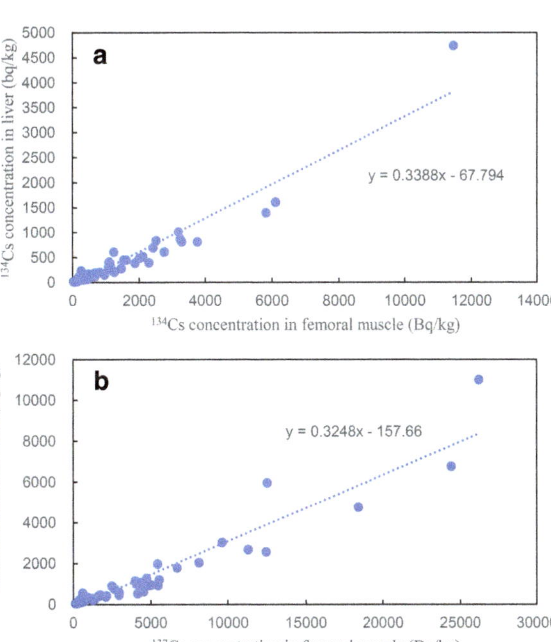

6.3.3 Environmental Half-Life of ^{134}Cs and ^{137}Cs

It is assumed that ^{134}Cs and ^{137}Cs concentrations in each organ reflect those in the environment. The temporal change of ^{137}Cs concentrations in the femoral muscle was examined in each capture area, and the period during which the concentration was reduced by half was defined as the environmental half-life, which was used to estimate internal radiation dose. The environmental half-life of ^{137}Cs and the concentration ratio of ^{134}Cs to ^{137}Cs were used to estimate the temporal change of ^{134}Cs concentration. Since the environmental half-life varies greatly depending on weather and the retention level in soil, it was estimated separately for four districts: Namie Town, Kashima Ward, Haramachi Ward, and Odaka Ward in Minamisoma City. For example, Fig. 6.6 shows the correlation between the time since the accident occurred and ^{137}Cs concentration in femoral muscle for Haramachi Ward. The environmental half-life of ^{137}Cs was shorter, roughly one-third compared to the physical half-life.

The environmental half-life of ^{134}Cs concentration was estimated from the ratio and the elapsed time since the accident, assuming that the activity ratio of ^{134}Cs to ^{137}Cs at the beginning of the accident was 1 [14]. Figure 6.7 shows the ratio of the measured data and the estimated curve as a function of time for Haramachi Ward. Table 6.3 summarizes the half-lives obtained. Different half-lives were used depending on the four sampling areas for deriving the internal doses.

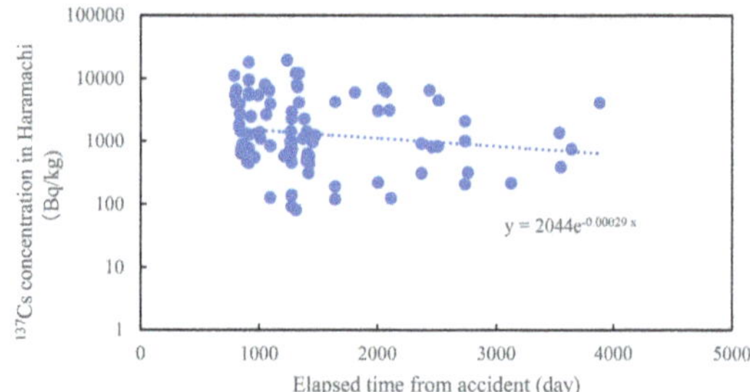

Fig. 6.6 Correlation between ^{137}Cs concentration in femoral muscle for Haramachi Ward and the elapsed time since the accident.

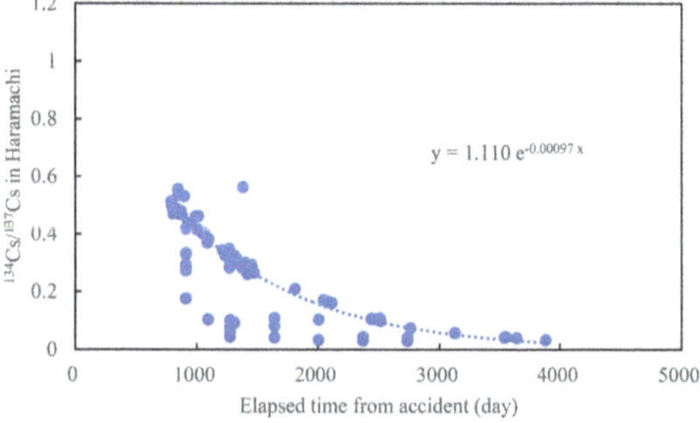

Fig. 6.7 Relation between the ratio of ^{137}Cs and ^{134}Cs at Haramachi Ward and the time elapsed since the accident.

Table 6.3 Environmental half-life of Japanese macaques.

	^{134}Cs(day)	^{137}Cs(day)
Namie Town	592	3,014
Minamisoma City		
Haramachi Ward	550	2,390
Kashima Ward	699	7,702
Odaka Ward	575	3,151

Table 6.4 Mean of internal doses.

	Mean dose (mGy)
Namie Town	191 ± 164
Odaka Ward	39.2 ± 23.3
Kashima Ward	10.1 ± 7.9
Haramachi Ward	35.2 ± 23.4

6.3.4 Internal Dose Calculation for ^{134}Cs and ^{137}Cs

Each internal organ dose was calculated from ^{134}Cs and ^{137}Cs concentrations in Japanese macaques and the internal organ dose-rate conversion coefficients using Eq. (6.2). The total internal radiation dose was calculated, including bone, bone marrow, and intestine for which measurements were not available, in other component. Table 6.4 shows means and standard deviations. The highest internal dose was estimated to be 191 mGy in Namie Town, while the lowest was 10.1 mGy in Kashima Ward, Minamisoma City. For humans, the total internal dose to ^{134}Cs and ^{137}Cs up to January 31, 2012, was reported to be less than 1 mSv [15]. To compare with human internal dose, the absorbed dose was converted to effective dose using the tissue weighting factors for humans. The calculated mean effective dose was estimated to be 158 mSv at maximum, which means that radiation doses to the affected macaques in this study are quite higher than those for humans. Macaques were exposed to such high levels of internal radiation because they consumed foods such as fruits, plant leaves, mushrooms, and insects in a natural environment contaminated by radioactive fallout from the FNPP accident. Currently, contamination is rapidly decreasing due to decontamination work, but it is thought that contamination of the macaques will continue for some time, and it remains to be seen whether the long-term effects of internal exposure, including intergenerational effects, will become clear.

6.4 Conclusion

In this study, voxel phantoms were created for six macaques of different body weights. Internal dose-rate conversion coefficients for ^{134}Cs, ^{137}Cs, ^{129}I, and ^{131}I were then estimated. The results showed that there is a correlation between body weight and the conversion coefficients. For each organ, a function of the conversion coefficient with respect to body weight was derived. This enabled the internal dose to be calculated for each organ according to body weight. The internal doses were also calculated from the measured ^{134}Cs and ^{137}Cs concentration data of 246 macaques. The results showed that the mean internal radiation dose was less than 191 mGy for absorbed dose and 158 mSv for effective dose (the whole-body internal dose for ^{134}Cs and ^{137}Cs in humans is reported to be less than 1 mSv), which is quite higher than that for humans.

Acknowledgments This work was supported by the Japan Atomic Energy Agency (JAEA) under the Intensive Support Project for Nuclear Science and Technology and Human Resources Development (Eichi-Centralized Grant No. JPJA19B19207322), IAEA Coordinated Research Project CRP-K41023 Research Agreement JPN 26529. Part of this research was also supported by a JSPS Postdoctoral Fellowship for Foreign Researchers (1st stage) in 2021 and JSPS Kakenhi 23K11429. Furthermore, this work was supported by Research Project on the Health Effects of Radiation organized by the Ministry of the Environment, Japan, under the research theme "Cross-disciplinary joint research to deepen our understanding of biological effects of Cs-bearing insoluble microparticles."

References

1. Gunningham K, Hinton TG, Luxton JJ (2021) Evaluation of DNA damage and stress in wildlife chronically exposed to low-dose, low-dose rate radiation from the Fukushima Dai-ichi Nuclear Power Plant accident. Environ Int 155. https://doi.org/10.1016/j.envint.2021.106675
2. Yamashiro H, Abe Y, Fukuda T (2013) Effects of radioactive caesium on bull testes after the Fukushima nuclear plant accident. Sci Rep 3:Article 2850. https://doi.org/10.1038/srep02850
3. Suzuki M, Suzuki H, Ishiguro H et al (2019) Correlation of radiocesium activity between muscle and peripheral blood of live cattle depending on presence or absence of radiocontamination in feed. Radiat Res 192:589–601
4. Takamura Y, Kajimoto T, Tanaka K et al (2023) Internal organ dose rate conversion coefficients of Japanese macaques to ^{134}Cs, ^{137}Cs and ^{131}I. J Radiat Res:1–7. https://doi.org/10.1093/jrr/rrad055
5. Sato T, Niita K, Matsuda N et al (2018) Feature of Particle and Heavy Ion Transport code System (PHITS) version 3.02. https://doi.org/10.1080/00223131.2017.1419890
6. Endo S, Ishii K, Suzuki M et al (2020) Dose estimation of external and internal exposure in Japanese macaques after the Fukushima nuclear power plant accident. In: Fukumoto M (ed) Low-dose radiation effects on animals and ecosystems. Springer Open, Tokyo, pp 165–178. https://doi.org/10.1007/978-981-13-8218-5
7. Fedorov A, Beichel R, Kalpathy-Cramer J et al 3D slicer as an image computing platform for the quantitative imaging network. Magn Imaging. https://www.slicer.org. Accessed 2021
8. PHITS website, PHITS Utility tool: DICOM2PHITS, https://phits.jaea.go.jp/index.html
9. NNDC (National Nuclear Center): search and plot nuclear structure and decay data interactively. https://www.nndc.bnl.gov/nudat3/
10. Endo S, Tanaka K, Kajimoto T et al (2014) Estimate of β-rays dose, in air and soil from Fukushima Daiichi power plant accident. J Radiat Res 55:476–483. https://doi.org/10.1093/jrr/rrt209
11. Endo S, Kajimoto T, Tanaka K et al (2015) Mapping of cumulative, β-ray dose on the ground surface surrounding the Fukushima area. J Radiat Res 56:i48–i55. https://doi.org/10.1093/jrr/rrv056

12. Nakamura S, Kajimoto T, Tanaka K et al (2018) Measurement of 90Sr radioactivity in cesium hot particles originating from the Fukushima Nuclear Power Plant Accident. J Radiat Res 59:i677–684. https://doi.org/10.1093/jrr/rry063
13. Endo S, Matsutani Y, Kajimoto T et al (2020) Internal exposure rate conversion coefficients and absorbed fractions of mouse for ^{137}Cs, ^{134}Cs and ^{90}Sr contamination in body. J Radiat Res 61(4):535–545. https://doi.org/10.1093/jrr/rraa030
14. Hayama S, Nakiri S, Nakahashi S et al (2013) Concentration of radiocesium in the wild Japanese monkey (Macaca fuscata) over the First15 months after the Fukushima Daiichi nuclear disaster. PLoS One 8(7):e68530. https://doi.org/10.1371/journal.pone.0068530
15. Momose T, Takada C, Nakagawa T et al (2012) Whole-body counting of Fukushima residents after the TEPCO Fukushima Daiichi nuclear power station accident NIRS-M-252, pp 67–82

Part III
Biological Impacts of the FNPP Accident on Japanese Macaques

Chapter 7
Why Do We Chase Macaques?

Manabu Fukumoto

Abstract In a nuclear disaster, the greatest concern is whether there are any effects on human health and on living organisms from long-term, low-dose-rate radiation exposure resulting from environmental contamination caused by leaked radioactive materials. Fieldwork on the Fukushima Daiichi Nuclear Power Plant (FNPP) accident is essential to address this issue. Since the accident occurred, we have continued to investigate the effects on livestock and wild animals, and have been studying wild Japanese macaques, the species most closely related to humans, in earnest since approximately two years after the accident. Part III outlines the benefits of analyzing wild macaques and the current status of our studies.

Keywords Nuclear disaster · Fukushima Daiichi Nuclear Plant (FNPP) accident · Japanese wild macaques · Fieldwork · Radiation effects · Comprehensive dose evaluation project concerning animals affected by the FNPP accident (Affected Animal Project)

In epidemiological studies, it is difficult to quantitatively evaluate the effects of low-dose and low-dose-rate radiation exposure due to the inherent uncertainty of the population being analyzed and statistical limitations. In particular, there are only limited data, including experimental data, on the biological effects of radiation at doses of tens of mGy or at dose rates of several µGy/day, which are relevant to the general public [1] (Fig. 7.1).

Even now, 15 years after the accident, the environment and wildlife around FNPP continue to be contaminated by cesium-137 (^{137}Cs). The latency period for liver cancer in Thorotrast patients caused by internal exposure to radioactive material, thorium dioxide, was more than 20 years [2], and the increase in pediatric thyroid cancer began 5 years after the Chernobyl (Chornobyl) nuclear accident, in which the amount of radioactive materials released was ten times that of the FNPP accident [3]. Considering these facts, it can be interpreted that roughly 30 years or

M. Fukumoto (✉)
International Research Institute of Disaster Science, Tohoku University, Sendai, Japan
e-mail: manabu.fukumoto.a8@tohoku.ac.jp

M. Fukumoto (ed.), *Low-Dose Radiation Effects on Animals and Ecosystems II*,
https://doi.org/10.1007/978-981-95-5559-8_7

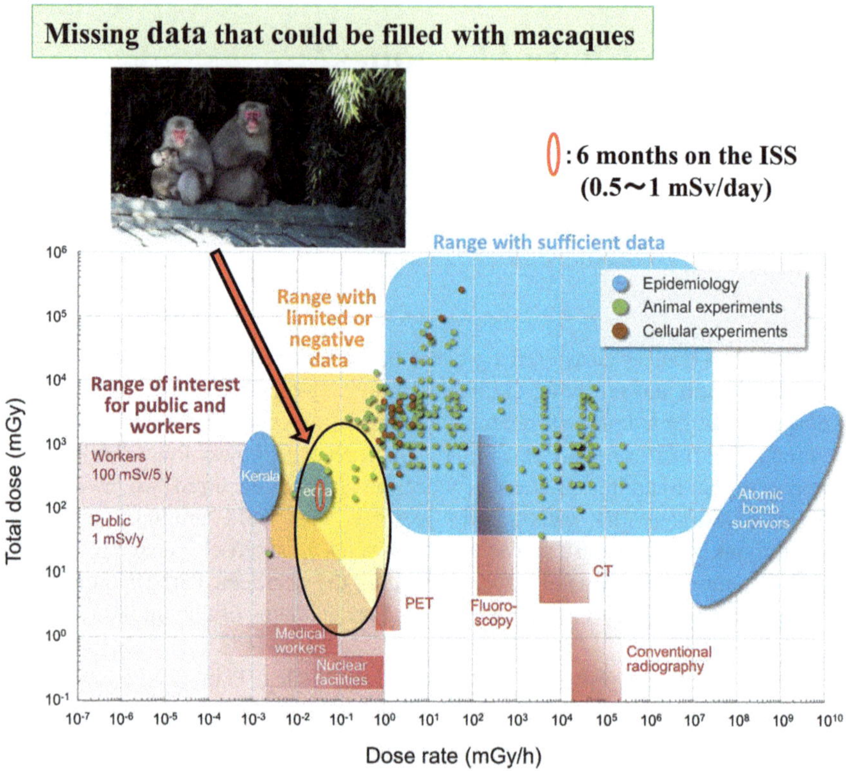

Fig. 7.1 Dose and dose-rate ranges that macaques are expected to fill. There are limited epidemiological and experimental data (indicated by dots) in the range of doses and dose rates that are crucial for protecting the public and workers from accidental radioactive releases into the environment and from medical exposure. Black oval: The macaques in the Comprehensive dose evaluation project concerning animals affected by the FNPP accident are expected to supplement these data. Red oval: radiation exposure during 6 months on the International Space Station (ISS). The macaque data may also help protect against radiation exposure during future space travel (Adapted from Fig. 1 of Ref [1]).

more of follow-up surveys of ecosystems and wild animals are needed to determine the biological effects of the FNPP accident. We believe that the analysis of wild Japanese macaques is the most important, and we are currently focusing on collecting samples from wild macaques (Fig. 7.2).

Japanese macaques are primates, so their genome structure is closest to that of humans among wild animals. What is happening and will happen to macaques that roam freely in contaminated environments without protection and consume contaminated wild foods? Once any changes are observed and it becomes clear whether they correlate with internal or external radiation dose/dose-rate, we can infer the effect on humans. The Chornobyl nuclear accident has raised a significant question as to whether radiation can have direct psychological and/or emotional effects.

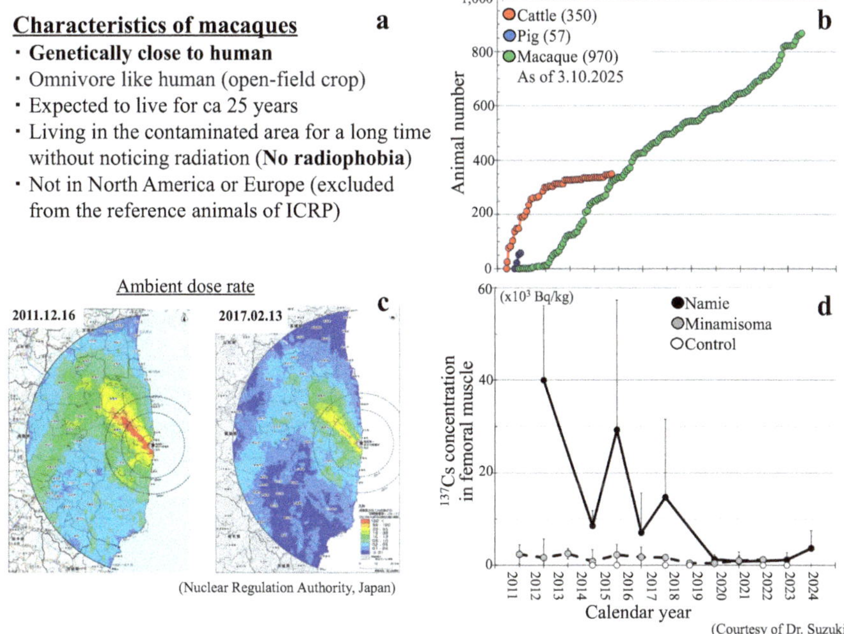

Fig. 7.2 Wild macaques (*Macaca fuscata*), an excellent resource for understanding radiation effects on both ecosystems and humans. (**a**) Characteristics of macaques, highlighting their genetic similarity to humans and their lack of radiophobia. (**b**) The cumulative number of macaques collected in the archive has been steadily increasing. (**c**) Ambient dose rate in Fukushima Prefecture from ^{137}Cs contamination has decreased dramatically in the 6 years since the accident. (https://radioactivity.nra.go.jp/en/results/land/airborne/survey-results) (**d**) ^{137}Cs contamination levels in macaques are still fluctuating, although they are on a downward trend.

Unlike humans, macaques are not aware of and unafraid of the presence of radiation. Therefore, studying them allows us to elucidate the pure biological effects of radiation, which may in turn provide clues to understanding its psychological effects. Macaques do not smoke or drink alcohol, which are always problematic confounding factors in epidemiological studies observing subtle differences in the effects of radiation. The reproductive age of Japanese macaques is 3.5 years or later, and their life span is about 25 years. Their chronological age and total radiation dose can be determined from their teeth. These characteristics make it possible to determine their age at the time of the accident and the impact on offspring. Macaques are not one of the reference organisms for environmental monitoring designated by the International Commission on Radiological Protection (ICRP) because all nuclear accident areas prior to the FNPP accident were not habitats for monkeys. Therefore, the Ministry of Education, Culture, Sports, Science and Technology, Japan, has judged that the results obtained from wild Japanese macaques are meaningless as subjects for analysis because they cannot be compared with research results from around the world, which is an extremely unfortunate decision for radiation protection. However, we are determined to continue the Affected Animal Project with sustained commitment and enthusiasm, convinced that the knowledge accumulated will ultimately serve as an invaluable scientific legacy for future generations.

References

1. Yamada Y, Imaoka T, Iwasaki T et al (2024) Establishment and activity of the planning and acting network for low dose radiation research in Japan (PLANET): 2016–2023. J Radiat Res 1–14. https://doi.org/10.1093/jrr/rrae049
2. Fukumoto M (2014) Radiation pathology: from thorotrast to the future beyond radioresistance. Pathol Int 64:251–262. https://doi.org/10.1111/pin.12170
3. Imanaka T (2019) Comparison of radioactivity release and contamination from the Fukushima and Chernobyl Nuclear Power Plant accidents. In: Fukumoto M (ed) Low-dose radiation effects on animals and ecosystems. Springer, Singapore. https://doi.org/10.1007/978-981-13-8218-5_20

Chapter 8
Analysis of Cementum Incremental Line Formation in the Teeth of Japanese Macaques Affected by the Fukushima Daiichi Nuclear Power Plant Accident

Hiroyuki Mishima, Masatoshi Suzuki, Hisashi Shinoda, Tohru Hayakawa, and Manabu Fukumoto

Abstract The purpose of this study was to analyze the effect of the Fukushima Daiichi Nuclear Power Plant (FNPP) accident on the incremental line formation of cementum in the teeth of Japanese macaques. Radioactive cesium-137 (^{137}Cs) concentration in the body was determined by γ-ray spectrum analysis of the femoral muscle using a germanium semiconductor detector. Tooth samples were fixed in 10% formalin solution, decalcified, sectioned at 4 μm thickness, and stained with hematoxylin and eosin (HE). Cementum incremental lines were observed under a light microscope and analyzed using the image analysis software WinROOF 2018. The age distribution of macaques was 2–25 years, as determined from the analysis of cementum incremental lines. In juveniles, the incremental lines of the affected group by the accident were unclear compared to those of the unaffected control group. In adults exposed to high concentrations of ^{137}Cs, the incremental lines were locally irregularly spaced and obscured. The tissue structure was disturbed by a mixture of cellular and acellular cementum. It is suggested that radiation exposure may affect the formation of incremental lines by cementoblasts.

Keywords Japanese macaque · Tooth cementum · Radioactive cesium (Cs) · Incremental lines · Biological rhythm

H. Mishima (✉)
School of Dental Medicine, Tsurumi University, Yokohama, Japan

Graduate School of Agricultural and Life Sciences, The University of Tokyo, Tokyo, Japan
e-mail: mishima6065@circus.ocn.ne.jp

M. Suzuki · M. Fukumoto
International Research Institute of Disaster Science, Tohoku University, Sendai, Japan

H. Shinoda
Graduate School of Dentistry, Tohoku University, Sendai, Japan

T. Hayakawa
School of Dental Medicine, Tsurumi University, Yokohama, Japan

M. Fukumoto (ed.), *Low-Dose Radiation Effects on Animals and Ecosystems II*,
https://doi.org/10.1007/978-981-95-5559-8_8

8.1   Introduction

The tissue structure of monkey molars (cheek teeth) is similar to that of human molars, composed of three hard tissues: enamel, dentin, and cementum [1]. Acellular cementum is distributed mainly in the cervical region, while cellular cementum is distributed in the apical region of the tooth [2]. In this study, we observed and analyzed the incremental lines of both cellular and acellular cementum from the cervical region to the root apex (Fig. 8.1).

Biological rhythms are cyclical patterns of biological activity that repeat over time. They are classified into the following hierarchies according to the length of their cycles: (1) ultradian rhythm (shorter than 20 h), (2) circatidal rhythm (12.4 h: tidal rhythm of about half a day), (3) circadian rhythm (diurnal cycle of 20–28 h), (4) rhythm of about 2 days, (5) infradian rhythm (longer than the circadian rhythm), (6) circalunar rhythm (lunar cycle of about 28 days), and (7) circannual rhythm (annual cycle of about 1 year) [3]. These rhythms are driven by the internal biological clock of each organism and are influenced by environmental factors like light and temperature. The periodic incremental lines are observed in the hard tissues of

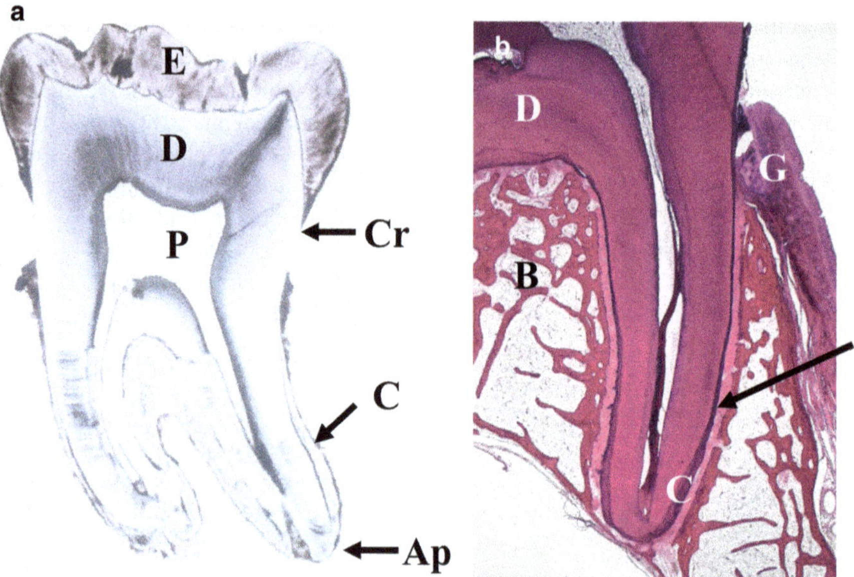

Fig. 8.1 Histological structure of a human molar. (**a**) Undemineralized section (polished section). (**b**) Demineralized section (HE staining). Enamel (E) is the hardest tissue covering the outermost portion of the tooth, while dentin (D) lies beneath the enamel and surrounds the pulp cavity (P). Cementum (C) is distributed from the tooth cervical region (Cr) to the tooth apex (Ap), covering the tooth root and connecting the tooth to the alveolar bone (B). Gingiva (G) covers the alveolar bone. The arrow in (**b**) indicates the area of cementum studied in this work.

the teeth [2]. In mammalian tooth enamel, incremental lines with diurnal cycles and 7–10-day cycles are observed. In the incremental lines of dentin, four cycles have been identified: circadian, lunar, seasonal, and annual cycles. In cementum, annual incremental lines are recognized [1, 4]. Analysis of cementum incremental lines has been performed in whales, deer, and monkeys to assess individual age and life history [1, 5]. There are two types of cementum: cellular cementum and acellular cementum. Incremental lines are observed in both of these types of cementum [6, 7]. Annual incremental lines have been reported in cementum of Japanese macaques [1, 5].

To date, studies have been conducted to determine the effects of long-term low-dose-rate radiation exposure on livestock, Japanese macaques, and other animals living in areas contaminated by radioactive material following the Fukushima Daiichi Nuclear Power Plant (FNPP accident) [8, 9]. Radioactive strontium-90, derived from contamination by the FNPP accident, was incorporated into the developing teeth of cattle abandoned in the ex-evacuation zone set within a 20-km radius of FNPP [10]. There are reports that radiation affects the composition and formation of hard tissues such as teeth and bones [11–13]. In order to investigate the biological effects of radiation, it is necessary to know the radiation dose and age of each individual. The age of an individual is determined by the annual incremental lines of cementum [1, 5]. In previous studies, the age of Japanese macaques affected by the FNPP accident was assessed based on the annual incremental lines of cementum. However, no study has been conducted on the effect of radiation on the incremental lines of the teeth of Japanese macaques. Nor have there been any reports examining the effects of radiation from the FNPP accident on biological rhythms [1, 3]. The aim of this study was to analyze whether the formation of cementum incremental lines is affected in the teeth of Japanese macaques exposed to radiation due to the FNPP accident.

8.2 Materials and Methods

8.2.1 Japanese Macaque Tooth Samples and Radioactive Cesium (^{137}Cs) Concentration Measurement

A total of 39 Japanese macaque tooth samples were analyzed, with 30 from the affected area (Minamisoma City and Namie Town, Fukushima Prefecture) and 9 from an unaffected area (Niigata Prefecture) as controls. Cesium-137 (^{137}Cs) concentration in femoral muscle was determined by γ-ray spectral analysis using a germanium semiconductor detector as previously described [9]. This study was approved by the Tohoku University Animal Ethics Committee (2016 Kado-043-1).

8.2.2 Sample Preparation and Age Assessment

The tooth sample was fixed in 10% formalin solution, demineralized in 10% formic acid solution for about 3–4 weeks, sectioned at 4 μm thickness, and stained with hematoxylin and eosin (HE) according to the standard method. Incremental lines of cementum were observed in HE-stained specimens under a light microscope (ECLIPSE Ni-E, Nikon, Japan) and analyzed using the image analysis software WinROOF 2018 (MITANI, Japan). The age of Japanese macaques was determined by analyzing the incremental lines of cementum [1, 5]. The number of annual incremental lines was measured at three sites for each sample, and the average value was taken as the age of the sample. Comparative analysis of the histological structure of cementum and the morphology of incremental lines was performed in Japanese macaques from the affected and the unaffected control areas.

8.3 Results

8.3.1 Age and ^{137}Cs Concentration Distributions

The distributions of age and ^{137}Cs concentrations for the affected group (Fig. 8.2a) and the unaffected group (Fig. 8.2b) are shown. Analysis of cementum incremental lines revealed that the age distribution of the 39 Japanese macaques ranged from 2 to 25 years. The mean age of the affected group was 11 years, and that of the unaffected group was 13 years. The average ^{137}Cs concentration in femoral muscle was 822 Bq/kg in the affected group and 6 Bq/kg in the unaffected group. In the affected group, ^{137}Cs concentration in adults (5 years or older) tended to be higher, exceeding 1,000 Bq/kg in three cases, but none were observed under 5 years of age. In the unaffected group, ^{137}Cs concentration did not exceed 25 Bq/kg, regardless of age.

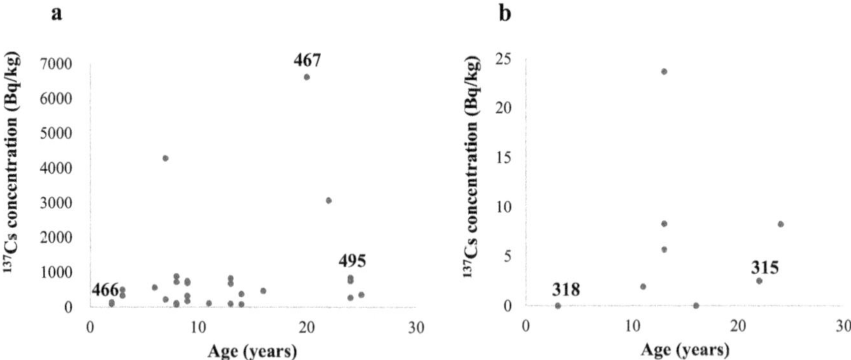

Fig. 8.2 Age and ^{137}Cs concentration in femoral muscle. (**a**) The affected group: The numbers in the figure indicate Macaque specimen numbers—Macaque No. 466 in Fig. 8.3a, Macaque No. 467 in Fig. 8.4a, and Macaque No. 495 in Fig. 8.5. (**b**) The unaffected group: Macaque No. 318 in Fig. 8.3b and Macaque No. 315 in Fig. 8.4b.

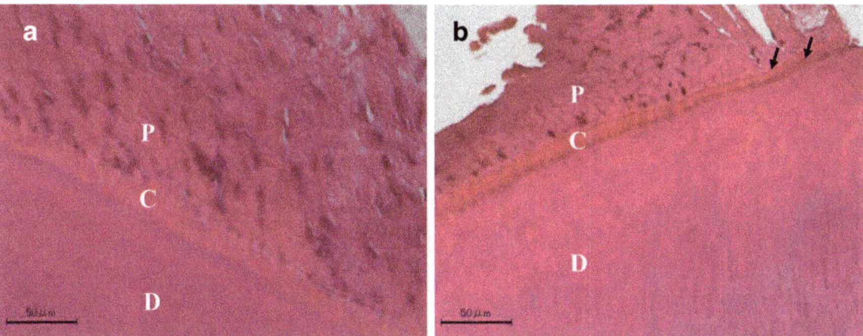

Fig. 8.3 Dental tissue image of juvenile macaques. (**a**) The affected group: Incremental lines are unclear (Macaque No. 466, 2 years old, ^{137}Cs concentration: 141.3 Bq/kg). (**b**) The unaffected control group: Incremental lines (arrows) are clearly observed (Macaque No. 318, 3 years old, ^{137}Cs concentration below detection limit). *P* periodontium, *C* cementum, *D* dentin. Scale: 50μm, HE staining.

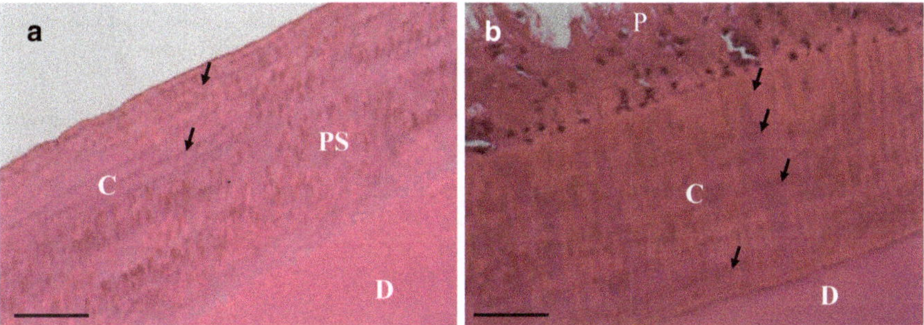

Fig. 8.4 Dental tissue image of adult macaques. (**a**) The affected group: Incremental lines (arrows) are observed only in a part of the surface layer (Macaque No. 467, 20 years old, ^{137}Cs concentration: 6619.8 Bq/kg). The patchy stained structure (PS) is distributed from the deep layer to the surface layer. (**b**) The unaffected group: Incremental lines (arrows) are observed (Macaque No. 315, 22 years old, ^{137}Cs concentration: 2.5 Bq/kg). No patchy stained structure is observed. *P* periodontium, *C* cementum, *D* dentin, *PS* patchy stained structure. Scale: 50μm, HE staining.

8.3.2   *Comparison of Incremental Lines Between the Affected Group and the Unaffected Group*

In juveniles, the incremental lines of the affected group (Fig. 8.3a) were unclear compared to those of the unaffected group (Fig. 8.3b).

In adults of the affected group, the spacing of incremental lines was locally irregular, and the incremental lines were unclear (17 out of 25 macaques) compared to the unaffected group (2 out of 7). Adults in the affected group (Fig. 8.4a) had patchy stained irregular structures and disorganized tissue structure (6 out of 25 macaques) compared to the unaffected group (1 out of 7) (Fig. 8.4b).

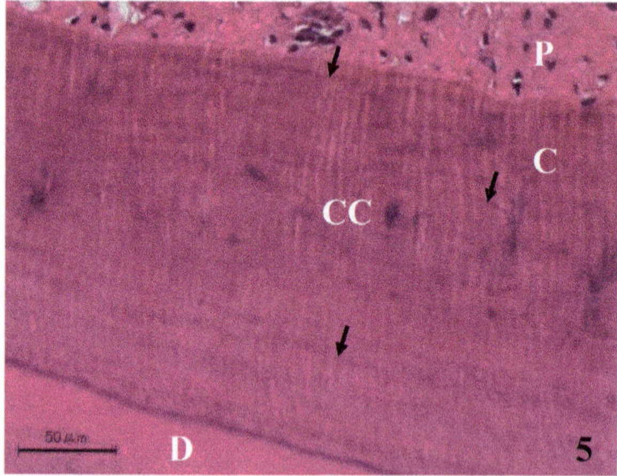

Fig. 8.5 Dental tissue image of an adult macaque from the affected group. The tissue structure of cementum in the affected group is disorganized with a mixture of cellular and acellular cementum. In cellular cementum, incremental lines are not straight and their spacing is irregular. (Macaque No. 495, 24 years old, ^{137}Cs concentration: 755.2 Bq/kg). *P* periodontium, *C* acellular cementum, *D* dentin, *CC* cellular cementum, *arrows* incremental lines. Scale: 50μm, HE staining.

Some adults in the affected group had a mixture of cellular and acellular cementum (Fig. 8.5). In the affected group (9 out of 25 macaques), the frequency of the appearance of mixed tissue structures was higher than in the unaffected group (1 out of 7).

8.4 Discussion

In this study, the annual incremental lines were identified in the cementum of Japanese macaques affected by the FNPP accident. The incremental lines of the affected group were unclear in juvenile macaques. In the affected adult group, the intervals between incremental lines were irregular in some areas, and the incremental lines were partially indistinct. Additionally, irregular structures stained in a patchy pattern were observed in cementum, and the tissue showed a mixture of cellular and acellular cementum, resulting in a disordered tissue structure.

Acellular cementum is usually present near the cervical region, while cellular cementum is well developed at the apex. A mixture of both acellular and cellular cementum is rarely seen in the central region of the root [2]. In both cellular cementum and acellular cementum, there are two types of collagen fibers: intrinsic fibers and extrinsic fibers (Sharpey's fibers) [6, 7]. The cellular and acellular cementum differ in the degree of calcification and the intrinsic fiber running [7]. Although the tissue structures of acellular cementum and cellular cementum are different, periodic annual incremental lines are present in both types of cementum [1, 5]. The age of many wild animals, including marsupials, insectivores, chiroptera, rodents, and primates, is assessed using the incremental lines of cementum. In this study, based on previous studies [1, 5, 14], we investigated cementum incremental lines of Japanese macaques as annual incremental lines. However, in artiodactyls that live in the tropics, there have been some reports of individuals exhibiting strong rhythms due to seasonal changes in addition to annual growth rhythms, resulting in the formation of two incremental lines in 1 year [1]. Furthermore, the dentin of the marine animal beluga whale develops two incremental lines per year [15]. Papagerakis et al. [16] reported that changes in the external environment affect the periodic rhythms of peripheral organs (e.g., body temperature, cardiovascular rhythm, hepatic metabolism, tooth mineralization, etc.) via central and peripheral circadian clocks. It is reported that the periodicity of the incremental lines of teeth and bones fluctuates due to changes in the external environment, changes in the body clock, and changes in the secretion of melatonin, a regulator of the body clock [4, 17, 18]. It remains a subject for future research to investigate whether environmental changes induce the formation of seasonal incremental lines in cementum, in addition to annual incremental lines, and whether such patterns vary among individuals.

There are reports that therapeutic radiation affects the hard tissues of teeth [11, 12]. Studies on coronal and root dentin results indicate that radiation has a major effect on the organic matrix [11]. It is possible that radiation directly alters mechanical properties, micromorphology, crystal properties, and chemical composition of dental hard tissues. Early destruction of enamel adjacent to the dentin–enamel junction and decreased enamel crystallinity under radiation exposure may be related to the formation of characteristic radiation caries [12]. It was concluded that γ-irradiation interferes with cytodifferentiation of the enamel organ and dental papilla and subsequently inhibits normal odontogenesis [13]. Furthermore, a study of the effects on hard tissues after the Chernobyl (Chornobyl) Nuclear Power Plant (CNPP) accident found that 78% of children living in radioactivity-contaminated areas had jawbone abnormalities [19].

Regarding the deposition of ^{137}Cs in the body, there are reports that its concentration is high in the muscles, but no studies on its deposition in teeth [20]. In the present study, the incremental lines were locally irregularly spaced and indistinct in adults exposed to high concentrations of ^{137}Cs. It is suggested that the FNPP accident may have affected the incremental line formation mechanism of cementoblasts in radiation-exposed Japanese macaques. However, in some cases, individuals did not show any change in the annual incremental lines or tissue structure of cementum. The radiation effects of individuals may differ depending on the variations in the time of fertilization and individual differences in the tissue formation and morphogenesis stages during radiation exposure [13]. ^{137}Cs in the body is constantly replaced, and the effects of external exposure must also be taken into account. The effects on the individual macaques are thought to vary depending on where they lived at the time the FNPP accident occurred and what they ate after the accident. It is not clear whether the tissue structure of cementum and the indistinct incremental lines are due to individual variation or regional differences in the mode of radiation exposure. Further studies are needed to clarify these issues.

8.5 Conclusions

The annual incremental lines were observed in cementum of Japanese macaques, and their ages were determined. The incremental lines of the affected group were unclear compared to those of the unaffected group. In adults exposed to high concentrations of ^{137}Cs due to the FNPP accident, the incremental lines were locally irregularly spaced and obscured. The structure of cementum was disturbed due to the mixture of cellular and acellular cementum. It is suggested that low-dose radiation exposure may have affected the rhythm of incremental line formation and the tissue structure of cementum, which will be studied in more detail in the future.

References

1. Klevezal GA (Miona MV, Oreshkin AV tr.) (1996) Recording structures of mammals determination of age and reconstruction of life history, Balkema AA, pp 53–61. ISBN 9054106212
2. Nanci A, Somerman MJ (2003) Periodontium. In: Nanci A (ed) Ten Cate's oral histology: development, structure, and function, 6th edn. Mosby, pp 240–274. ISBN 0-323-01614-6
3. Koukkari WL, Sothern RB (2006) Introducing biological rhythms. Springer, pp 19–65. ISBN 978-1-4020-3691-0
4. Mishima H, Hattori A (2022) A study on the relationship between the periodicity of tooth dentin incremental lines and the circadian rhythm synchronizing factor melatonin. Relationship between the periodicity of tooth dentin incremental lines and melatonin. Col Mem Pa Prof Michihei Hoshino, EG Service, pp 95–102
5. Wada K, Ohtaishi N, Hachiya N (1978) Determination of age in the Japanese Monkey from growth layers in the dental cementum. Primates 19(4):775–784
6. Yamamoto T, Hasegawa T, Yamamoto T et al (2016) Histology of human cementum: its structure, function, and development. Jpn Dent Sci Rev 52:63–74. https://doi.org/10.1016/j.jdsr.2016.04.002
7. Takahashi S, Yamamoto T, Takahashi T et al (2023) Incremental lines in human cellular cementum: a histological study. J Oral Biosci 65:55–61. https://doi.org/10.1016/j.job.2022.12.001
8. Fukumoto M (ed) (2020) Low-dose Radiation effects on animals and ecosystems. Long-term study on the Fukushima nuclear accident. Springer open, pp 113–165. ISBN 978-981-13-8218-5 (eBook) https://doi.org/10.1007/978-981-13-8218-5
9. Urushihara Y, Suzuki T, Shimizu Y et al (2018) Haematological analysis of Japanese macaques (*Macaca fuscata*) in the area affected by the Fukushima Daiichi Nuclear Power Plant accident. Sci Rep 8:16748. https://doi.org/10.1038/s41598-018-35104-0
10. Koarai K, Kino Y, Takahashi A et al (2016) ^{90}Sr in teeth of cattle abandoned in evacuation zone: record of pollution from the Fukushima-Daiichi Nuclear Power Plant accident. Sci Rep 6:24077. https://doi.org/10.1038/srep24077
11. Douchya L, Gauthier R, Abouelleil-Sayed H et al (2022) The effect of therapeutic radiation on dental enamel and dentin: a systematic review. Dental Materials 38:E181–E201. https://doi.org/10.1016/j.dental.2022.04.014
12. Lu H, Zhao Q, Guo J et al (2019) Direct radiation-induced effects on dental. hard tissue. Radiat Oncol 14. https://doi.org/10.1186/s13014-019-1208-1
13. Saad AY, Abdelazim AA, El-Khasab MM et al (1991) Effects of gamma radiation on incisor development of the prenatal albino mouse. J Oral Pathol Med 20:385–388. https://doi.org/10.1111/j.1600-0714.1991.tb00949.x

14. Tajima Y, Yamada TK, Koike H, Kasuya T (2014) Estimating the ages of mammals captured in the wild-methods and significance. Mammal Sci 55:89–91. https://doi.org/10.11238/mammalianscience.55.89
15. Stewart REA, Campana SE, Jones CM et al (2006) Bomb radiocarbon dating calibrates beluga (Delphinapterus leucas) age estimates. Canad J Zool 84:1840–1852. https://doi.org/10.1139/z06-182
16. Papagerakis S, Zheng L, Schnell S et al (2014) The circadian clock in oral health and diseases. J Dent Res 93:27–35. https://doi.org/10.1177/0022034513505768
17. Mishima H, Tanabe S, Hattori A et al (2018) The relationship between the structure and calcification of dentin and the role of melatonin. In: Endo K, Kogure T, Nagasawa H (eds) Biomineralization: from molecular and nano-structural analysis to environmental science. Springer open, pp 199–209. ISBN 978-981-13-1002-7 (eBook) https://doi.org/10.1007/978-981-3-1002-7
18. Mishima H, Ishikawa N, Hattori A et al (2022) Relation of bone morphology and bone quality with melatonin intake in rats. J Oral Tissue Eng 20(1):1–10. https://doi.org/10.11223/jarde.20.1
19. Sevbitov AV, Persin LS, Slabkobskaia AB et al (1999) The morphological status of the maxillodental system in children living in an area contaminated by radionuclides as a result of the accident at the Chernobyl Atomic Electric Power Station. Stomatologiia 78(6):41–42
20. Persson BRR, Gjelsvik R, Holm E (2018) Radioecological modelling of Polonium-210 and Caesium-137 in lichen-reindeer-man and top predators. J Environ Radioact 186(2018):54–62. https://doi.org/10.1016/j.jenvrad.2017.08.006

Chapter 9
A Histopathological Analysis of the Cardiovascular System of Low-Dose-Rate Radiation-Exposed Japanese Macaques from the Area Affected by the Fukushima Daiichi Nuclear Power Plant Accident

Sohsuke Yamada, Suzuki Masatoshi, and Manabu Fukumoto

Abstract According to several large studies, there are significant dose-related increases after radiation exposure in the incidence of cardiovascular diseases, such as stroke or myocardial infarction, and circulatory disease/dysfunction, including chronic kidney disease. However, no basic in vivo studies have described the detailed pathological and/or molecular features or mechanisms underlying the development of radiation-induced cardiovascular diseases. In "a comprehensive dose evaluation project concerning animals affected by the FNPP accident" (Affected Animal Project), our group focused on the histopathological findings of the cardiovascular system in Japanese macaques with persistent whole-body exposure to low-dose-rate radiation in the area affected by the Fukushima Daiichi Nuclear Power Plant (FNPP) accident. We found that none of the 320 macaques affected by the accident showed any histopathologically severe atherosclerotic changes or overt myocardial infarctions. Furthermore, 12 macaques (12/320; 3.75%) revealed very mild intimal thickening in the relatively peripheral small coronary arteries, and in one case, the stenotic rate was only as high as approximately 15%. It may be too early to detect any significant findings of cardiovascular disease, such as atherosclerosis, in radiation-exposed Japanese macaques. Therefore, we propose that this project be continued as consecutive, multidisciplinary investigations, including molecular analyses, over the next 15–30 years.

S. Yamada (✉)
Department of Pathology, Kanazawa Medical University Hospital, Uchinada, Ishikawa, Japan

Department of Pathology and Laboratory Medicine, Kanazawa Medical University, Uchinada, Ishikawa, Japan
e-mail: sohsuke@kanazawa-med.ac.jp

S. Masatoshi · M. Fukumoto
International Research Institute of Disaster Science, Tohoku University, Sendai, Japan

M. Fukumoto (ed.), *Low-Dose Radiation Effects on Animals and Ecosystems II*,
https://doi.org/10.1007/978-981-95-5559-8_9

Keywords Japanese macaques · Low-dose-rate radiation · Cardiovascular diseases · Atherosclerosis · Intimal thickening

9.1 Introduction

Since 1950, the Radiation Effects Research Foundation (RERF) has conducted the Life Span Study (LSS) on the health of atomic bomb (A-bomb) survivors in Hiroshima and Nagasaki [1] and the Adult Health Study (AHS) consisting of biennial clinical and laboratory studies of approximately 15% of the LSS cohort members [2]. Both of these large cohort studies show significant dose-related increases in the incidence of cardiovascular diseases (CVD), such as stroke or myocardial infarction, as well as circulatory disease/dysfunction, including chronic kidney disease. In addition, based on previous meta-analyses of epidemiological data, exposure to low and moderate doses of ionizing radiation appears to result in significantly elevated risks of incident and mortality rates of human cardiovascular diseases [3, 4].

Epidemiologic studies of radiation exposure and CVD have used data from radiation therapy, occupational exposure, or environmental exposure. In most radiotherapy studies in which local rather than whole-body exposure was used, the incidence of myocardial infarction was not significantly increased at doses of less than 1.5 Gy, while an increased risk of CVD was reported for A-bomb survivors exposed to doses greater than 0.5 Gy [1, 2].

However, no basic human studies have described the detailed pathological and/ or molecular features and mechanisms of radiation-induced cardiovascular diseases. Therefore, whether circulatory disease or dysfunction after radiation exposure is caused by gene mutations, epigenetic alterations, or both remains unclear.

Several experimental studies on the effects of exposure to ionizing radiation using rodent models have revealed that concentrated irradiation results in the significant development of cardiac hypertrophy, myocardial remodeling with fibrosis, or atherosclerosis [5]. However, these evaluations in animal models have all had study limitations, since each radiation dose was abnormally high, and no studies in larger animal models that might more closely resemble the human cardiovascular system or better reflect the biological processes and pathogenesis of human cardiovascular diseases have yet been conducted.

9.2 Materials and Methods

In this Affected Animal Project, our group focused on the histopathological findings of the cardiovascular system in 320 Japanese macaques with persistent whole-body exposure to low-dose-rate radiation in the area affected by the Fukushima Daiichi Nuclear Power Plant (FNPP) accident on March 12, 2011. In particular, we focused on the tissue of the heart in each macaque, allowing us to pathologically observe not only large to small arteries (i.e., aortic bulb to coronary arteries) but also cardiac muscles.

The heart was cut at the level of its maximal short-axis diameter, and histological sections at 4 μm were prepared using standard methods and then stained with hematoxylin and eosin (H&E) and elastica van Gieson (EVG) in sequential sections. EVG staining revealed both internal and external elastic laminae of the coronary arteries.

9.3   Results and Discussion

In conclusion, none of the 320 FNPP radiation-exposed macaques showed any histopathologically severe atherosclerotic changes or overt myocardial infarctions (Fig. 9.1a). However, in a few cases, the attachment of inflammatory cells (such as monocytes) to the arterial endothelium was rarely recognized as very early-phase atherosclerosis, a nonsignificant finding.

According to the classically established hypothesis known as the "response to injury theory" proposed by Russell Ross [6], after the migration of monocytes with subsequent differentiation into macrophages from the peripheral blood into the intima via degradation of the endothelial cells to the basement membrane, early atherosclerotic lesions (mainly fatty streaks) occur.

Notably, 12 out of 320 macaques (3.75%) revealed very mild intimal thickening in the relatively peripheral small coronary arteries, and in one case, the stenotic rate was as high as approximately 15% (Fig. 9.1b). These atherosclerotic lesions were histologically composed mainly of migrating and proliferating spindled smooth

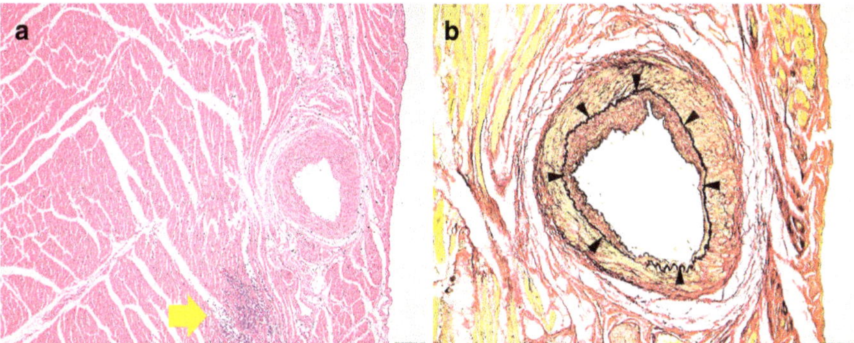

Fig. 9.1 Histopathological findings of the heart of a Japanese macaque with persistent whole--body exposure to low-dose-rate radiation in the area affected by the FNPP accident (Macaque No. 631). (**a**) In the low-power view, H&E staining revealed very mild intimal thickening in the relatively peripheral small coronary artery. The heart contains a focus of patchy and mild chronic inflammatory infiltrates around this small coronary artery. Lymphocytes (yellow arrow) are observed. However, we noted no severe atherosclerotic changes or overt myocardial infarction. Scale bar = 200 μm. (**b**) Elastica van Gieson (EVG) staining reveals the stenotic rate of the vessel lumen as being as high as approximately 15%, showing both the internal elastic lamina (arrowheads) and the external elastic lamina. The atherosclerotic lesion is composed mainly of migrating and proliferating spindled smooth muscle cell-like cells, very similar to the mild intimal hyperplasia of the human coronary artery. Scale bar = 100 μm.

muscle cell-like cells, very similar to mild intimal hyperplasia of the human coronary arteries [6], and were not considered to be genuinely pathologic changes. In fact, in our thorough observations, there were no aggregated cholesterol-phagocytosing foamy macrophages, necrotic central lipid cores, or calcifications, which are truly histopathological atherosclerotic changes [6]. Furthermore, among the 12 abovementioned macaques, the hearts in six histologically revealed patchy and mild chronic inflammatory infiltrate around the small coronary arteries (Fig. 9.1a), although the possibility of agonal, nonspecific findings could not be excluded. Similarly, scattered and mild subendocardial fibrosis in very few cases may result from aging-related nonspecific histological changes. Nevertheless, we will investigate the relationship between the abovementioned histopathological features and the dose rate of radioactive cesium or the age of each radiation-exposed Japanese macaque in the near future.

More than 12 years have passed since the FNPP accident in 2011, but it still seems too early to detect any significant findings of cardiovascular diseases, such as atherosclerosis, in these radiation-exposed Japanese macaques. Atherosclerosis is a complex multifactorial disease that affects glucose/lipid/bile acid metabolism, insulin resistance, inflammatory cell infiltration, cytokine levels and/or apoptotic activities in various organs, translocation of either intestinal bacteria or microbial cell components, oxidative stress, and other factors [7, 8]. Therefore, we propose that this project be continued as consecutive, multidisciplinary investigations, including molecular analyses, over the next 15–30 years. Furthermore, we need to perform detailed examinations of circulatory diseases induced by fetal exposure to low-dose-rate radiation and their heritable/hereditary effects on Japanese macaques after the FNPP accident.

References

1. Shimizu Y, Kodama K, Nishi N et al (2010) Radiation exposure and circulatory disease risk: Hiroshima and Nagasaki atomic bomb survivor data, 1950–2003. BMJ 340:b5349. https://doi.org/10.1136/bmj.b5349
2. Yamada M, Naito K, Kasagi F et al (2005) Prevalence of atherosclerosis in relation to atomic bomb radiation exposure: an RERF Adult Health Study. Int J Radiat Biol 81:821–826. https://doi.org/10.1080/09553000600555504
3. Little MP, Azizova TV, Bazyka D et al (2012) Systematic review and meta-analysis of circulatory disease from exposure to low-level ionizing radiation and estimates of potential population mortality risks. Environ Health Perspect 120:1503–1511. https://doi.org/10.1289/ehp.1204982
4. Baselet B, Rombouts C, Benotmane AM et al (2016) Cardiovascular diseases related to ionizing radiation: the risk of low-dose exposure (Review). Int J Mol Med 38:1623–1641. https://doi.org/10.3892/ijmm.2016.2777
5. Meerman M, Bracco Gartner TCL, Buikema JW et al (2021) Myocardial disease and long-distance space travel: solving the radiation problem. Front Cardiovasc Med 8:631985. https://doi.org/10.3389/fcvm.2021.631985
6. Ross R (1999) Atherosclerosis—an inflammatory disease. N Engl J Med 340:115–126. https://doi.org/10.1056/NEJM199901143400207

7. Yamada S, Tanimoto A, Sasaguri Y (2016) Critical in vivo roles of histamine and histamine receptor signaling in animal models of metabolic syndrome. Pathol Int 66:661–671. https://doi.org/10.1111/pin.12477
8. Yamada S, Guo X (2018) Peroxiredoxin 4 (PRDX4): Its critical in vivo roles in animal models of metabolic syndrome ranging from atherosclerosis to nonalcoholic fatty liver disease. Pathol Int 68:91–101. https://doi.org/10.1111/pin.12634

Chapter 10
Effects of Low-Dose Radiation Exposure on the Crystalline Lens of the Japanese Macaque Eye

Naoki Yamamoto, Noriko Hiramatsu, Yu Kato, Yumika Kuno, Kana Aihara, Natsuko Hatsusaka, Hiroshi Sasaki, Noriaki Nagai, Yosuke Nakazawa, Masatoshi Suzuki, and Manabu Fukumoto

Abstract In order to assess the effects of long-term exposure to low-dose-rate radiation in the crystalline lens, eyes of 114 wild Japanese macaques inhabiting the vicinity of Fukushima Daiichi Nuclear Power Plant (FNPP) were examined 3–11.4 years after the accident that caused a massive release of radioactive materials in 2011. Histological examinations revealed dissection of the superficial cortex along the Y-shaped sutures (water cleft) and the presence of vacuoles, typical of early-stage cataracts. Unlike diabetic cataract rats, aquaporin 0 (AQP0) and AQP5 did not accumulate around these vacuoles, suggesting that the cataracts observed in this study arise from a mechanism distinct from diabetic cataracts. Internal doses and dose rates were higher in the group with cataractous changes in the lens than in the group without such changes. However, it should be noted that these changes do not immediately lead to visual impairment or the development of cataracts. Despite the limitations inherent in fieldwork, the findings in this study contribute insights into the impact of cumulative low-dose-rate radiation on the lens and underscore the

N. Yamamoto (✉)
Center for Society-Academia Collaboration, Research Promotion Headquarters, Fujita Health University, Toyoake-city, Aichi, Japan

Faculty of Engineering, Sanyo-Onoda City University, Sanyo-Onoda-city, Yamaguchi, Japan
e-mail: naokiy@fujita-hu.ac.jp

N. Hiramatsu · Y. Kato
Center for Society-Academia Collaboration, Research Promotion Headquarters, Fujita Health University, Toyoake-city, Aichi, Japan

Y. Kuno · K. Aihara · Y. Nakazawa
Faculty of Pharmacy, Keio University, Tokyo, Japan

N. Hatsusaka · H. Sasaki
Department of Ophthalmology, Kanazawa Medical University, Kahoku-gun, Ishikawa, Japan

N. Nagai
Faculty of Pharmacy, Kindai University, Higashi-Osaka-city, Osaka, Japan

M. Suzuki · M. Fukumoto
International Research Institute of Disaster Science, Tohoku University, Sendai, Japan

© The Author(s) 2026

M. Fukumoto (ed.), *Low-Dose Radiation Effects on Animals and Ecosystems II*,
https://doi.org/10.1007/978-981-95-5559-8_10

need for continued vigilance to protect both wildlife and humans from radiation-induced injury.

Keywords Low-dose/low-dose-rate radiation · Crystalline lens · Japanese macaques · Fukushima Daiichi Nuclear Power Plant (FNPP) · Radiation cataract · Aquaporins

10.1 Introduction

The Great East Japan Earthquake and Tsunami of March 11, 2011, led to the accident at Tokyo Electric Power Company's (TEPCO) Fukushima Daiichi Nuclear Power Plant (FNPP), resulting in significant radioactive contamination over a wide area of eastern Japan. The evacuation zone and its surrounding areas have been home to wild Japanese macaques (*Macaca fuscata*) since before the FNPP accident. The lifespan of macaques, a nonhuman primate species, exceeds 20 years in the wild. Their average habitat range spans 8.99 km^2 (0.29–39.7 km^2), and they typically form troops comprising several dozen individuals. Therefore, wild macaques, living in the vicinity of FNPP (affected macaques), serve as a useful surrogate model to evaluate the effects of long-term exposure to low-dose-rate radiation in humans [1].

The lens of the eye is recognized as one of the most radiosensitive organs in the human body, and radiation exposure is recognized to induce cataracts. Cataracts that cause clinical visual impairment are classified into three main types according to the location of the lesion in the lens: nuclear cataracts, cortical cataracts, and posterior subcapsular cataracts. Ionizing radiation is generally, but not exclusively, associated with cortical and posterior subcapsular opacities, with the latter being particularly dependent on radiation dose [2]. The lens is enclosed in a capsule containing collagen type IV. Lens epithelial cells (LECs) utilize the lens capsule as their basement membrane, forming a single-layer arrangement within the capsule. In the proliferative zone located slightly anterior to the equator of the lens, LECs proliferate toward both the anterior pole and the equator. As LECs proliferate and migrate toward the equator, they differentiate into lens fiber cells (LFCs) [3]. LFCs that have initiated differentiation elongate along the anterior–posterior axis of the lens, and the lens grows as these LFCs cover the old lens fiber core. In addition, during the maturation process of LFCs, the cell nucleus disappears, and intracellular organelles such as the endoplasmic reticulum, Golgi apparatus, and mitochondria also disappear. The disappearance of these intracellular organelles is thought to be important in achieving lens transparency (Fig. 10.1a). Cataracts are a condition in which the lens becomes clouded due to various causes, making it difficult for light to pass through and causing symptoms such as blurred vision. Based primarily on their location, cataracts are classified into three major types: cortical, nuclear, and posterior subcapsular cataracts. Additionally, several subtypes exist, including water clefts, retrodots, and vacuoles. It is generally accepted that radiation damages dividing cells, that is, dividing LECs are damaged by radiation, differentiate into

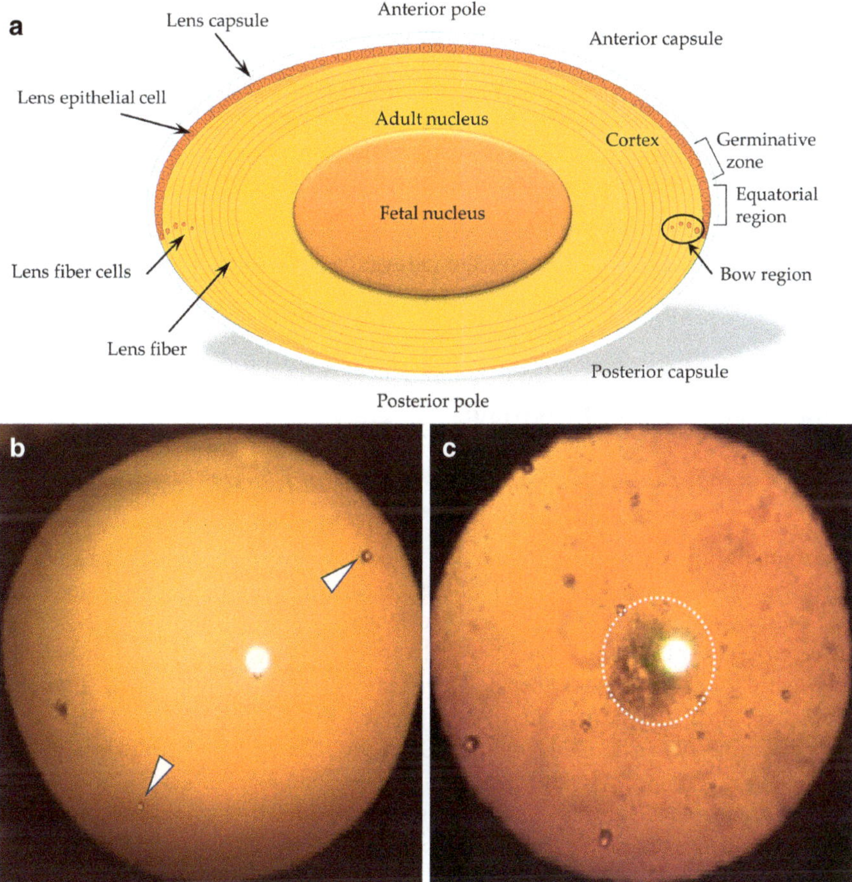

Fig. 10.1 Crystalline lens and findings in human radiation cataracts. (**a**) Schematic diagram of the crystalline lens. (**b**) Vacuoles (arrowheads), early lesions observed in human cataract, are depicted. (**c**) Posterior subcapsular cataract (within circular dotted lines) were observed as the human cataract progressed (Reproduced with approval from Japanese Society for Cataract Research homepage, with some modifications).

LECs with damage which migrate to the posterior pole, resulting in light refraction and opacity of the lens [4, 5]. In the early stages of human cataracts, microopacities such as vacuoles (Fig. 10.1b) and the dissection of the superficial layers of the lens cortex along the Y-shaped suture (water cleft) are observed. As these changes progress, they are thought to develop into posterior subcapsular (Fig. 10.1c) and cortical cataracts [6].

Recently, it was reported that vacuoles are observed in the lens of a rat model of diabetic cataract and that the expression of aquaporin 0 (AQP0) and AQP5, important regulators of ion and water microcirculation, is increased around these vacuoles [7]. Controlling the transport of ions and water in the lens is thought to be important in keeping its optical properties constant and preventing cataracts. It has been suggested that the transient receptor potential vanilloid channels, TRPV1 and TRPV4 function as mechanosensors converting alteration in lens volume and internal hydrostatic pressure into activation of signal transduction pathways in LECs [8]. Therefore, we searched for vacuoles in the lens of affected macaques and, when found, examined the expression of AQP0 and AQP5 around the vacuoles in the lens tissue. Furthermore, we investigated the expression of TRPV1 and TRPV4 proteins in the early stages of cataractous changes. In this study, we summarize the results of histological observations of the crystalline lens of macaques exposed for a long time to low-dose-rate radiation emitted from radioactive material dispersed by the FNPP accident.

10.2 Materials and Methods

10.2.1 Observation of Japanese Macaque Lenses

The animals utilized in this study were individuals captured and culled as part of the Japanese macaque management plan, designed to prevent crop damage under the Act on the Protection of Wildlife and the Management of Hunting. Of these, 114 macaques, captured from September 2016 to July 2022, underwent both external and internal exposure assessments. This study was approved by the Institutional Animal Control Committee of the Center for Experimental Animal Research, Tohoku University (Approval Number: 2014 IDAC-037). All experiments were carried out in accordance with the relevant guidelines and regulations [1]. To examine the crystalline lens in situ in macaques, a simplified transillumination camera (LOVEOX Co., Ltd., Tokyo, Japan) [7] was used.

10.2.2 External and Internal Exposure Doses

Evaluation of external and internal radiation doses from radioactive cesium (^{134}Cs + ^{137}Cs) was performed as previously described [9]. Modeling macaques as ellipsoids, external exposure was assumed to occur from uniformly contaminated ground, and internal exposure was from radioactive Cs uniformly distributed within the body. External dose was calculated using radioactive Cs concentration in soil at the capture sites from data published by the Ministry of Education, Culture, Sports, Science and Technology of Japan [10]. The conversion factor for internal dose was calculated using radioactive Cs concentration in femoral muscle. For calculating dose from dose rates, we assumed that macaques were continuously exposed to radioactive Cs from birth to capture at the same site because the habitat range of the macaques studied was limited.

10.2.3 Preparation and Staining of Tissue Specimens

Lenses were removed from eyeballs and fixed using Super Fix (Kurabo Industries Ltd., Osaka, Japan) [3]. Following fixation, crystalline lenses were processed into paraffin blocks using standard procedures, sectioned, and used for hematoxylin–eosin (H&E) staining or immunostaining. For immunostaining, as primary antibodies for aquaporins, anti-AQP0 (sc-376445, Santa Cruz Biotechnology, Santa Cruz, CA, USA) and anti-AQP5 (AB15858, Merck Millipore, Billerica, MA, USA) were used. Primary antibodies for TRPV proteins, anti-TRPV1 (ab39260, Abcam plc, Cambridge, UK) and anti-TRPV4 (ACC-034, Alomone Labs, Jerusalem, Israel), were employed. Subsequently, slides were incubated with goat anti-mouse or anti-rabbit Alexa Fluor 488 (A-11008, Thermo Fisher Scientific, Inc., Waltham, MA, USA) secondary antibody in a blocking solution with 4′,6-diamidino-2-phenylindole (DAPI), followed by incubation with wheat germ agglutinin (WGA)–Alexa Fluor 594 (W11262, Thermo Fisher Scientific) to label the cell membrane. Image observation was performed under a laser scanning confocal microscope (FV3000, Olympus, Japan) after mounting coverslips using VECTASHIELD HardSet™ (Vector Laboratories, Burlingame, CA, USA) antifade mounting medium. Additionally, we confirmed the presence or absence of α-smooth muscle actin (α-SMA) as an indicator of epithelial–mesenchymal transition (EMT), a phenomenon observed in the abnormal proliferation of LECs such as posterior capsule opacification [11]. The primary antibody used was anti-α-SMA antibody (ab7817, Abcam), and the secondary antibody was Simple Stain MAX PO MULTI (for mouse and rabbit primary antibodies; Nichirei, Tokyo, Japan). Observation was performed under a light microscope after coloration with 3,3′-diaminobenzidine tetrahydrochloride (DAB).

10.2.4 Statistical Analysis

The comparison between pairs of groups was performed by the Mann–Whitney U test. The Statistical Package for the Social Sciences (SPSS Statistics 24, IBM Corporation, New York, NY, USA) was used for data analysis.

10.3 Results

10.3.1 Observation of the Macaque Lens with a Simplified Transillumination Camera

Macaque crystalline lenses were photographed using a transillumination camera. In some lenses, water clefts and the Y-shaped suture were observed in the center of the posterior capsule (Fig. 10.2).

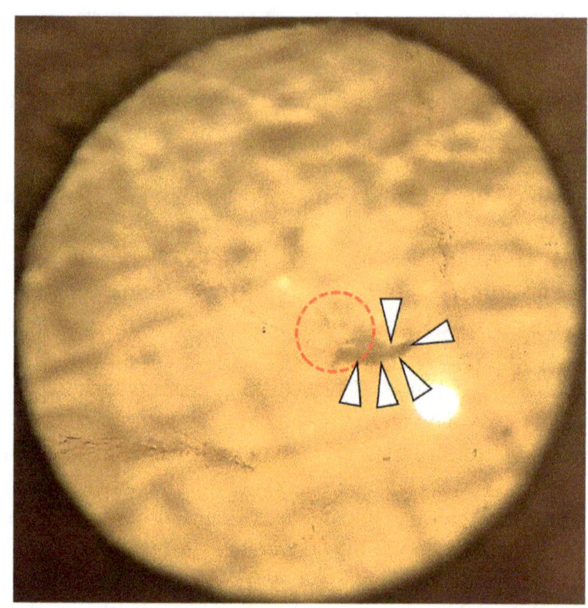

Fig. 10.2 Transillumination photograph of an affected macaque lens. The Y-suture (circular dotted line) and water cleft (white arrowheads) were observed at the early stage of cataract in the center of the posterior capsule (Macaque No. 683).

10.3.2   Histological Observations of the Lens Fiber Cell Layer

We could calculate dose and make histological observations of the lenses for 74 of the 114 macaques sampled. In some lenses, we observed a backward shift of cell nuclei in the LFC layer (Fig. 10.3a). Multiple vacuoles were observed between the LFCs in the subsurface portion of the lens from the equatorial region to the posterior pole (Fig. 10.3a). Cell membrane staining with WGA revealed vacuoles in the intercellular cleft of LFCs (Fig. 10.3b, c). However, immunostaining of the same region did not show any accumulation of AQP0, AQP5, TRPV1, or TRPV4 around the vacuoles (Fig. 10.3d–k).

10.3.3   Lens with Posterior Subcapsular Opacity

Examination of the removed lens revealed opacities in the posterior capsule and cortex, corresponding to the areas that appeared opaque on the transillumination image (Fig. 10.4a). In H&E-stained tissue sections, a distinct difference in staining was observed in the medial region of the posterior capsule, consistent with the area of macroscopic opacity. Additionally, areas where the tips of LFCs were not joined were observed at the posterior pole (Fig. 10.4b, c). Within the lens cortex, a backward migration of LFC nuclei toward the posterior polar side was observed

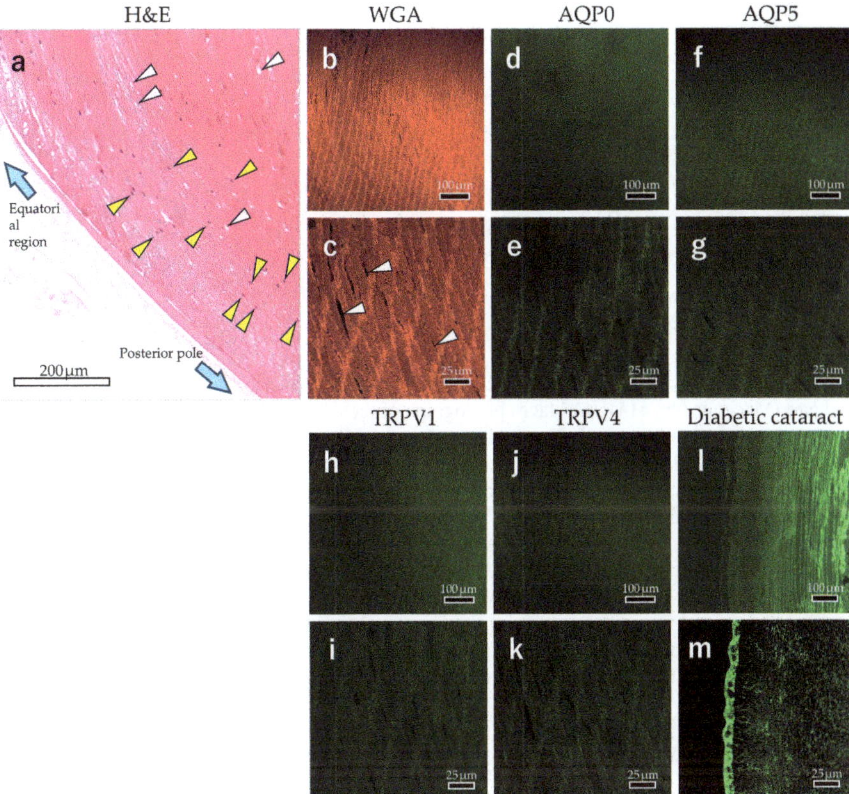

Fig. 10.3 A lens in which vacuoles were observed (Macaque No. 414, external dose 355.4 mGy, internal dose 69.2 mGy). (**a**) H&E-stained specimen showing the nuclei of LFCs moving backward to the posterior pole (yellow arrowheads) and vacuoles observed between LFCs (white arrowheads). Vacuoles appear more oval than spherical with fragile intercellular adhesions. (**b**) WGA staining of the cell membrane. (**c**) Enlarged view of the central area of **b** showing vacuoles in the intercellular spaces of LFC (white arrowheads). (**d**) Immunostaining for AQP0. (**e**) Enlarged view of the central area of **d**. (**f**) Immunostaining for AQP5. (**g**) Enlarged view of the central area of **f**. (**h**) Immunostaining for TRPV1. (**i**) Enlarged view of the central area of **h**. (**j**) Immunostaining for TRPV4. (**k**) Enlarged view of the central area of **j**. (**l**) Immunostaining for AQP0 in diabetic cataract model rat. (**m**) Immunostaining for AQP5 at diabetic cataract model rat.

(Fig. 10.4d). Negative α-SMA staining in this region indicated that EMT from LECs to LFCs had not occurred (Fig. 10.4e). The tips of LFCs at the posterior pole were not joined, exhibiting signs of melting or voiding (Fig. 10.4f), and were also negative for α-SMA staining (Fig. 10.4g). Furthermore, immunostaining showed no accumulation of AQP0, AQP5, TRPV1, or TRPV4 around the posterior pole and surrounding LFCs (Fig. 10.5a–e).

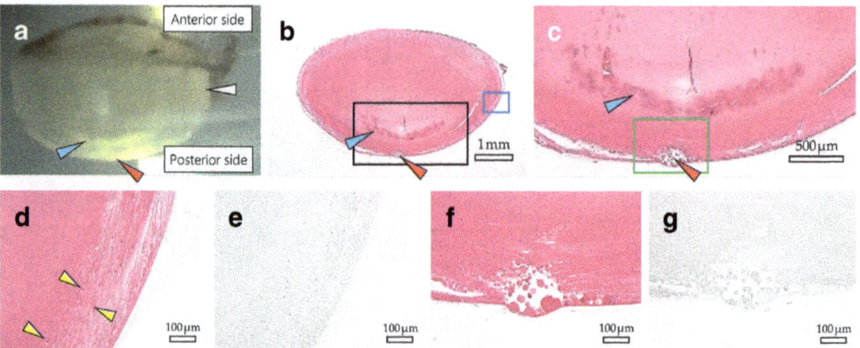

Fig. 10.4 Macaques lens with slight opacity observed on the posterior side and around the equatorial part (Macaque No. 414). (**a**) Macro photograph of the extracted crystalline lens showing slight opacities in the posterior capsule area (red arrowhead) and around the equatorial area (white arrowheads). Opacity behind the lens nucleus (adult nucleus) on the posterior side is also observed (blue arrowhead). (**b**) Lens tissue specimen shown in **a**. Visual observation reveals the clear difference corresponding to the opacified area near the posterior pole of the lens nucleus (blue arrowhead, H&E stain). Areas where the tips of LFCs were not joined were observed at the posterior pole (red arrowhead). (**c**) Enlarged view of the black square area in **b**. A void is observed at the posterior pole (green square, H&E stain). (**d**) Enlarged view of the blue square area in **b**. Cell nuclei of the LFCs are directed toward the posterior pole of the lens compared to normal (Yellow arrowheads). (**e**) Immunostaining of α-SMA in sequential sections of **d**. (**f**) Enlarged view of the green square area in **c** (H&E stain). (**g**) Immunostaining of α-SMA in sequential sections of **f**.

10.3.4 Exposure Dose and Lens Findings

Both radiation doses and dose rates received by the macaques were biased toward the low end. The total dose in the group with cataractous changes (cataract group) was 3.2–643.6 mGy (median: 25.7 mGy), which was not significantly different from the group without cataractous changes (non-cataract group) (3.3–199.3 mGy, median: 16.6 mGy). Compared with the non-cataract group, the internal dose was significantly, and the internal dose rate was sub-significantly, higher in the cataract group (Fig. 10.6).

Within the cataract group, there is a good correlation between ambient dose rate and the internal dose rate, that is, radioactive Cs concentration in the body ($r = 0.84$) (Fig. 10.7a). Similarly calculated external and internal doses are also well correlated in the cataract group ($r = 0.90$). However, these correlations were not observed in the non-cataract group (Fig. 10.7b). Figure 10.7a, b shows that these strong correlations are due to the contribution of individuals with relatively high doses and dose rates. Interestingly, though the number was small, cataractous changes were observed in macaques exposed to internal dose rate of 50 μGy/day or higher.

The most frequently observed cataractous change was the posterior transition of the cell nuclei of LFCs, but the presence or absence of this change in LFCs was not related to dose/dose rate. Cataracts can also develop as a result of aging, but in this

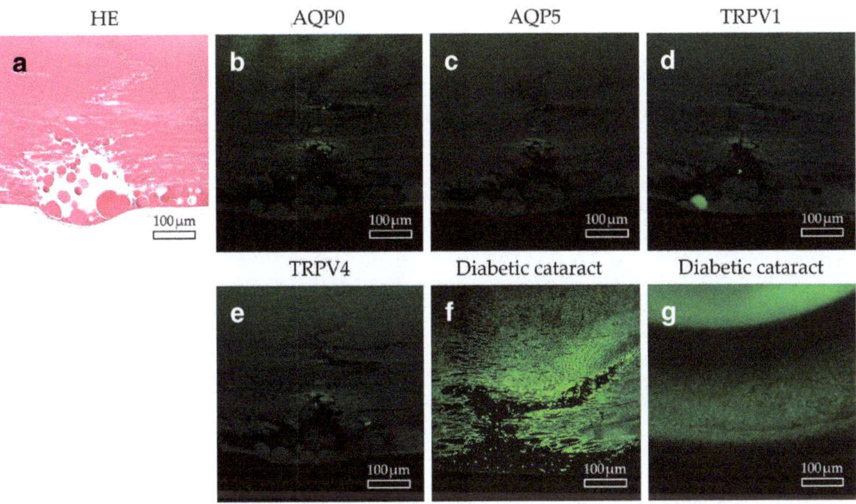

Fig. 10.5 Void in the posterior pole of the crystalline lens (Macaque No. 414). (**a**) H&E stained specimen of the posterior pole of the crystalline lens. (**b**) Immunostaining for AQP0. (**c**) Immunostaining for AQP5. (**d**) Immunostaining for TRPV1. (**e**) Immunostaining for TRPV4. (**f**) Immunostaining for AQP0 at diabetic cataract model rat. (**g**) Immunostaining for AQP5 at diabetic cataract model rat.

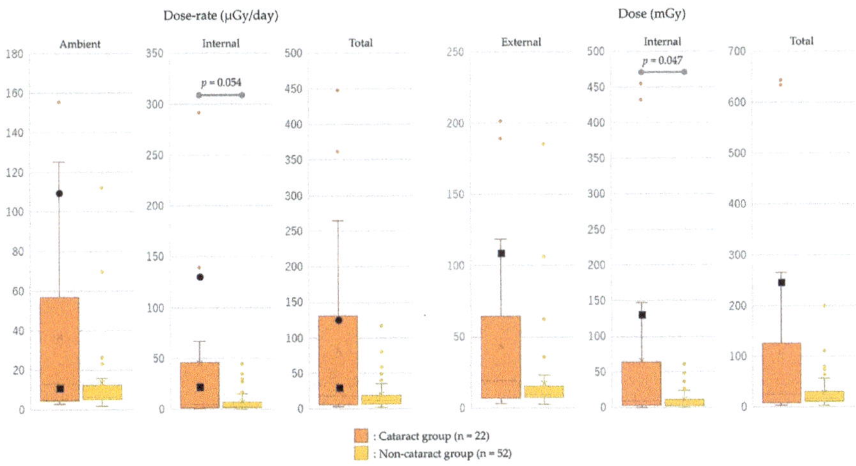

Fig. 10.6 Comparison of exposure dose-rate and dose distributions between cataract and non-cataract groups. ●: Macaque No. 414, ■: Macaque No. 683.

study the age distribution of the cataract group ranged from 3 to 19.5 years (median: 7 years), and that of the non-cataract group ranged from 2.5 to 20.0 years (median: 6.5 years), suggesting that the onset of cataracts was unrelated to age. No gender-specific differences in cataract incidence were observed (Table 10.1).

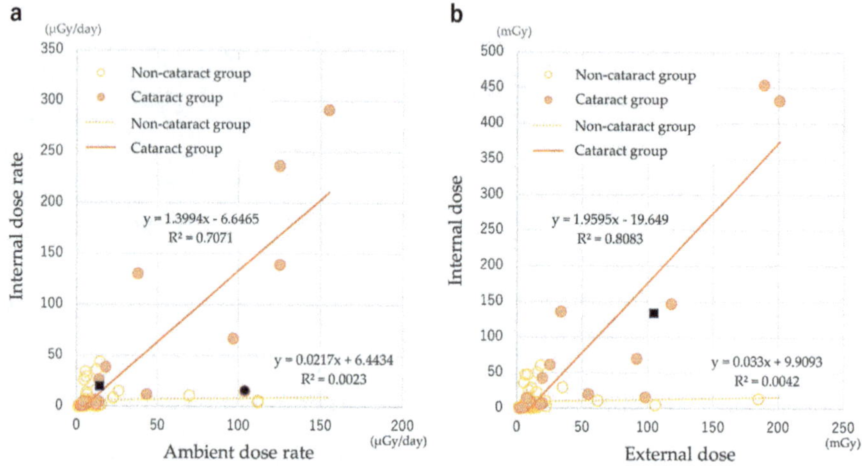

Fig. 10.7 Correlation between external and internal exposure stratified into cataract and non-cataract groups. (**a**) Ambient dose rate and internal dose rate. (**b**) External dose and internal dose. ●: Macaque No. 414, ■: Macaque No. 683.

Table 10.1 Characteristics of macaques classified by the presence or absence of cataractous changes.

	Cataract (+)		Cataract (−)		
	Min, Max	Median	Min, Max	Median	p
	mGy				
External dose	2.7, 201.2	19.2	2.2, 185.4	9.4	0.081
Internal dose	0.5, 454.2	8.7	0.5, 60.6	4.3	0.047
Total dose	3.2, 643.6	25.7	3.3, 199.3	16.6	0.06
	µGy/day				
Ambient (external) dose rate	2.7, 155.5	13.1	1.7, 112.5	6.5	0.142
Internal dose rate	0.5, 291.8	4.6	0.3, 44.2	2.4	0.054
Total dose rate	3.2, 447.3	18.5	2.0, 118.6	12.3	0.139
	Years				
Age	3, 19.5	7	2.5, 20	6.5	0.730
Duration	3, 10.9	6.1	2.5, 11.4	5.7	0.771
	No.				Total
M	11		32		43
F	11		20		31

Posterior subcapsular cataract, a characteristic change of radiation, was seen in four macaques, consistent with individuals with vacuole formation, a possible early change. All of them received higher internal dose and dose rate than the median for the non-cataract group, but external dose and dose rate were not necessarily lower than the median of the non-cataract group.

10.4 Discussion

The exact mechanism of radiation-induced cataract formation is unknown. The lens comprises actively dividing cells, including lens epithelial stem/progenitor cells (LECs in the proliferative or germinative zone), quiescent cells activated by stimulation (LECs under the anterior capsule), and nondividing cells (LFCs differentiated from LECs) [3]. The pathogenesis of cataracts is thought to be due to induction of abnormal cell division and differentiation rather than cell death of LFCs due to genomic damage.

It has been suggested that the accumulation and fusion of microopacities within the damaged LFC population leads to the formation of larger lens defects and ultimately to clinical opacification [4].

Epidemiological studies of atomic bomb survivors suggest that there is a threshold dose of 0.1–0.7 Gy for the development of cataracts due to acute exposure [12, 13]. Although the majority of cases were only early-stage cataracts, threshold dose estimates for long-term exposure were derived from the Chernobyl (Chornobyl) survivor data and ranged from 0.34 to 0.50 Gy (95% confidence interval [CI], 0.17–0.69 Gy) [14]. In this study, we observed that LFC nuclei at the lens equator were displaced posteriorly and that LFCs were unable to fully elongate near the posterior pole, resulting in poor intercellular connections such as vacuole formation. In order to determine whether there is a threshold dose, we are working to accumulate the number of specimens so that a precise analysis can be performed for early cataract changes.

The strong correlation between external and internal exposure observed in this study suggests that radioactive Cs is dynamically transferred from soil to plants and from plant foods to macaques. Furthermore, the similarity in the profile of the relationship between external and internal exposure, both in terms of dose and dose rate, suggests that ingestion of contaminated food over a period of time, rather than total dose, is responsible for causing cataract changes. It is interesting to note that internal, but not external, dose and dose rate were higher in the cataract group than in the non-cataract group, although this is an unlikely situation to occur in a human exposure accident.

It is known that there is a long latency period between radiation exposure and the development of cataracts [15]. In epidemiologic studies, cataracts are not recognized unless symptoms appear or surgery is performed. However, in affected macaques, initial lesions can be accurately analyzed by acquiring transillumination images and dissection. Furthermore, the 20-year lifespan of the macaques is considered to be a sufficient period to observe the development of cataracts. In this study, we found that the expression of AQP0 and AQP5, regulators of lens ions and water microcirculation, did not accumulate around the vacuoles. This is in contrast to observations in diabetic cataract model rats where AQP0 and AQP5 are strongly localized around the vacuoles [7]. These results suggest different origins for vacuoles in radiation-induced and diabetic cataract. Backward transition of LFC nuclei and abnormal arrangement of the arcuate region were observed in some macaques, but immunostaining for α-SMA to detect EMT was negative. These findings suggest that the observed posterior migration and abnormal arrangement are likely due to abnormal differentiation of LECs into LFCs rather than promotion of extracellular matrix overgrowth by LECs.

During the first year of restoration work following the FNPP, six TEPCO employees were exposed to doses exceeding the then-effective dose limit of 250 mSv, with a maximum lens equivalent dose of 199.42 mSv [16]. It will be necessary to conduct follow-up surveys of employees to take into account early cataract changes such as vacuole and water cleft formation.

This study has the following limitations. The condition of the macaque lens prior to the FNPP accident could not be investigated, so the impact of the accident on the lens cannot be genuinely assessed. The age at capture was calculated from the growth ring of tooth enamel, which lacks accuracy on a monthly basis. Total radiation exposure over time was estimated but not directly measured. Since the animals lived in wild conditions and the crystalline lens was observed after capture, it was difficult to rule out that some observed minor lens findings captured by the transillumination camera were due to scratches and dryness of the cornea. Furthermore, since internal exposure calculations were based on radioactive cesium concentration at the time of capture, it was impossible to determine whether an animal had been exposed to higher dose in the past than at the time of capture.

10.5   Conclusions

This study investigated the effects of long-term, low-dose-rate radiation exposure on the lens of wild macaques affected by the FNPP accident. Some lens tissues showed water clefts and vacuoles, which are observed in the early stages of human cataract. The fact that AQP0 and AQP5 accumulation was not observed around the vacuoles in this study suggests that the vacuoles observed in radiation-induced cataract are formed by a different mechanism than in diabetic cataracts. The presence or absence of findings on the crystalline lens was associated with internal radiation exposure, but no findings were found that would immediately lead to visual impairment or the development of cataract. The long-term observation of the effects of low-dose-rate exposure on the crystalline lens conducted in this study is crucial in providing scientific insight into how to protect the lenses of radiation workers.

Acknowledgments We are indebted to Masato Morikawa for editing and reviewing this manuscript for technical support and to David Price for English proofreading. This work was partly supported by JSPS Kakenhi 20K12173 and 23K11429.

References

1. Urushihara Y, Suzuki T, Shimizu Y et al (2018) Haematological analysis of Japanese macaques (Macaca fuscata) in the area affected by the Fukushima Daiichi Nuclear Power Plant accident. Sci Rep 8:16748. https://doi.org/10.1038/s41598-018-35104-0
2. Ainsbury EA, Bouffler SD, Dorr W et al (2009) Radiation cataractogenesis: a review of recent studies. Radiat Res 172:1–9. https://doi.org/10.1667/RR1688.1
3. Yamamoto N, Majima K, Marunouchi T (2008) A study of the proliferating activity in lens epithelium and the identification of tissue-type stem cells. Med Mol Morphol 41:83–91. https://doi.org/10.1007/s00795-008-0395-x
4. Sparrow JM, Bron AJ, Brown NA et al (1986) The Oxford clinical cataract classification and grading system. Int Ophtalmol 9:207–225. https://doi.org/10.1007/BF00137534
5. Terasima T, Tolmach LJ (1963) Variations in several responses of HeLa cells to x-irradiation during the division cycle. Biophys J 3(1):11–33. https://doi.org/10.1016/s0006-3495(63)86801-0. PMID: 13980635; PMCID: PMC1366421.
6. International Commission on Radiological Protection (ICRP) (2012) ICRP publication 118: ICRP statement on tissue reactions and early and late effects of radiation in normal tissues and organs—threshold doses for tissue reactions in a radiation protection context. Ann ICRP 41:1–322. https://doi.org/10.1016/j.icrp.2012.02.001
7. Aihara K, Nakazawa Y, Takeda S et al (2023) Aquaporins contribute to vacuoles formation in Nile grass type II diabetic rats. Med Mol Morphol 56:274–287. https://doi.org/10.1007/s00795-023-00365-w
8. Nakazawa Y, Donaldson PJ, Petrova RS (2019) Verification and spatial mapping of TRPV1 and TRPV4 expression in the embryonic and adult mouse lens. Exp Eye Res 186:107707. https://doi.org/10.1016/j.exer.2019.107707
9. Endo S, Ishii K, Suzuki M et al (2020) Dose estimation of external and internal exposure in Japanese Macaques after the Fukushima Nuclear Power Plant accident. In: Fukumoto M (ed) Low-dose radiation effects on animals and ecosystems. Springer Singapore, Singapore, pp 179–193
10. MEXT (in Japanese). https://www.rcnp.osaka-u.ac.jp/dojo/. Accessed on 14 Oct 2025
11. Urakami C, Kurosaka D, Tamada K et al (2012) Lovastatin alters TGF-beta-induced epithelial-mesenchymal transition in porcine lens epithelial cells. Curr Eye Res 37:479–485. https://doi.org/10.3109/02713683.2012.665121
12. Nakashima E, Neriishi K, Minamoto A (2006) A reanalysis of atomic−bomb cataract data, 2000–2002: a threshold analysis. Health Phys 90:154–160. https://doi.org/10.1097/01.hp.0000175442.03596.63
13. Neriishi K, Nakashima E, Minamoto A et al (2007) Postoperative cataract cases among atomic bomb survivors: radiation dose response and threshold. Radiat Res 168:404–408. https://doi.org/10.1667/RR0928.1
14. Worgul BV, Kundiyev YI, Sergiyenko NM et al (2007) Cataracts among Chernobyl clean-up workers: implications regarding permissible eye exposures. Radiat Res 167:233–243. https://doi.org/10.1667/rr0298.1
15. Wolf N, Pendergrass W, Singh N et al (2008) Radiation cataracts: mechanisms involved in their long delayed occurrence but then rapid progression. Mol Vis 14:274–285
16. Hayashida T, Tsubota K, Sasaki H (2018) Situation of radiation protection at Fukushima Daiichi Nuclear Power Station – based on radiation protection of the lens of the eye – [Japanese]. J Jpn Soc Cataract Res 30:54–56. https://doi.org/10.14938/cataract.10-009

Chapter 11
Estimation of Iodine-131 Thyroid Dose Using Iodine-129 Concentration and Thyroid Lesions in Macaques Affected by the Fukushima Daiichi Nuclear Power Plant Accident

Somei Ohtsuki, Satoru Endo, Masatoshi Suzuki, Kina Satoh, Hiroyuki Mishima, Toshihiko Suzuki, Kosei Yamada, Takumi Urayama, Tsuyoshi Kajimoto, Yasushi Kino, Miwa Uzuki, Hideaki Yamashiro, Takeshi Ohno, and Manabu Fukumoto

Abstract Epidemiological studies have reported an increase in childhood thyroid cancer due to milk and foods contaminated with Iodine-131 (^{131}I) from the Chernobyl (Chornobyl) Nuclear Power Plant (CNPP) accident. Despite successful

Authors Somei Ohtsuki and Satoru Endo have equally contributed to this chapter.

S. Ohtsuki
IMS Fujimi General Hospital, Fujimi City, Saitama, Japan

S. Endo · K. Yamada · T. Urayama · T. Kajimoto
Graduate School of Advanced Science and Engineering, Hiroshima University, Higashi-Hiroshima, Hiroshima, Japan

M. Suzuki · M. Fukumoto (✉)
International Research Institute of Disaster Science, Tohoku University, Sendai, Japan
e-mail: manabu.fukumoto.a8@tohoku.ac.jp

K. Satoh · T. Ohno
Faculty of Science, Gakushuin University, Tokyo, Japan

H. Mishima
School of Dental Medicine, Tsurumi University, Yokohama, Japan

T. Suzuki
Graduate School of Dentistry, Tohoku University, Sendai, Japan

Y. Kino
Faculty of Science and Graduate School of Science, Tohoku University, Sendai, Japan

M. Uzuki
School of Health Sciences, Fukushima Medical University, Fukushima, Japan

H. Yamashiro
Faculty of Agriculture, Niigata University, Niigata, Japan

M. Fukumoto (ed.), *Low-Dose Radiation Effects on Animals and Ecosystems II*,
https://doi.org/10.1007/978-981-95-5559-8_11

food control measures implemented immediately after the Fukushima Daiichi Nuclear Power Plant (FNPP) accident, it has become clear that the incidence of thyroid cancer among young people in Fukushima Prefecture is much higher than previously thought. Because ^{131}I has a short half-life and the number of thyroid monitoring devices was insufficient at the time of the accident, only a very limited number of Fukushima residents had their thyroid ^{131}I measured immediately after the accident. Therefore, we attempted to reconstruct ^{131}I concentration in macaque thyroid glands from the ^{129}I concentration measured by triple quadrupole inductively coupled plasma mass spectrometry (ICP-MS). By plotting the decrease of ^{129}I concentration over time, we were able to estimate the ^{131}I concentration in the thyroid gland of affected wild Japanese macaques at the time of the FNPP accident. The thyroid doses of macaques born before the FNPP accident due to ^{131}I were estimated to be between 34 and 1,145 (median: 173) mGy. In comparison, the doses from ^{129}I were three orders of magnitude lower than from ^{131}I and were negligible. Four out of 449 macaques were found to have microscopic thyroid lesions. None of the cases were diagnosed as malignant. One macaque had not yet been born at the time of the accident and therefore clearly had no exposure to ^{131}I, while the other three macaques were already adults at that time. Furthermore, no relationship was found with the level of exposure to radioactive cesium (^{134}Cs + ^{137}Cs). More than 10 years after the FNPP accident, we were able to reconstruct the thyroid dose from ^{131}I derived, using ^{129}I concentration in the thyroid as a surrogate indicator, and no obvious radiation-related thyroid lesions were observed in the affected macaques examined.

Keywords FNPP accident · Macaque · Thyroid · The Fukushima Health Management Survey · iodine-129 (^{129}I) · iodine-131 (^{131}I) · cesium-134 (^{134}Cs) · cesium-137 (^{137}Cs) · Triple quadrupole inductively coupled plasma mass spectrometry (ICP-MS)

11.1 Introduction

The thyroid gland is known to be highly sensitive to the carcinogenic effect of radiation exposure during childhood and adolescence. Epidemiological studies of atomic bomb survivors have shown that the risk of developing thyroid cancer decreases rapidly with increasing age at the time of exposure, and there is little evidence of an increase in people exposed after the age of 20 [1]. Iodine is an essential component of thyroid hormones, which control metabolism, growth, and many other bodily functions. Therefore, because iodine has a high affinity for the thyroid gland, ingested radioactive iodine accumulates in the thyroid, resulting in localized radiation exposure. Iodine-131 (^{131}I) is the radionuclide of greatest concern for radiation hazards in nuclear accidens due to its high fission yield, high volatility, and high emission of moderately high-energy β and γ rays. The incidence of pediatric thyroid cancer in the heavily contaminated areas increased about 4–5 years after the Chernobyl (Chornobyl) Nuclear Power Plant (CNPP) accident. The increase of thyroid cancer is generally accepted to be attributable to the consumption of milk and foods contaminated with ^{131}I, and is the only confirmed health effect of radiation from the CNPP accident on the general population [2]. A large amount of radioactive iodine was released into the environment following the Fukushima Daiichi Nuclear Power Plant (FNPP) accident in 2011. Immediately after the accident, food control measures were implemented, including the disposal of all contaminated raw milk [3]. Based on these facts, 7 months after the FNPP accident, the Fukushima Health Management Survey, including ultrasound examinations of the thyroid gland, was initiated [4]. A particularly striking finding from the survey is that the incidence of thyroid cancer among people 18 years or younger at the time of the accident was 100 times higher than the previously thought rate of about 2 cases per million among Japanese people aged 19 or younger [5]. This condition, referred to as "Fukushima thyroid cancer," has ignited vigorous discussions about the causal relationship with direct radiation exposure from the accident. While individual radiation doses have been estimated from behavioral surveys [6], internal thyroid dose from ^{131}I could not be directly measured at the time of the accident, due to its short half-life of 8.0 days and the limited availability of measurement equipment. One of the fission products, [129]I, has a very long half-life of about 15.7 million years and has the same chemical properties as [131]I. In addition, a study on the deposition of radioactive materials dispersed by the FNPP accident on soil has reported that the ^{131}I/[129]I ratio is almost similar regardless of the sampling site [7]. We, therefore, hypothesized that [129]I could serve as a surrogate for reconstructing the thyroid dose from [131]I. Japanese macaques, non-human primates closely related to humans, are culled each year by local authorities to control their population size. The macaques living in areas affected by the FNPP accident have been continually exposed to radiation both externally from ontaminated soil and internally through the consumption of food contaminated with radionuclides, particularly radioactive cesium ([134]Cs and ^{137}Cs) [8]. They are, therefore, ideal for assessing the effects of long-term exposure to low-dose-rate radiation in humans. In this study, by measuring [129]I concentration in the thyroid gland and radioactive Cs concentration in the body of wild Japanese macaques, we estimated the thyroid radiation dose, and assessed thyroid histopathology in relation to the estimated dose.

11.2 Materials and Methods

In accordance with the Act on the Protection and Management of Wildlife, and the Optimization of Hunting, the population of Japanese macaques is being controlled to prevent damage to crops. Macaques were captured using box traps and euthanized by licensed hunters at the request of each local government. Japanese macaques inhabiting the areas of this study were not listed as endangered species in the Red List revised by the Ministry of the Environment in 2020. This entire study was approved by the Institutional Animal Care and Use Committee of the Center for Laboratory Animal Research, Tohoku University. All experiments were performed in accordance with relevant guidelines and regulations. The macaques analyzed in this study were captured from May 2013 to January 2019. Thyroid histopathological examination was performed on 449 macaques captured in Fukushima Prefecture (affected group). Of these, 44 macaques were evaluated for radiation doses (25 born before the FNPP accident and 19 born after the accident). The group unaffected by the FNPP accident (control) consisted of five macaques from Niigata Prefecture, located just west of Fukushima Prefecture, separated by mountain ranges. Macaque age was estimated from cementum increment lines on the demineralized tooth specimen [9,10].

11.2.1 Iodine Measurement

The organ samples were stored in a deep freezer at −80 °C until use. Pretreatment of the thawed samples was performed according to the pyrohydrolysis method. Briefly, 0.01 g of the lyophilized thyroid gland tissue was placed in a quartz glass tube and heated at 1,000 °C in the tube oven for 30 min under a flow of oxygen containing water vapor, and the vaporized iodine was trapped as much as possible in 10 ml of 0.5% tetramethylammonium hydroxide (TMAH) and 0.1% Na_2SO_3 solution. The sample solution was subjected to measurements of $^{129}I/^{127}I$ by a triple quadrupole inductively coupled plasma–octopole reaction system–quadrupole mass spectrometer (ICP-ORS-QMS) (Agilent 7700x, Agilent Technologies Inc., Santa Clara). Details of the instrument and the operating parameters are described previously [11].

11.2.2 ^{129}I Concentration in the Thyroid Gland

The ^{129}I concentration in the thyroid gland was determined from the total iodine (^{127}I + ^{129}I)concentration, ρ_I, in the thyroid gland and the $^{129}I/^{127}I$ atomic ratio determined by ICP-ORS-QMS. The ^{129}I concentration, that is, the number of ^{129}I atoms per gram of thyroid (^{129}I (atom/g-thyroid)) was obtained as follows:

$$\rho_I\left(g\,/\,g-\text{thyroid}\right)=\left[\,^{129}I\left(g\,/\,g-\text{thyroid}\right)+\,^{127}I\left(g\,/\,g-\text{thyroid}\right)\right] \quad (11.1)$$

$$
\begin{aligned}
^{127}I&\left(g\,/\,g-\text{thyroid}\right)\\
&=\rho_I\left(g\,/\,g-\text{thyroid}\right)/\left[1+\left(^{129}I\left(g\,/\,g-\text{thyroid}\right)/^{127}I\left(g\,/\,g-\text{thyroid}\right)\right)\right]\\
&=\rho_I\,/\left[1+\left(^{129}I\left(\text{atom}\,/\,g-\text{thyroid}\right)\right)/^{127}I\left(\text{atom}\,/\,g-\text{thyoroid}\right)\times\left(129\,/\,127\right)\right]\\
&=\rho_I\,/\left[1+\left(^{129}I\left(\text{atom}\right)/^{127}I\left(\text{atom}\right)\times\left(129\,/\,127\right)\right)\right]
\end{aligned}
\quad (11.2)
$$

$$^{127}I\left(\text{atom}\,/\,g-\text{thyroid}\right)=\,^{127}I\left(g\,/\,g-\text{thyroid}\right)\times N_A\,/\,127 \quad (11.3)$$

$$^{129}\mathrm{I}\left(\mathrm{atom}\,/\,g-\mathrm{thyroid}\right)=\left(^{129}\mathrm{I}\,/^{127}\mathrm{I}\right)\times^{127}\mathrm{I}\left(\mathrm{atom}\,/\,g-\mathrm{thyroid}\right) \qquad (11.4)$$

where (g/g-thyroid) represents the weight of iodine (g) per g of thyroid. N_A is Avogadro's number. To estimate $^{129}\mathrm{I}$ attributed to the FNPP accident, the $^{129}\mathrm{I}$ atomic concentration of the affected macaque was subtracted by the averaged $^{129}\mathrm{I}$ atomic concentration of the control samples using the decay constant of $^{129}\mathrm{I}$: $\lambda_{129} = 1.3990 \times 10^{-15}$ (s^{-1}). The radioactivity concentration of $^{129}\mathrm{I}$ per g of thyroid can be obtained by

$$^{129}\mathrm{I}\left(Bq\,/\,g-\mathrm{thyroid}\right)=\lambda_{129}[\left(^{129}\mathrm{I}\left(\mathrm{atom}\,/\,g-\mathrm{thyroid}\right)\right)_{\mathrm{affected}}$$
$$-\left(^{129}\mathrm{I}\left(\mathrm{atom}\,/\,g-\mathrm{thyroid}\right)\right)_{\mathrm{control}}] \qquad (11.5)$$

where subscripts "affected" and "control" refer to the measured value in an affected macaque and the mean thyroid value of control macaques, respectively.

11.2.3 Estimation of Environmental Decay Constant for ^{129}I

The highly sensitive triple quadrupole ICP-MS used in this study was able to measure $^{129}\mathrm{I}$ concentration with an accuracy comparable to that of accelerator mass spectrometry (AMS), and 100 mg wet weight of thyroid tissue from macaques affected by the FNPP accident was sufficient for measurement.

The effective half-life of $^{129}\mathrm{I}$ in the macaque thyroid gland was calculated by plotting the $^{129}\mathrm{I}/^{127}\mathrm{I}$ ratio from the day of maximum radioactive material release from the FNPP accident (March 15, 2011) to the date of collection for each individual, according to the region where they were captured. In this study, we assumed that environmental iodine was continuously ingested orally and that environmental $^{129}\mathrm{I}$ concentration decreased with the environmental half-life, which includes the physical half-life and attenuation due to environmental factors including weathering. Therefore, in this study, to calculate the thyroid radiation dose, we defined the environmental decay constant λ_{env} in the thyroid by fitting the decline in thyroid radioactivity concentration as a function of days elapsed from the accident to sampling.

11.2.4 Thyroid Dose Estimation from ^{129}I and ^{131}I

Under the above assumptions, the ingested $^{129}\mathrm{I}$ changes as $A_0 e^{-\lambda_{\mathrm{env}}^{129}t}$ where A_0 is the initial intake of $^{129}\mathrm{I}$, $\lambda_{\mathrm{env}}^{129}$ is the environmental decay constant of $^{129}\mathrm{I}$, and $\lambda_{\mathrm{eff}}^{129}$ is the effective decay constant of $^{129}\mathrm{I}$. The effective decay constant $\lambda_{\mathrm{eff}}^{129}$ in this study was defined as $\ln(2)/(1/T_{\mathrm{biol}} + 1/T_{\mathrm{env}})$ using the biological half-life T_{biol} and the environmental half-life T_{env}. Since there are no data on the biological half-life of iodine in macaques, we decided to use human values for this study. Iodine is a mineral found in abundance in seaweed and seafoods, and the biological half-life of iodine is known to be short in Japanese people who consume large amounts of seaweed. In contrast, Westerners tend to have a longer biological half-life for iodine. Because macaques living in Fukushima Prefecture consume foods low in iodine, the biological half-life of iodine is estimated to be relatively long. Therefore, we assumed that the biological half-life of iodine in macaques was 138 days, the same as the longest value for humans [12].

The rate of change of thyroid ^{129}I concentration(A_{129}) is given by follows,

$$\frac{dA_{129}}{dt} = -\lambda_{\text{eff}}^{129} A_{129} + A_0 e^{-\lambda_{\text{env}}^{129} t} \tag{11.6}$$

The solution of this differential equation with the initial condition of $A_{129}(t=0)=0$ is expressed by

$$A_{129}(t) = \frac{A_0}{\lambda_{\text{eff}}^{129} - \lambda_{\text{env}}^{129}} \left[e^{-\lambda_{\text{env}}^{129} t} - e^{-\lambda_{\text{eff}}^{129} t} \right] \tag{11.7}$$

The time course of ^{129}I concentration, $A_{129}(t)$, after a long period of time longer than the biological half-life, almost depends on $e^{-\lambda_{\text{env}}^{129} t}$, which is consistent with the measured data in thyroid. We determined thyroid ^{131}I concentration from the ^{129}I radioactivity concentration using the $(^{131}\text{I}/^{129}\text{I})_{t=0}$ radioactivity ratio in soil as $A_0{}^{131}$ (Bq/g) $= A_0{}^{\text{meas}}$ (Bq/g) $(^{131}\text{I}/^{129}\text{I})_{t=0}$. The $(^{131}\text{I}/^{129}\text{I})_{t=0}$ radioactivity ratio on March 15, 2011, was set to 2.44×10^8, corrected from the reported value of 9.37×10^3 on June 14, 2011 [7]. Thyroid doses D_{131} and D_{129} for ^{131}I and ^{129}I, respectively, are estimated by

$$D_{131} = \eta_{131} \int_{2011/3/15\,\text{or date of birth}}^{\text{sampling date}} A_{131}(t)\,dt$$

$$= \eta_{131} \int_{2011/3/15\,\text{or date of birth}}^{\text{sampling date}} \left(\frac{^{131}\text{I}}{^{129}\text{I}}\right)_{t=0} \frac{A_0^{\text{meas}}}{\lambda_{\text{eff}}^{131} - \lambda_{\text{phy}}^{131}} \left[e^{-\lambda_{\text{phy}}^{131} t} - e^{-\lambda_{\text{eff}}^{131} t} \right] dt \tag{11.8}$$

$$D_{129} = \eta_{129} \int_{2011/3/15\,\text{or date of birth}}^{\text{sampling date}} A_{129}(t)\,dt$$

$$= \eta_{129} \int_{2011/3/15\,\text{or date of birth}}^{\text{sampling date}} \frac{A_0^{\text{meas}}}{\lambda_{\text{eff}}^{129} - \lambda_{\text{env}}^{129}} \left[e^{-\lambda_{\text{env}}^{129} t} - e^{-\lambda_{\text{eff}}^{129} t} \right] dt \tag{11.9}$$

where η_i ($i = 131$ or 129) denotes the conversion factor from the radioactivity concentration (Bq/kg) of ^{131}I or ^{129}I to thyroid dose, $\lambda_{\text{phy}}^{131}$ is the physical decay constant of ^{131}I (0.8641655 d^{-1}), $\lambda_{\text{env}}^{129}$ is the environmental decay constant of ^{129}I discussed in the Results section, and $\lambda_{\mathrm{eff}}^{i}$ (i = 131 or 129) are the effective decay constants of ^{131}I (0.9143936 day^{-1}) or ^{129}I (0.0072464 day^{-1}). The conversion coefficient of ^{131}I and ^{129}I were taken from Ref. [13].

11.2.5 Thyroid Dose Estimation from Radioactive Cs

Since radioactive Cs has also contributed to the thyroid dose, the thyroid dose attributable to radioactive Cs was estimated from its concentration in the femoral muscle measured as previously described [14]. Using the effective decay constant $\lambda_{\mathrm{eff}}^{i}$ (i = ^{134}Cs or ^{137}Cs) calculated from the environmental half-lives [13] for Namie, Kashima, and Odaka, the measured ^{137}Cs concentration (Bq/kg) in femoral muscle was decay-corrected to March 15, 2011. Since no effective decay constant $\lambda_{\mathrm{eff}}^{i}$ for Iitate was available, the same value as that for Namie was used. Assuming that radioactive Cs concentration in the thyroid gland $A_{i}^{h}(t)$ is 1/3 that in femoral muscle [14] and that the concentration in the body tissue $A_{i}^{t}(t)$ to the same as that in femoral muscle, radioactive Cs concentrations in the thyroid gland and in the body tissue were calculated. For this estimation, ^{134}Cs concentration was equal to ^{137}Cs concentration on March 15, 2011. Using femoral muscle and thyroid radioactivity concentrations calculated from the measurements as $A_{i}^{t}(t)$ and $A_{i}^{h}(t)$, respectively, and conversion coefficients η_{i}^{t} (body tissue to thyroid) and η_{i}^{h} (thyroid to thyroid), (i = ^{134}Cs or ^{137}Cs) [14], the cumulative thyroid dose from ^{134}Cs or ^{137}Cs is expressed by

$$
\begin{aligned}
D_{i} &= \int_{\text{sampling date}}^{\text{2011/3/15 or date of birth}} \eta_{i}^{t} A_{i}^{t}(t) + \eta_{i}^{h} A_{i}^{h}(t)\, dt \\[2mm]
&= \int_{\text{sampling date}}^{\text{2011/3/15 or date of birth}} \frac{\eta_{i}^{t} A_{i}^{\text{meas},t}(0) + \eta_{i}^{h} A_{i}^{\text{meas},h}(0)}{\lambda_{\mathrm{eff}}^{i} - \lambda_{\mathrm{env}}^{i}} \left[e^{-\lambda_{\mathrm{env}}^{i} t} - e^{-\lambda_{\mathrm{eff}}^{i} t} \right] dt \\[2mm]
&\approx \int_{\text{sampling date}}^{\text{2011/3/15 or date of birth}} \frac{\eta_{i}^{t} A_{i}^{\text{meas},t}(0) + \eta_{i}^{h} A_{i}^{\text{meas},h}(0)}{\lambda_{\mathrm{eff}}^{i}} \left[e^{-\lambda_{\mathrm{env}}^{i} t} \right] d \quad \left(i = ^{137}\text{Cs or } ^{134}\text{Cs} \right)
\end{aligned}
\tag{11.10}
$$

11.3 Histological Examination

During dissection, care was taken to select an area of the thyroid gland that appeared slightly elevated above the surrounding tissue. Otherwise, sections were cut so as to maximize the cross-sectional area. After fixing in 10% neutralized formalin, histological sections were prepared according to the standard procedure and observed under a microscope after hematoxylin and eosin staining.

11.4   Results

11.4.1   Environmental Half-Life

The ^{129}I/^{127}I elemental concentration ratio in the thyroid gland of the affected macaques even those born after the FNPP accident (3.5×10^{-8}–6.8×10^{-7}) was significantly higher than that of the control group (5.6×10^{-9}–1.5×10^{-8}), indicating that they have been continuously ingesting ^{129}I released from the FNPP accident. The temporal changes of ^{129}I concentration in the thyroid gland of macaques are shown in Fig. 11.1. Since ^{131}I decays to 0.56% of its original amount within 2 months, its concentration in macaques born more than a few months after the accident was expected to be negligible. Therefore, thyroid doses from radioactive iodine in macaques born more than a few months after the accident were calculated for ^{129}I only. The data of the ^{129}I/^{127}I ratio were fitted using an exponential function to estimate the environmental half-life. Thyroid ^{129}I concentration declined slowly

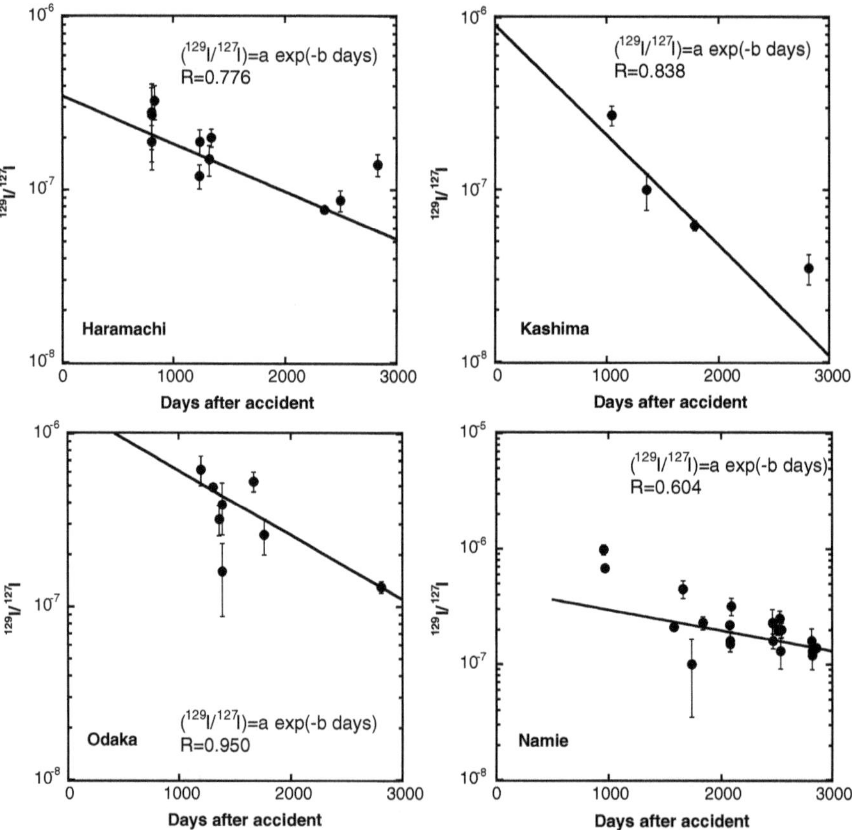

Fig. 11.1 Temporal change of the ^{129}I/^{127}I concentration ratio in the macaque thyroid gland since March 15, 2011. The plot is stratified by administrative unit (ward of city, town, and village).

Table 11.1 Estimated half-life of thyroid ^{129}I concentration by administrative unit.

	Half-life (days)	Error (days)
Namie	1,690	178
Kashima	471	68
Odaka	811	55
Haramachi	1,091	109

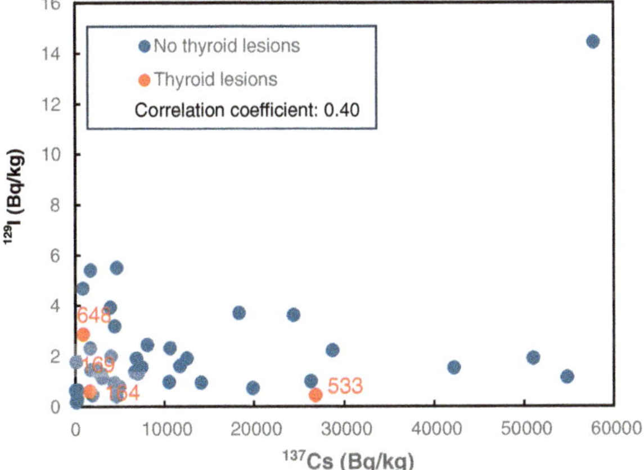

Fig. 11.2 Correlation between ^{137}Cs and ^{129}I concentrations in the thyroid glands of macaques. Red circles: macaques with the thyroid lesion; blue ccircles: those without; numbers; individual IDs.

over time, with the estimated half-life of 471 to 1,690 days, varying among municipalities (Table 11.1).

Since the inventory at the time of the accident was constant, we plotted radioactivity concentrations of ^{137}Cs and ^{129}I for each macaque to see if there was any relationship; however, no correlation was found between them (Fig. 11.2).

11.4.2   Thyroid Dose

The estimated thyroid doses resulting from the ingestion of radioactive iodine and cesium are summarized in Table 11.2. The radiation dose from ^{129}I was less than 1/1,000 of that from ^{131}I, indicating that its effects are considered negligible. The estimated thyroid doses due to ^{131}I ranged from 34 to 1,145 mGy (median: 173 mGy) for macaques born before the accident.

Figure 11.3a shows the thyroid doses from ^{137}Cs and ^{131}I in macaques born before the accident. In 19 out of the 23 macaques, thyroid doses were above 100 mGy, with a maximum of 1,145 mGy from ^{131}I, while those in four macaques were below 100 mGy from ^{131}I. There was no correlation between the doses from ^{137}Cs, which has a relatively long half-life, and those from ^{131}I. The thyroid doses from ^{137}Cs and

Table 11.2 Summary of ages, duration, and the estimated doses of macaques by ^{131}I, [129]I, and [134+137]Cs.

Macaques born			Location				Iitate	Total
			Namie Town	Minamisoma City			Village	
				Kashima	Odaka	Haramachi		
Before the accicdent								
No		M/F (total)	5/1 (6)	1/2 (3)	5/2 (7)	4/4 (8)	1/0 (1)	16/9 (25)
Age (years old)		Min, max (median)	5.5 – 18.5 (13)	7.5 – 18.5 (14)	4.5 – 9.5 (6.5)	2.5 – 22.5 (8.5)	20.5	2.5 – 22.5 (7.5)
Duration (days)			958 – 2,089 (1786)	1,046 – 1,784 (1354)	1,200 – 1,765 (1,395)	804 –3,634 (1,033.5)	1,351	804 – 3,634 (1,354)
Thyroid dose (Gy)	[131]I ($\times 10^{-3}$)		34 – 853 (142)	173 – 453 (362)	103 – 877 (363)	64 – 1,145 (139)	58.2	34 – 1,145 (173)
	[129]I ($\times 10^{-6}$)		0.72 – 10.41(3.02)	1.50 – 3.46 (3.45)	1.34 – 12.95 (4.73)	0.84 – 28.46 (1.64)	1.0	0.72 – 28.46 (2.81)
	[134+137]Cs		41.8 – 576.7 (195.3)	2.2 – 43.4 (11.3)	1.1 – 36.1 (21.5)	15.0 – 136.4 (26.1)	12.2	1.1 – 576.7 (31.3)
After the accicdent								
No		M/F (total)	7/6 (13)	0/1 (1)	1/0 (1)	2/2 (4)	0/0 (0)	10/9 (19)
Age (years old)		Min, max (median)	1.2 – 6.3 (2.7)	2.7	2.7	2 – 5.5 (2.25)		1.2 – 6.3 (2.7)
Duration (days)			438 – 2,301 (986)	986	986	731 – 2,006 (822)		438 – 2,301 (986)
Thyroid dose (Gy)	[131]I ($\times 10^{-3}$)		–	–	–	–	–	–
	[129]I ($\times 10^{-6}$)		0.24 – 4.08 (1.15)	0.23	1.21	0.16 – 2.74 (1.16)		0.16 – 4.08 (1.15)
	[134+137]Cs		5.18 – 409.07 (52.75)	0.7	21.84	0.12 – 89.99 (16.43)		0.12 – 409.07 (27.00)

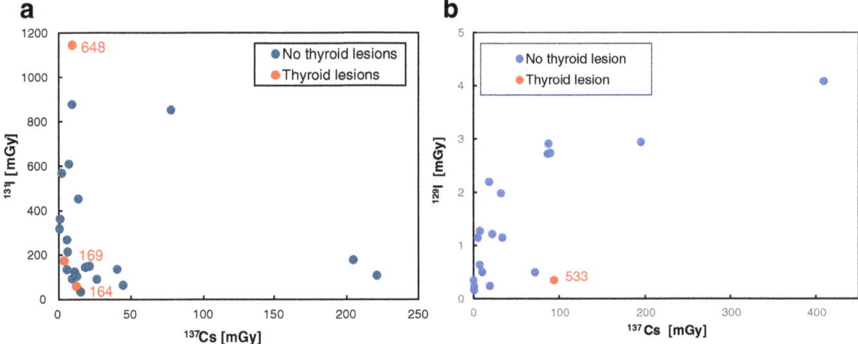

Fig. 11.3 (a) Correlation between thyroid doses from ^{137}Cs and ^{131}I in macaques born before the FNPP accident; (b) thyroid doses from ^{137}Cs and ^{129}I in macaques born after the accident. Red circles: macaques with the thyroid lesion; blue circles: those without; numbers: individual IDs.

^{129}I in macaques born after the accident is shown in Fig. 11.3b. The estimated thyroid doses from ^{129}I in all macaques were less than 4.1 µGy, and those from radioactive Cs exceeded 100 mGy only in two of the 19 macaques. These suggest that if significant changes were to be observed in the thyroid gland of macaques born before the accident, they would be related to ^{131}I exposure.

11.4.3 Thyroid Lesions

Of the 449 macaques whose thyroids were analyzed under a microscope, four showed epithelial lesions with high cell density, corresponding to the incidence of 0.89%. Macaques No.164 and 169 showed papillary growth, while No. 533 showed a luminal-like structure with blood vessels but no papillary structures. The histological feature of the lesion in macaque No. 648 was similar to that in No. 533, but both the vascular and epithelial structures were more dense than in No. 533. All lesions were small, less than 0.5 mm, and did not invade the surrounding tissue. In all of the lesions, cells were uniform in size and nuclear atypia was unremarkable. Furthermore, ground-glass nuclear appearance, characteristic of papillary carcinoma, was not observed (Fig. 11.4).

The location where each macaque was captured is shown in Fig. 11.5. The capture sites were located within approximately 10–35 km northwest to north-northwest of FNPP. No clear relationship was observed between the ^{129}I concentration in macaque thyroid glands and either the distance from FNPP or the ^{131}I deposited in soil. Although the number of macaques examined was small, no clear relationship was found between macaques with thyroid lesions and radiation dose or their location relative to FNPP. Thyroid doses in the macaques with thyroid lesion are shown in Table 11.3.

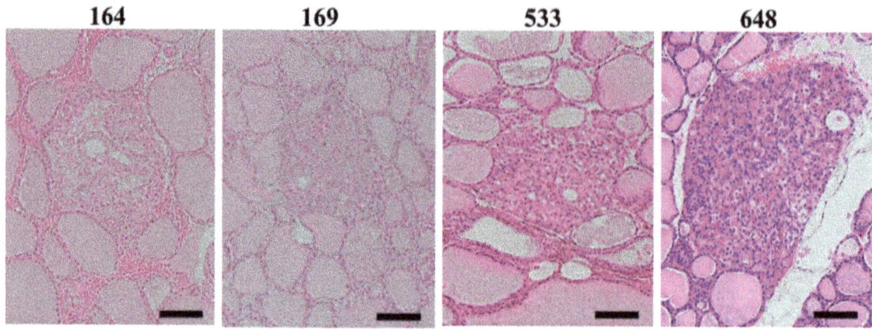

Fig. 11.4 Epithelial lesions found in the thyroid glands of macaques. Numbers: individual IDs; H&E staining.

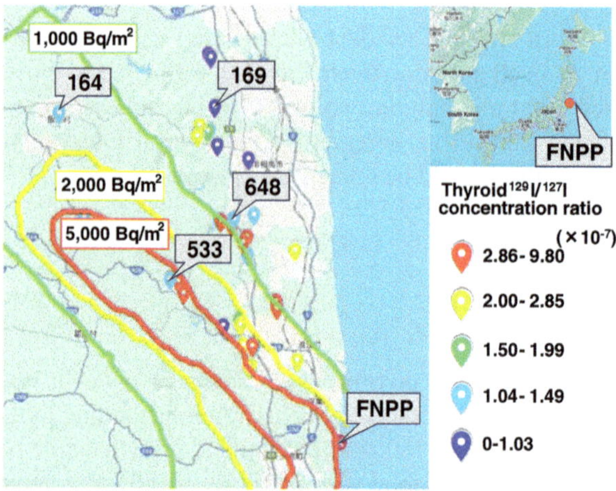

Fig. 11.5 Location of macaque capture sites and ^{131}I concentrations in soil. Marks: capture sites of individual macaques with color coding according to thyroid ^{129}I concentration; numbers: individual IDs with the thyroid lesion; contour: concentration of ^{131}I deposited in soil as of June 14, 2011. The figure of Ref. [22] was modified and traced onto Google Maps.

Table 11.3 Age, sex, and thyroid dose of macaques showing thyroid epithelial lesions.

Macaque No		164	169	533	648
Sex		M	M	F	M
Age (years)		20.5	15.5	2.7	15.5
Thyroid dose (mGy)	^{131}I	58.2	173.2	–	1,145.4
	$^{134+137}$Cs	12.2	24.8	94.0	20.4

11.5   Discussion

Using ^{129}I concentrations measured by accelerator mass spectrometry (AMS), the estimated thyroid doses from ^{131}I in cattle at two ranches in Okuma Town, where FNPP is located, have been reported to be 85 ± 48 mGy and 34 ± 4 mGy, respectively [15]. The mean thyroid dose of 305 ± 294 mGy (Haramachi: 269 ± 361 mGy, Kashima: 329 ± 143 mGy, Odaka: 423 ± 280 mGy, Namie: 242 ± 303 mGy) from ^{131}I in the macaques in this study was approximately threefold higher than that in the cattle, presumably because macaques are omnivorous whereas cattle are herbivorous. The biological half-life is estimated to be 138 days in humans but is unknown in macaques and cattle. Furthermore, age estimation in wild animals based on teeth lacks precision at the day level. Consequently, these factors may introduce significant uncertainty into dose evaluation.

The Fukushima Health Management Survey has revealed that the incidence of thyroid cancer is much higher than previously known. However, whether the large number of morbidity cases is attributable to radioactive ^{131}I dispersed by the FNPP accident is a major social problem that has not yet been conclusively determined. Recently, because of the improved quality of ultrasound imaging, thyroid nodules smaller than 10 mm are detected more frequently than larger nodules. An epidemiological study of Hiroshima and Nagasaki atomic-bomb survivors (Hibakusha) also revealed that the prevalence of thyroid nodules smaller than 10 mm in diameter is higher than that of large nodules greater than 10 mm. In Hibakusha, thyroid nodules with a diameter of 10 mm or more are known to be significantly associated with thyroid radiation dose, whereas nodules smaller than 10 mm in diameter are not [16]. In this study, thyroid lesions in macaques were detected at a fairly high frequency. However, the lesions found in this study were all microscopic, less than 0.6 mm in diameter, and could not be diagnosed as cancer. Macaque thyroid glands are small, based on our experience, weighing about one-eighth of those of humans per unit body weight. Therefore, similar lesions in humans may be larger than those identified in this study, however, it remains unclear whether such lesions would be detectable by ultrasonography. Careful observation during our dissections has, so far, not revealed any macaques exhibiting thyroid enlargement. Therefore, the microscopic sections were obtained almost randomly, and it is highly likely that the lesions found in this study would be observed more frequently if serial sections were performed on the thyroid glands of all macaques. Macaque No. 533, which had the thyroid lesion, was born 7 years after the accident, making exposure to ^{131}I extremely unlikely. Since male macaques are considered to reach sexual maturity by around 9 years of age and females by around 6 years, it can be assumed that the remaining three macaques (No. 164, 169, and 648) with thyroid lesions in this study were considered to have reached sufficient maturity at the time of the accident. Considering that radiation-induced thyroid cancer is characteristic of young people, it is unlikely that the thyroid lesions found in this study are related to radiation. It is assumed that there are some thyroid lesions in humans that do not grow larger [17], which could be supported by the lesions found in this study.

Immediately after the FNPP accident, measurements of ^{131}I deposited in the thyroid of Fukushima residents were conducted. However, only a limited people were examined and several approaches were devised to estimate thyroid exposure doses from [131]I. Using [134]Cs measured whole-body counters, the most conservative equivalent thyroid dose was calculated based on the ^{131}I/[134]Cs activity ratio, resulting in an estimated maximum equivalent thyroid dose of 18 mSv [18]. Thyroid ^{131}I concentration was measured with a scintillation survey meter placed on the neck, and the maximum thyroid doses for children and adults were estimated to be 23 mSv and 33 mSv, respectively, with mean values ranging from 3.5 to 4.2 mSv [19]. Based on urine samples, equivalent doses to the thyroid gland were estimated to be in the range of 27–66 mSv, albeit for five residents 37 km northwest of FNPP [20]. Compared with these human data, thyroid doses in the present study for macaques were much higher. There are two possible processes for the uptake of radioactive iodine: inhalation and ingestion. For the people surveyed, the main cause of thyroid exposure is thought to be ^{131}I, inhaled only once over a short period of time as a component of the radioactive plume released due to the accident. In this study, radiation dose was estimated from the dynamics of the concentration of radioactive iodine in the thyroid gland released by the accident. For single inhalation, the physical half-life of [129]I is so long that the effective half-life of [129]I in the thyroid gland is considered to be approximately equal to the biological half-life of iodine in humans of 80 to 138 days [12]. However, [129]I concentration in the thyroid gland of macaques decreased slowly with half-lives longer than 400 days, which is thought to be due to continuous oral ingestion of [129]I from the contaminated environment. Unlike people in Fukushima Prefecture, where food radiation was controlled, wild macaques have been outside throughout the day and continued to eat contaminated foods in the environment. Thus, it is quite reasonable that the thyroid dose in macaques could be much higher than that of people followed by the Fukushima Health Management Survey. Furthermore, we confirmed that it was not possible to estimate ^{131}I concentration from ^{137}Cs concentration in the body or the environment long after the accident.

We report in the present study that minute thyroid lesions that would not grow larger with age were found with a certain frequency in wild macaques affected by the FNPP accident. It will be necessary to continue field research to determine whether these lesions will grow large enough to be detected by detailed thyroid examinations. We are continuing to accumulate samples and to make careful observations. From the results of this study on macaques, it is suggested that the high incidence of thyroid cancer in the Fukushima survey is mainly attributed to vigilant observation with high sensitivity of ultrasound imaging. Traditionally, AMS-based analytical methods have been used to measure trace amounts of [129]I. However, those methods have various issues such as the lack of general accessibility due to the large size of the equipment, the long measurement time per sample, and the complicated preprocessing of samples needed [21]. In this study, we could measure [129]I concentration in the macaque thyroid gland using a benchtop high-sensitivity ICP-MS, which clearly indicates that [129]I in human urine can be measured in a similar manner. In the event of a future nuclear accident, it may be possible to assess thyroid doses by measuring ^{129}I concentrations in urine and in resected thyroid tumors, even if it is too late to measure ^{131}I due to the passage of time.

11.6 Conclusions

Using highly sensitive ICP-MS, ^{129}I concentration was successfully measured in a small amount of the thyroid tissue from Japanese macaques in Fukushima Prefecture, and ^{131}I concentration in the thyroid was further reconstructed. Epithelial microlesions were frequently observed in the macaque thyroid gland regardless of radiation dose.

Acknowledgments This work was supported by for Scientific Research from JSPS (KAKENHI 20K12173, 23K11429), Nuclear Energy S & T and Human Resource Development Project through concentrating wisdom Grant Number JPJA19B19207322. We greatly appreciate Mr. Abiru, Kyoto University, for preparing the sections of the tooth specimen.

References

1. Furukawa K, Preston D, Funamoto S et al (2013) Long-term trend of thyroid cancer risk among Japanese atomic-bomb survivors: 60 years after exposure. Int J Cancer 132:1222–1226. https://doi.org/10.1002/ijc.27749
2. Sources and effects of ionizing radiation (2010) UNSCEAR 2008 report. https://www.unscear.org/unscear/uploads/documents/unscear-reports/UNSCEAR_2008_Report_Vol.I-CORR.pdf
3. Emergency Notice (March 17, 2011) from the Ministry of Health, Labour and Welfare of Japan. in Japanese Emergency (In Japanese). https://www.mhlw.go.jp/stf/houdou/2r985200000015lgh-img/2r98520000016mf2.pdf. Accessed on 21 Aug 2025
4. Radiation Medical Science Center, The Fukushima Health Management Survey. https://fhms.jp/en/fhms/. Accessed on 8 Aug 2025
5. Sokawa Y (2024) Radiation-induced childhood thyroid cancer after the Fukushima Daiichi Nuclear Power Plant accident. Int J Environ Res Public Health 21:1162. https://doi.org/10.3390/ijerph21091162
6. Ohba T, Ishikawa T, Nagai H et al (2020) Reconstruction of residents' thyroid equivalent doses from internal radionuclides after the Fukushima Daiichi nuclear power station accident. Sci Rep 10:3639. https://doi.org/10.1038/s41598-020-60453-0
7. Muramatsu Y, Matsuzaki H, Toyama C et al (2015) Analysis of ^{129}I in the soils of Fukushima Prefecture: preliminary reconstruction of ^{131}I deposition related to the accident at Fukushima Daiichi Nuclear Power Plant (FDNPP). J Environ Radioact 139:344–350. https://doi.org/10.1016/j.jenvrad.2014.05.007
8. Urushihara Y, Suzuki T, Shimizu Y et al (2018) Haematological analysis of Japanese macaques (Macaca fuscata) in the area affected by the Fukushima Daiichi Nuclear Power Plant accident. Sci Rep 8:16748. https://doi.org/10.1038/s41598-018-35104-0
9. Klevezal GA (Miona MV and Oreshkin AV tr.) (1996) Recording structures of mammals: determination of age and reconstruction of life history. A.A. Balkema, Rotterdam, 53–61
10. Wada K, Ohtaishi N, Hachiya N et al (1978) Determination of age in the Japanese monkey from growth layers in the dental cementum, Primates, 19:775–784

11. Ohno T, Muramatsu Y, Shikamori Y et al (2013) Determination of ultratrace [129]I in soil samples by Triple Quadrupole ICP-MS and its application to Fukushima soil samples. J Anal At Spectrom 28:1283. https://doi.org/10.1039/c3ja50121c

12. International Commission on Radiological Protection (ICRP) (1959) ICRP (1960) Report of committee II on permissible dose for internal radiation. ICRP Publication 2. Pergamon Press, London. https://journals.sagepub.com/doi/pdf/10.1177/ANIA_OS_2_1

13. Urayama T, Takamura Y, Yamada K et al (2025) Evaluation of organ doses to Japanese macaques for internal dose using voxel phantom (Chapter 6 of this book)

14. Fukuda T, Kino Y, Abe, Y et al (2013) Distribution of artificial radionuclides in abandoned cattle in the evacuation zone of the Fukushima Daiichi nuclear power plant. PLoS One 8(1):e54312. https://doi.org/10.1371/journal.pone.0054312

15. Horikami D, Sayama N, Sasaki J et al (2022) The effect of exposure on cattle thyroid after the Fukushima Daiichi nuclear power plant accident. Sci Rep 12:21754. https://doi.org/10.1038/s41598-022-25269-0

16. Imaizumi M, Ohishi W, Nakashima E et al (2015) Association of radiation dose with prevalence of thyroid nodules among atomic bomb survivors exposed in childhood (2007–2011). JAMA Intern Med 175:228–236. https://doi.org/10.1001/jamainternmed.2014.6692

17. Welch HG, Black WC (2010) Overdiagnosis in Cancer. J Natl Cancer Inst 102:605–613. https://doi.org/10.1093/jnci/djq099

18. Hosoda M, Tokonami S, Akiba S et al (2013) Estimation of internal exposure of the thyroid to ^{131}I on the basis of [134]Cs accumulated in the body among evacuees of the Fukushima Daiichi Nuclear Power Station accident. Environ Int 61:73–76. https://doi.org/10.1016/j.envint.2013.09.013

19. Tokonami S, Hosoda M, Akiba S et al (2012) Thyroid doses for evacuees from the Fukushima nuclear accident. Sci Rep 2:507. https://doi.org/10.1038/srep00507

20. Kamada N, Saito O, Endo S et al (2012) Radiation doses among residents living 37 km northwest of the Fukushima Dai-ichi Nuclear Power Plant. J Environ Radioact 110:84–89. https://doi.org/10.1016/j.jenvrad.2012.02.007

21. Muramatsu Y, Takada Y, Matsuzaki H et al (2008) AMS analysis of [129]I in Japanese soil samples collected from background areas far from nuclear facilities. Quat Geochronol 3:291–297. https://doi.org/10.1016/j.quageo.2007.08.002

22. Fukushima Research and Engineering Institute, Japan Atomic Energy Agency. (In Japanese) https://fukushima.jaea.go.jp/fukushima/try/pdf/pdf05/04-1.pdf

Chapter 12
Effects of Chronic Radiation on the Testes of Wild Japanese Macaque (*Macaca fuscata*) After the Fukushima Daiichi Nuclear Power Plant Accident

Masamichi Kurohmaru, Toshiyasu Matsui, Ikki Mitsui, Yuki Ishii, Kanon Doi, Masatoshi Suzuki, Hideaki Yamashiro, and Manabu Fukumoto

Abstract Effects of radioactive cesium (Cs) derived from the Fukushima Daiichi Nuclear Power Plant (FNPP) accident on the testes of the wild Japanese macaque were investigated from a morphological viewpoint. Cesium-137 (^{137}Cs) concentration in the skeletal muscle of macaques in Fukushima Prefecture (affected group) ranged from 64.2 to 693.7 Bq/kg, which was clearly higher than that in Niigata Prefecture (unaffected group, 5.6 Bq/kg). Testicular tissue sections stained with hematoxylin and eosin were compared between the affected and unaffected groups under a light microscope. As a result, active spermatogenesis was clearly observed in the testicular tissues of both groups, and no definite differences were recognized. The distribution of vimentin in Sertoli cells was also similar in both groups. We then immunohistochemically determined the stage of the seminiferous epithelium and studied the proliferating and apoptotic spermatogenic cells and their specific cell types after type B spermatogonia at each stage in comparison between the affected and the unaffected groups. Consequently, proliferating spermatogenic cells of both macaque groups were type B spermatogonia at stages I–VI, preleptotene primary spermatocytes at stages VII and VIII, leptotene primary spermatocytes at stage IX, zygotene primary spermatocytes at stages X and XI, and pachytene primary spermatocytes at stages XII–VII. Meanwhile, apoptotic spermatogenic cells were type B spermatogonia at stages I–VI, preleptotene primary spermatocytes at stages VII and VIII, and leptotene primary spermatocytes at stage IX in both groups, though the

M. Kurohmaru (✉) · T. Matsui · I. Mitsui · Y. Ishii · K. Doi
Faculty of Veterinary Medicine, Okayama University of Science, Imabari, Japan

M. Suzuki · M. Fukumoto (✉)
International Research Institute of Disaster Science, Tohoku University, Sendai, Japan
e-mail: manabu.fukumoto.a8@tohoku.ac.jp

H. Yamashiro
Faculty of Agriculture, Niigata University, Niigata, Japan

M. Fukumoto (ed.), *Low-Dose Radiation Effects on Animals and Ecosystems II*,
https://doi.org/10.1007/978-981-95-5559-8_12

spermatogenic cells above were not always cleaved caspase-3-positive apoptotic cells. Thus, no concrete differences were confirmed between the affected and the unaffected macaque groups in either proliferating or apoptotic spermatogenic cells at any stage of the seminiferous epithelium or in any specific cell type, though ^{137}Cs concentrations in muscles were definitely different between these two groups. In conclusion, Japanese macaques currently inhabiting the area affected by radioactive materials from the FNPP accident possess normal activity of sperm reproduction.

Keywords Apoptosis · Caspase-3 · Japanese macaque · PCNA · Proliferating cell · Spermatocyte · Spermatogonium · Stage · Testis · Vimentin

12.1 Introduction

The activity of the seminiferous tubules is dynamic. The cyclical changes of spermatogenesis involve the slow movement of adjacent parts in a wave-like manner. The main cells that make up the seminiferous tubules are spermatogenic cells and the Sertoli cells that support them. Spermatogenic cells begin as (differentiating) type A spermatogonia derived from undifferentiated A spermatogonia, undergo mitotic cell divisions, and become type B spermatogonia. After the mitotic division of type B spermatogonia, primary spermatocytes appear. After chromosome duplication (preleptotene and leptotene stages), primary spermatocytes enter meiotic prophase, where they undergo pairing of homologous chromosomes (zygotene stage), crossover and partial exchange of chromosomes (pachytene stage), and separation of chromosomal pairs (diplotene stage) and then become secondary spermatocytes after the first meiotic division. Secondary spermatocytes quickly divide (the second meiotic division), and haploid cells (round spermatids) appear through these two meiotic divisions. The round spermatids become elongated, and when the maturation process is complete, they leave the epithelium of the seminiferous tubules as spermatozoa. During this maturation process, after a certain period has passed since the start of maturation, maturation of the next generation begins again (cycle of the seminiferous epithelium). In this way, 4–5 generations of spermatogenic cells coexist together in the seminiferous tubule. Since all germ cells mature at the same rate, the maturation stages of spermatogenic cells that coexist in a certain area of the seminiferous tubule are not random but show cell associations in a vertical line toward the lumen of the seminiferous tubule. The typical cell associations are called stages.

Meanwhile, it has been reported that large amounts of radioactive materials were released into the environment by the Fukushima Daiichi Nuclear Power Plant (FNPP) accident, which was caused by the tsunami following the Great East Japan Earthquake [1–3]. Radioactive cesium-137 (^{137}Cs), one of the main radionuclides released by the accident, has a long half-life of about 30 years. Therefore, even now, more than 14 years after the accident, there are concerns about the long-term effects on ecosystems, including various animals. It has long been widely accepted that the testes are sensitive to radiation [4–11]. Therefore, after the FNPP accident, the effect of radioactive materials on the testes of mammals such as large Japanese field mice [12–14], bulls [15], boars [16], inobuta (a hybrid of *Sus scrofa* and *Sus scrofa domesticus*) [16], and raccoons [17] have been investigated. Different from these terrestrial mammals, wild Japanese macaques (*Macaca fuscata*) are arboreal (not terrestrial), living on trees in forests, and, more importantly, are the only nonhuman wild primate mammals in Japan. The changes in ^{137}Cs concentration [18–21] and hematological findings [22, 23] have already been reported for Japanese macaques around FNPP. However, no such study has yet been carried out on the testes of wild Japanese macaques. In addition, the previous studies on testicular tissues mentioned above did not focus on specific cell types, such as preleptotene, leptotene, pachytene, or zygotene primary spermatocytes, nor on the appearance at the stages of the seminiferous epithelium of proliferating and/or apoptotic spermatogenic cells. In the present study, we measured ^{137}Cs concentration in organs of each macaque and subsequently investigated the effect of chronic low-dose-rate radiation on the testes from a morphological viewpoint. We then attempted to clarify the appearance of proliferating and apoptotic spermatogenic cells at each stage of the seminiferous epithelium and their specific cell types after type B spermatogonia in the groups affected and unaffected by the FNPP accident.

Vimentin, one of the intermediate filaments, is often used as a marker to identify Sertoli cells. In Sertoli cells, vimentin is distributed around the nucleus and further radiates toward the cell periphery, playing a role in positioning the nucleus and maintaining cell shape [24]. The intracellular distribution of vimentin is also one of the indicators of normal/abnormal Sertoli cells [25–27]. In the present study, we attempted to determine differences in vimentin distribution in Sertoli cells of the affected group compared to the unaffected control. We believe it is important to analyze the effects of chronic exposure to low-dose-rate radiation from ^{137}Cs on the testes of wild Japanese macaques living around FNPP.

12.2 Materials and Methods

12.2.1 Specimens

All wild Japanese macaques analyzed in the present study were euthanized by licensed hunters at the request of Fukushima [28] and Niigata Prefectures [29] for the control of their numbers. The method of capture and sacrifice was carried out in accordance with the guidelines published by the Primate Research Institute of Kyoto University [30]. All experiments were approved by the Institutional Animal

Table 12.1 Collection date, capture area, and ^{137}Cs concentration in each Japanese macaque. [137]Cs concentration of the macaque captured in Niigata Prefecture is quite low (5.6 Bq/kg). Those of the macaques captured in Fukushima Prefecture are relatively high and vary from 64.2 to 693.7 Bq/kg.

Collection date	Capture area		[137]Cs (Bq/kg)
2018.11.14	Niigata Pref.	Shibata City	5.6
2018.12.14	Fukushima Pref.	Minamisoma City	64.2
2019.11.06	Fukushima Pref.	Minamisoma City	75.0
2019.11.19	Fukushima Pref.	Minamisoma City	220.5
2019.11.25	Fukushima Pref.	Minamisoma City	693.7
2020.06.16	Fukushima Pref.	Minamisoma City	360.1
2020.06.25	Fukushima Pref.	Minamisoma City	195.3
2020.08.24	Fukushima Pref.	Minamisoma City	379.5
2020.09.24	Fukushima Pref.	Minamisoma City	642.8

Care and Use Committee of the Center for Laboratory Animal Research, Tohoku University (approved number: 2016 IDAC-043-1). The data (collection date, capture area, and ^{137}Cs concentration in the femoral muscles) on Japanese macaques used in this study are presented in Table 12.1. Four populations of Japanese macaques are known to inhabit Fukushima Prefecture, designated the Haramachi, Minami-Ou/Iide-minami, Shiga/Nikko, and Tadami populations [28]. The affected macaques in this study were from the Haramachi population, located in the area where soil deposition of ^{137}Cs was most severe after the FNPP accident [31]. The macaque captured in Niigata Prefecture (the unaffected area) served as the unaffected control.

12.2.2 *[137]Cs Concentration*

To measure the radioactivity of the samples, γ-ray spectrometry with three high-purity germanium detectors (ORTEC, Oak Ridge, TN) was used, as previously reported [16]. In cases where characteristic photopeaks greater than 3σ were recognized above the baseline in the spectrum, we identified a nuclide. Then, we calculated the concentration of the radionuclides (Bq/kg sample), based on the count rate from each sample. Efficiency curves for the detectors were obtained by using standard gel sources containing known amounts of [137]Cs.

12.2.3 *Hematoxylin and Eosin Staining*

The testes were fixed in a refrigerator with ½-diluted Bouin's fixative overnight, and 4-µm-thick sections for microscopic examination were prepared in the ordinary manner and stained with hematoxylin and eosin.

12.2.4 Vimentin Immunohistochemistry

Mouse monoclonal anti-vimentin antibody (diluted 1:300, clone LN-6; Sigma-Aldrich, St. Louis, MO) was used as the primary antibody. The sections were rinsed in phosphate-buffered saline (PBS; pH 7.4), blocked with a TNB blocking buffer (0.1 M Tris-HCl, 0.15 M NaCl, 0.5% Blocking Reagent, pH 7.5; PerkinElmer, Waltham, MA), and then treated with a tyramide signal amplification (TSA) biotin system kit (PerkinElmer, Waltham, MA). The sections were incubated with the primary antibody overnight at 4 °C and were incubated with the secondary antibody, biotinylated goat anti-mouse IgG (1:400, Vector Laboratories), for 1 h at room temperature, followed by the avidin–biotin peroxidase complex (VECTASTAIN ABC kit, Vector Laboratories) treatment. The immunoreaction was visualized with 0.05% 3,3′-diaminobenzidine (DAB) and H_2O_2 in PBS. The cell nuclei were stained with hematoxylin.

12.2.5 Soybean Agglutinin (SBA) Staining for Stage Determination

SBA specifically stains the acrosome of spermatids. For SBA staining, sections were treated with 1% bovine serum albumin (BSA) in 10 mM PBS and incubated with biotinylated SBA lectin (Vector Laboratories, Burlingame, CA, USA, 20 µg/ml) in PBS overnight at 4 °C. After washing with PBS, the sections were treated with the ABC kit and DAB.

12.2.6 Proliferating Cell Nuclear Antigen (PCNA) Staining to Detect Proliferating Spermatogenic Cells

After antigen retrieval by heating in a microwave oven for 10 min in 0.01 M citrate buffer (pH 6.0), sections were blocked with a TNB blocking buffer and incubated with mouse anti-PCNA antibody (1:1000, PC10, Santa Cruz Biotechnology, Dallas, TX) for 12 h at 4 °C, then washed with PBS and incubated with the secondary antibody for 1 h at room temperature. This reaction was enhanced and visualized with the ABC kit and DAB solution. For a negative control, the incubation step with the primary antibody was omitted.

12.2.7 Cleaved Caspase-3 Staining to Detect Apoptotic Spermatogenic Cells

Immunostaining for activated caspase-3 (cleaved caspase-3), one of the key mediators of apoptosis, was performed to detect apoptotic spermatogenic cells. As the primary antibody, rabbit polyclonal antibody (1:200; NB600–1235; Novus Biologicals, Centennial, CO, USA) was used. The staining procedure performed was similar to the PCNA staining method mentioned above.

12.3 Results

12.3.1 ^{137}Cs Concentration

The ^{137}Cs concentration of the unaffected control was quite low (5.6 Bq/kg), whereas those of the affected group were relatively high and varied from 64.2 to 693.7 Bq/kg (average: 238.8, standard error: 84.4) (Table 12.1).

12.3.2 Hematoxylin and Eosin Staining

In spite of the difference in ^{137}Cs concentrations between the two groups, active spermatogenesis was observed in the affected Japanese macaques (Fig. 12.1a), as well as in the unaffected one (Fig. 12.1b). Furthermore, the epididymal duct of the affected group was filled with spermatozoa (Fig. 12.1c). Thus, it appears that no definite differences in spermatogenesis were recognized between both groups, and it was also confirmed that all wild Japanese macaques used in this study were sexually mature and in a breeding season.

12.3.3 Vimentin Immunohistochemistry

Similar to the unaffected control (Fig. 12.2a), in the testicular epithelium of the affected group, vimentin was detected around the cell nucleus of the Sertoli cells and from the basal to the apical regions (Fig. 12.2b).

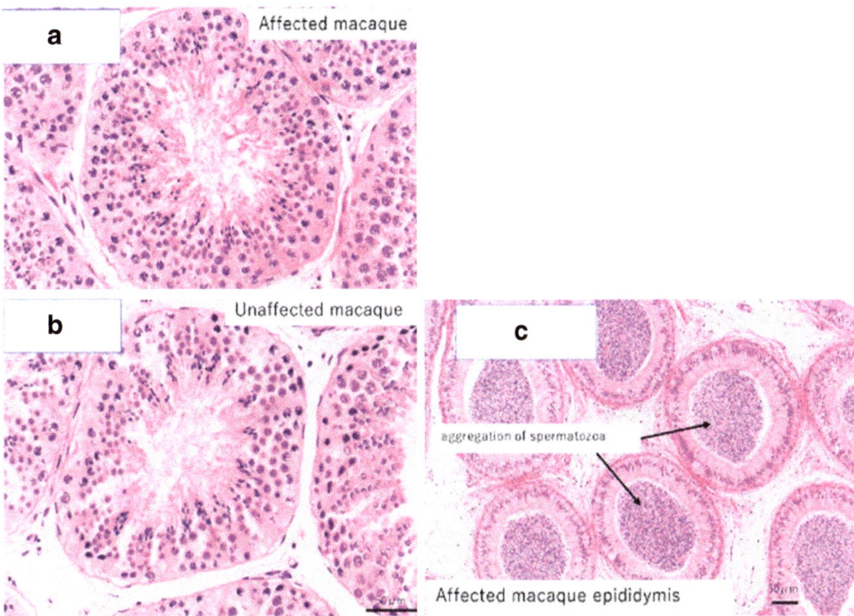

Fig. 12.1 Cross sections of seminiferous tubules in unaffected and affected Japanese macaques and of the epididymis in affected Japanese macaque stained with hematoxylin and eosin. Scale bar = 50 μm (**a**) Active spermatogenesis is observed in seminiferous tubules of an affected Japanese macaque. (**b**) Active spermatogenesis is observed in seminiferous tubules of the unaffected Japanese macaque. (**c**) Epididymal duct of the affected Japanese macaque is filled with spermatozoa.

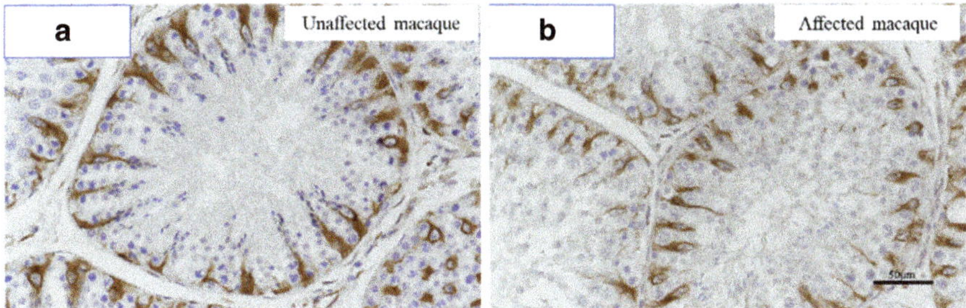

Fig. 12.2 Vimentin distribution in cross sections of seminiferous tubules in unaffected and affected Japanese macaques. Scale bar = 50 μm. (**a**) Vimentin (stained brown) is found around the Sertoli cell nucleus and from the basal region to the apical region of the Sertoli cell in the seminiferous epithelium of the unaffected Japanese macaque. (**b**) Vimentin is also observed from the basal to the apical regions of the Sertoli cell in the seminiferous epithelium of affected Japanese macaques.

12.3.4 Stage Determination

After determining the stage of the seminiferous epithelium in Japanese macaques, we attempted to compare proliferating and apoptotic spermatogenic cells and their specific cell types following differentiation into type B spermatogonia between the affected and the unaffected macaque. Generally, the cycle of the seminiferous epithelium of macaques, such as *Macaca mulatta* [32], *Macaca speciosa* [33], and *Macaca fascicularis* [34–36], has been divided into 12 stages. In the present study, therefore, we assigned the results to 12 stages of the seminiferous epithelium and 14 steps of developing spermatids in the Japanese macaque testes (Figs. 12.3 and 12.4). In general, at stage II, proacrosomal vesicles first appear and are not in contact with the spermatid nucleus. Then, at stage III, they make a contact with the nucleus [26]. In the present study, however, it was very difficult to judge whether proacrosomal vesicles make a contact with the nucleus at the light microscopic level. Therefore, we designated stage II–III as one stage, as in mice and rats [26]. In addition, since primary spermatocytes in the basal region of the seminiferous epithelium at stage VIII are thought to be in contact with the basement membrane of the seminiferous epithelium, as well as those at stage VII, we determined these primary spermatocytes at stage VIII to be preleptotene primary spermatocytes.

Other than the above, we determined the stage of the seminiferous epithelium, using SBA staining, with particular reference to the literature on *Macaca fascicularis* [34] (Fig. 12.3). These characteristics of each stage were found in both the affected and the unaffected macaques. Thus, we made the 12-stage diagram of the Japanese macaque seminiferous epithelium (Fig. 12.4). In this diagram, we show spermatogenic cells after type B spermatogonia at stage I.

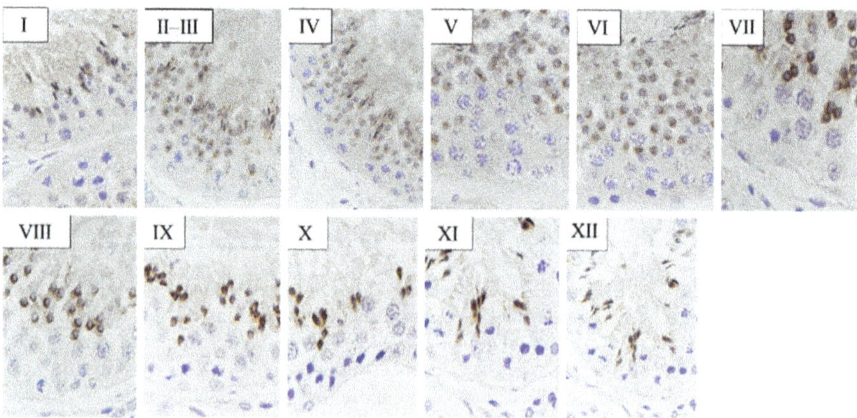

Fig. 12.3 Twelve stages of the Japanese macaque seminiferous epithelium stained with soybean agglutinin (SBA) obtained from unaffected and affected Japanese macaques. Acrosomes of spermatids appearing at all stages are stained brown.

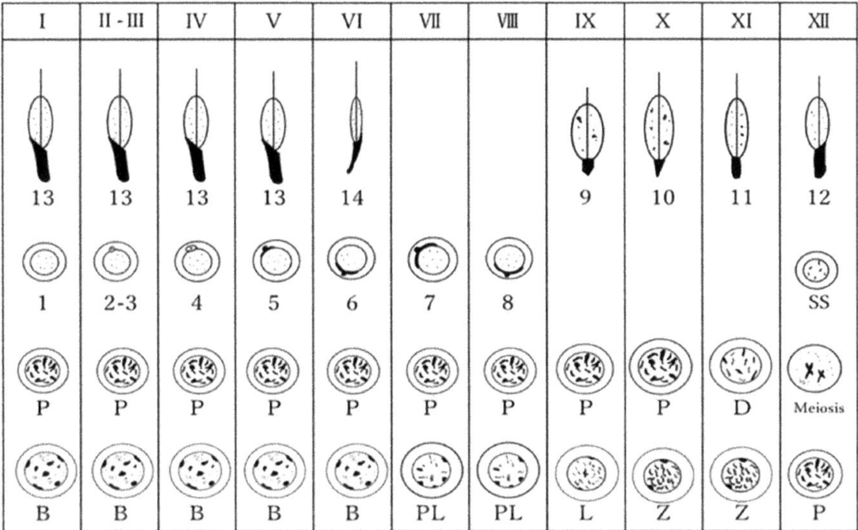

Fig. 12.4 Staging scheme of Japanese macaque seminiferous epithelium. This scheme contains spermatogenic cells after type B spermatogonia at stage I. Developing spermatids are divided into 14 steps. B: type B spermatogonium; PL: preleptotene primary spermatocyte; L: leptotene primary spermatocyte; Z: zygotene primary spermatocyte; P: pachytene primary spermatocyte; D: diplotene primary spermatocyte; SS: secondary spermatocyte; 1–14: step 1–14 spermatid.

12.3.5   Proliferating Spermatogenic Cells

In sections immunolabeled by anti-PCNA antibody, in addition to the staging scheme (Fig. 12.4) obtained in the present study from SBA-stained sections, we assigned the stage number of each seminiferous epithelium by evaluating the location of developing spermatids in the seminiferous epithelium using the following features: characteristics of the nuclear chromatin in each primary spermatocyte; each primary spermatocyte being in contact or not in contact with the basement membrane of the seminiferous epithelium, coadjacent seminiferous epithelia being the successive stages, and so on.

Figure 12.5a–c shows the cross sections of the unaffected Japanese macaque seminiferous epithelia immunolabeled by anti-PCNA antibody. At stage VIII (Fig. 12.5a), only preleptotene primary spermatocytes were positive (proliferating spermatogenic cells), and at stage X (Fig. 12.5b), only zygotene primary spermatocytes were positive, but other spermatogenic cells (including pachytene primary spermatocytes) were negative at stages VIII and X. On the other hand, at stages IV and V (Fig. 12.5c), pachytene primary spermatocytes were positive.

Figure 12.6a–d shows the cross sections of the seminiferous epithelia of the affected group immunolabeled by anti-PCNA antibody. At stage II–III (Fig. 12.6d), type B spermatogonia and pachytene primary spermatocytes were positive.

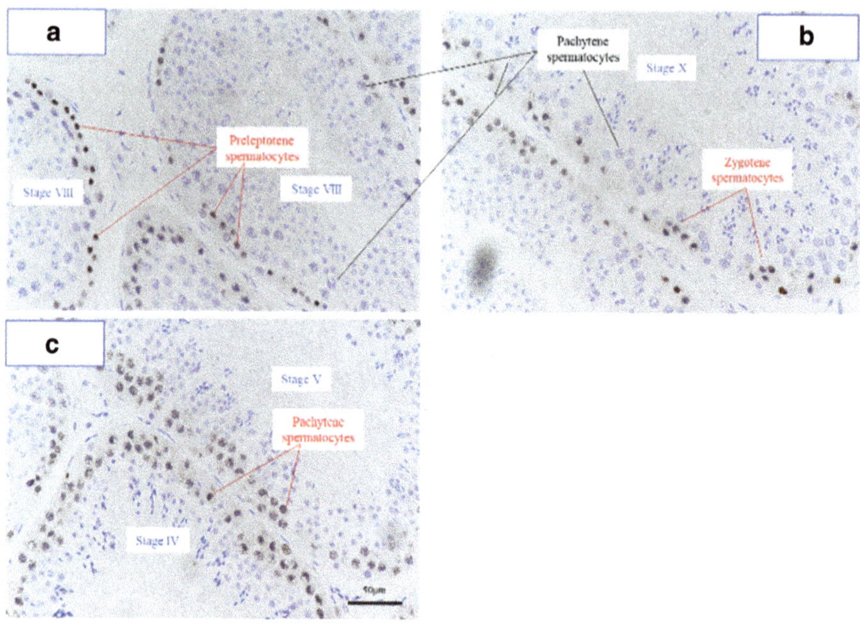

Fig. 12.5 Cross sections of seminiferous tubules in the unaffected Japanese macaque by PCNA labeling. Red letters: positive cell types; black letters: negative cell types; brown-stained cells: positive cells; scale bar = 50 μm. (**a**) At stage VIII, preleptotene primary spermatocytes are positive, but pachytene primary spermatocytes are negative. (**b**) At stage X, zygotene primary spermatocytes are positive, but pachytene primary spermatocytes are negative. (**c**) At stages IV and V, pachytene primary spermatocytes are positive.

Similarly, at stage VI (Fig. 12.6a), type B spermatogonia and pachytene primary spermatocytes were positive, while at stage VII (Fig. 12.6a), preleptotene and pachytene primary spermatocytes were positive. At stage VIII (Fig. 12.6b–d), preleptotene primary spermatocytes were positive, but pachytene primary spermatocytes were negative. At stage IX (Fig. 12.6b), only leptotene primary spermatocytes were positive, but pachytene primary spermatocytes were negative. At stage XI (Fig. 12.6c), only zygotene primary spermatocytes were positive. In addition to the abovementioned results (stages II–III, VI–IX, and XI), through the observation in seminiferous epithelia at stages I, IV, V, X, and XII, no differences in immunolabeling of spermatogenic cells with anti-PCNA antibody were recognized in the affected group compared to the unaffected control. Therefore, the present results made clear that proliferating spermatogenic cells in Japanese macaque testes were type B spermatogonia at stages I–VI, preleptotene primary spermatocytes at stages VII and VIII, leptotene primary spermatocytes at stage IX, zygotene primary spermatocytes at stages X and XI, and pachytene primary spermatocytes at stages XII-VII.

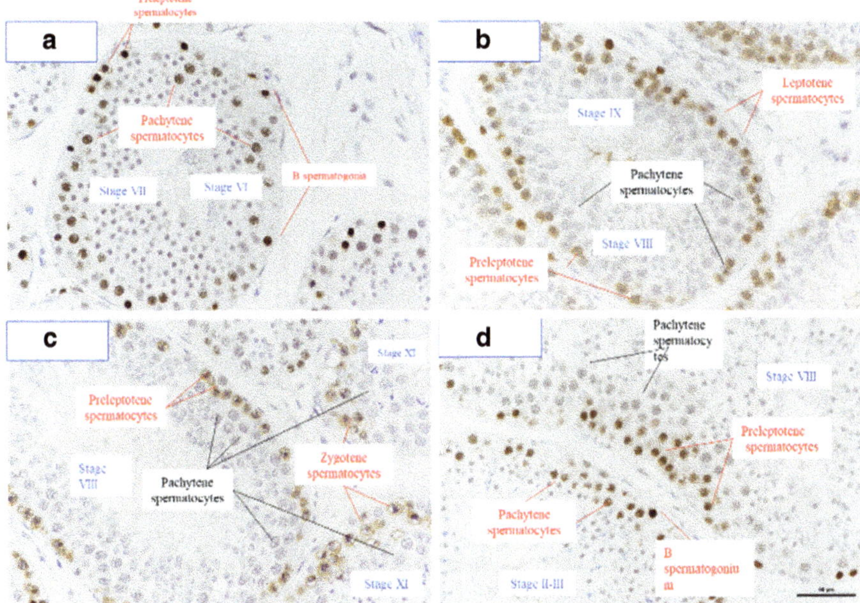

Fig. 12.6 Cross sections of seminiferous tubules in affected Japanese macaques by PCNA labeling. Red letters: positive cell types; black letters: negative cell types; brown-stained cells: positive cells; scale bar = 50 μm. (**a**) At stage VI, type B spermatogonia are positive, while at stage VII, preleptotene primary spermatocytes are positive. At both stages, pachytene primary spermatocytes are positive. (**b**) At stage VIII, preleptotene primary spermatocytes are positive, while at stage IX, leptotene primary spermatocytes are positive. At both stages, pachytene primary spermatocytes are negative. (**c**) At stage VIII, preleptotene primary spermatocytes are positive, while at stage XI, zygotene primary spermatocytes are positive. At both stages, pachytene primary spermatocytes are negative. (**d**) At stage II–III, type B spermatogonia and pachytene primary spermatocytes are positive. At stage VIII, preleptotene primary spermatocytes are positive, but pachytene primary spermatocytes are negative.

Figure 12.7 represents the distribution of PCNA-positive cells (proliferating spermatogenic cells; red area) on the stages of the seminiferous epithelium, common to both the affected and unaffected groups.

12.3.6   *Apoptotic Spermatogenic Cells*

To determine the stage number of the seminiferous epithelium in the cleaved caspase-3-stained sections, we used the same criteria used in the PCNA-stained sections as mentioned above. Different from the case in PCNA-positive cells, apoptotic spermatogenic cells were scarcely distributed in the seminiferous epithelium of the Japanese macaque testes analyzed in this study. Although some type B

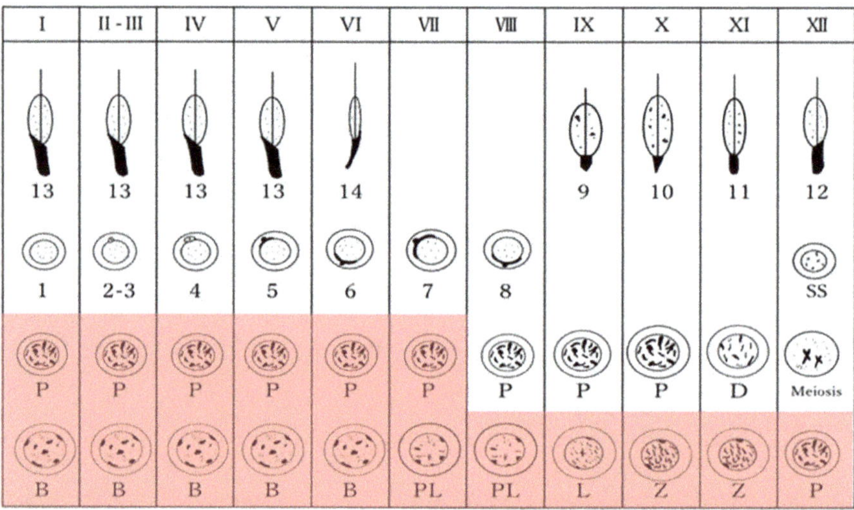

Fig. 12.7 Distribution of PCNA-positive cells (proliferating spermatogenic cells; red area) across the stages of the seminiferous epithelium in unaffected and affected Japanese macaques. type B spermatogonia at stages I–VI, preleptotene primary spermatocytes at stages VII and VIII, leptotene primary spermatocytes at stage IX, zygotene primary spermatocytes at stages X and XI, and pachytene primary spermatocytes at stages XII–VII in unaffected and affected Japanese macaques are PCNA-positive. B: type B spermatogonium; PL: preleptotene primary spermatocyte; L: leptotene primary spermatocyte; Z: zygotene primary spermatocyte; P: pachytene primary spermatocyte; D: diplotene primary spermatocyte; SS: secondary spermatocyte; 1–14: step 1–14 spermatid.

spermatogonia and primary spermatocytes were positive for cleaved caspase-3, these were not always positive in macaque testes in both groups.

Figure 12.8a–c shows cross sections of the unaffected control seminiferous epithelia stained with cleaved caspase-3. At stage V (Fig. 12.8a), some type B spermatogonia were positive; at stage VII (Fig. 12.8c), some preleptotene primary spermatocytes were positive; and at stage XI (Fig. 12.8b), some leptotene primary spermatocytes were positive. On the other hand, Fig. 12.9a–c shows cross sections of the seminiferous epithelia of the affected group stained with cleaved caspase-3. At stages V (Fig. 12.9c) and VI (Fig. 12.9a), some type B spermatogonia were positive. At stage VII (Fig. 12.9a), some preleptotene primary spermatocytes were positive, and at stage IX (Fig. 12.9b), some leptotene primary spermatocytes were positive. Thus, in both the affected and unaffected groups, some type B spermatogonia and some preleptotene and leptotene primary spermatocytes underwent apoptosis, with no differences observed between the groups.

Figure 12.10 depicts the distribution of cleaved caspase-3-positive apoptotic spermatogenic cells (blue areas) at each stage of the testicular epithelium, which is common to both the affected and unaffected groups.

From the above results, no differences were found in proliferating and apoptotic spermatogenic cells at each stage of the seminiferous epithelium and their specific cell types between the affected and unaffected groups.

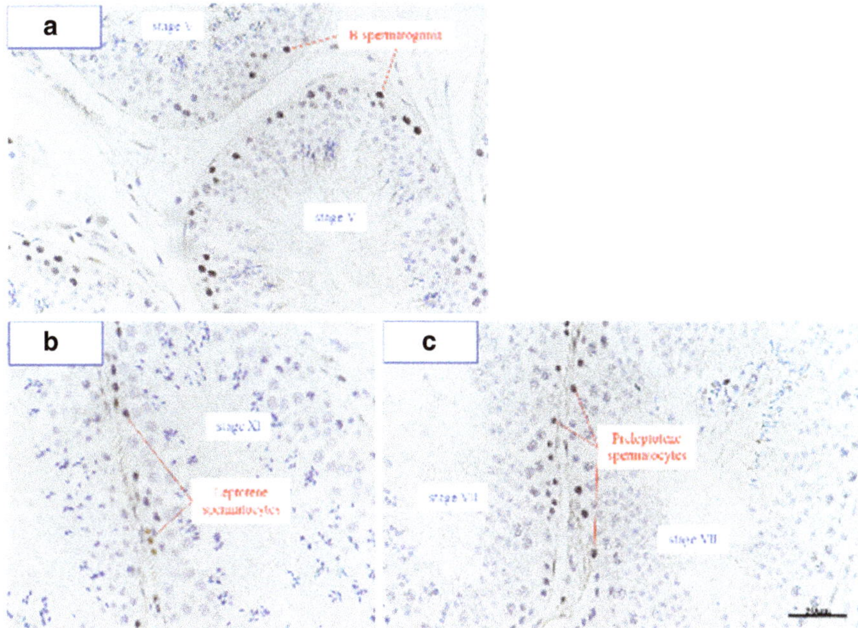

Fig. 12.8 Cross sections of seminiferous tubules in unaffected Japanese macaque, stained with caspase-3. Red letters: positive cell type; brown-stained cells: positive cells: scale bar = 50 µm. (**a**) At stage V, type B spermatogonia are positive. (**b**) At stage XI, leptotene primary spermatocytes are positive. (**c**) At stage VII, preleptotene primary spermatocytes are positive.

12.4   Discussion

In the present study, we first measured ^{137}Cs concentration in femoral muscles of both the affected and unaffected macaque groups. As a result, ^{137}Cs concentration in the affected group (64.2–693.7 Bq/kg) varied widely, but even the lowest level was ten times higher than that of the unaffected control (5.6 Bq/kg), confirming a clear difference between the two groups. Next, we observed the testicular tissues stained with hematoxylin and eosin under a light microscope. The result showed that spermatogenesis was active in both testicular tissues, and, at a glance, no specific differences were recognized between the affected group and the unaffected control. Even in the individual showing the highest ^{137}Cs concentration (693.7 Bq/kg), active spermatogenesis was clearly found. In order to compare the testicular tissues of both macaque groups in more detail, we performed histochemical examinations. Vimentin was clearly detected from the basal to the apical regions of Sertoli cells in the affected group, as well as in the unaffected control. This fact might show the normal state of Sertoli cells in the affected Japanese macaque testes.

We determined the stage of the seminiferous epithelium and assigned 12 stages according to previous reports on the stages of the testicular epithelium in the rhesus macaque [32] and the crab-eating macaque [34–36], which belong to the same

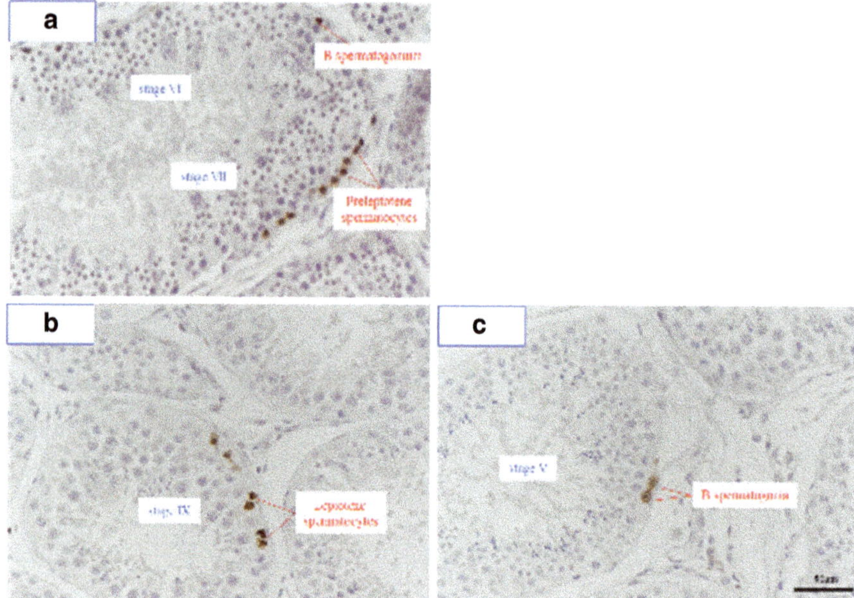

Fig. 12.9 Cross sections of seminiferous tubules in affected Japanese macaque, stained with caspase-3. Red letters: positive cell types; brown-stained cells: positive cells; scale bar = 50 μm. (**a**) At stage VI, type B spermatogonia are positive, and at stage VII, preleptotene primary spermatocytes are positive. (**b**) At stage IX, leptotene primary spermatocytes are positive. (**c**) At stage V, type B spermatogonia are positive.

primate order as Japanese macaques, *Macaca, fuscata*. PCNA immunostaining was then performed to compare the appearance of proliferating spermatogenic cells at different stages of the seminiferous epithelium and specific cell types between the affected and unaffected groups. Consequently, type B spermatogonia at stages I–VI, preleptotene primary spermatocytes at stages VII and VIII, leptotene primary spermatocytes at stage IX, zygotene primary spermatocytes at stages X and XI, and pachytene primary spermatocytes at stages XII–VII were proliferating spermatogenic cells in both groups. Furthermore, no obvious qualitative differences were observed in the proliferating cells of the stage and proliferating cell type between the affected and unaffected groups. In normal mice, PCNA-positive spermatogenic cells are type B spermatogonia, leptotene and zygotene primary spermatocytes, and pachytene primary spermatocytes at stages I–VII, whereas preleptotene primary spermatocytes are negative [37]. The distribution of PCNA-positive cells in Japanese macaque testes is very similar to that of normal mice, with the exception of preleptotene primary spermatocytes (positive in Japanese macaques, negative in mice). Therefore, it is supposed that the present data on the distribution of PCNA-positive proliferating cells in Japanese macaques reveal a normal state of testicular tissues.

Cleaved caspase-3 immunostaining was performed to compare the appearance of apoptotic spermatogenic cells and the types of apoptotic cells at each stage of the

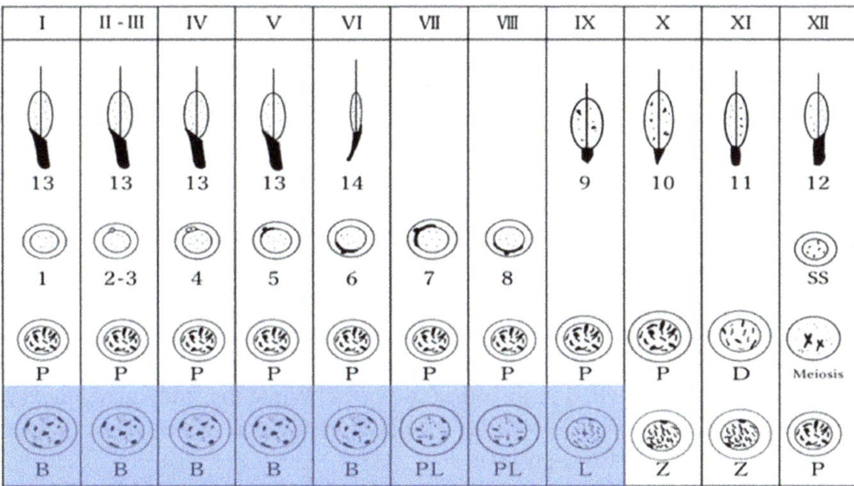

Fig. 12.10 Distribution of caspase-3-positive cells (apoptotic spermatogenic cells; blue area) on stages of seminiferous epithelium in unaffected and affected Japanese macaques. type B spermatogonia at stages I–VI, preleptotene primary spermatocytes at stages VII and VIII, and leptotene primary spermatocytes at stage IX are positive in unaffected and affected Japanese macaques. B: type B spermatogonium; PL: preleptotene primary spermatocyte; L: leptotene primary spermatocyte; Z: zygotene primary spermatocyte; P: pachytene primary spermatocyte; D: diplotene primary spermatocyte; SS: secondary spermatocyte; 1–14: step 1–14 spermatid.

seminiferous epithelium in the affected and unaffected Japanese macaques. As a result, some type B spermatogonia at stages I–VI, some preleptotene primary spermatocytes at stages VII and VIII, and some leptotene primary spermatocytes at stage IX were apoptotic spermatogenic cells in both macaque groups. Several studies [6, 38–40] have shown that radiation causes apoptosis in spermatogonia and spermatocytes. The stage-specific apoptosis in the rat seminiferous epithelium (14 stages in total) has been reported [39]. In that study, intermediate- and B-spermatogonia at stages II–IV, primary spermatocytes at stage I, diakinetic spermatocytes at stage XIII, and preleptotene–zygotene primary spermatocytes at stages VII–XII were sensitive to irradiation. In the present study, type B spermatogonia, preleptotene primary spermatocytes at stages VII–VIII, and leptotene primary spermatocytes at stage IX were also apoptotic; however, the frequency was smaller compared to the above study, and the same observations were obtained in both the affected and the unaffected Japanese macaques. It is well accepted that apoptosis is an essential process in normal spermatogenesis. For example, in the normal stallions [41], apoptotic spermatogenic cells are type B spermatogonia and primary spermatocytes at stages IV–VI (eight stages in total). The distribution of apoptotic spermatogenic cells in the present study on the Japanese macaque was similar to that of the normal stallion. Thus, it is suggested that the present study on the distribution of apoptotic spermatogenic cells in the affected Japanese macaques shows spontaneous apoptosis, namely a normal state of testicular tissues.

Active spermatogenesis was clearly observed in the testes of Japanese macaques exposed to chronic low-dose-rate radiation, and no obvious differences were found between the affected and the unaffected macaques in proliferating and apoptotic spermatogenic cells at each stage of the seminiferous epithelium and their specific cell types.

Although ^{137}Cs concentration in muscles was different between the two groups, this difference did not appear to affect the testicular tissues. Studies on the testes of other animal species inhabiting Fukushima Prefecture, such as bulls [15], wild boars [16], field mice [12, 13], and raccoons [17], have shown that these mammals possess the morphologically normal testicular tissues and normal spermatogenic activity. On the other hand, Takino et al. [14] showed that in Fukushima Prefecture, the testes of Japanese field mice captured in one area had more PCNA-positive cells compared to those captured in the other two areas. While the study quantitatively analyzed the number of PCNA-positive cells, it is not clear which types of spermatogenic cells were PCNA-positive.

In conclusion, the present study revealed that Japanese macaques living in the affected areas of the FNPP accident exhibit normal testicular tissue. From the perspective of extrapolation to humans, we believe that the present information on male ability of reproduction in Japanese macaques is of great importance.

References

1. González AJ, Akashi M, Boice JD Jr et al (2013) Radiological protection issues arising during and after the Fukushima nuclear reactor accident. J Radiol Prot 33:497–571. https://doi.org/10.1088/0952-4746/33/3/497
2. Kinoshita N, Sueki K, Kitagawa J et al (2011) Assessment of individual radionuclide distributions from the Fukushima nuclear accident covering central-east Japan. Proc Natl Acad Sci U S A 108:19526–19529. https://doi.org/10.1073/pnas.1111724108
3. Zheng J, Tagami K, Watanabe Y et al (2012) Isotopic evidence of plutonium release into the environment from the Fukushima DNPP accident. Sci Rep 2:304. https://doi.org/10.1038/srep00304
4. Cordelli E, Fresegna AM, Leter G et al (2003) Evaluation of DNA damage in different stages of mouse spermatogenesis after testicular X irradiation. Radiat Res 160:443–451. https://doi.org/10.1667/rr3053
5. Gong EJ, Shin IS, Son TG et al (2014) Low-dose-rate radiation exposure leads to testicular damage with decreases in DNMT1 and HDAC1 in the murine testis. J Radiat Res 55:54–60. https://doi.org/10.1093/jrr/rrt090
6. Hasegawa M, Wilson G, Russell LD et al (1997) Radiation-induced cell death in the mouse testis: relationship to apoptosis. Radiat Res 147:457–467. https://doi.org/10.2307/3579503
7. Liu G, Gong P, Zhao H et al (2006) Effect of low- level radiation on the death of male germ cells. Radiat Res 165:379–389. https://doi.org/10.1667/rr3528.1
8. Meistrich ML, Hunter NR, Suzuki N et al (1978) Gradual regeneration of mouse testicular stem cells after exposure to ionizing radiation. Radiat Res 74:349–362. https://doi.org/10.2307/3574894
9. Rakici SY, Guzel AI, Tumkaya L et al (2020) Pelvic radiation-induced testicular damage: an experimental study at 1 gray. Syst Biol Reprod Med 66:89–98. https://doi.org/10.1080/19396368.2019.1679909

10. Sapp WJ, Philpott DE, Williams CS et al (1992) Comparative study of spermatogonial survival after x-ray exposure, high LET (HZE)CC irradiation or spaceflight. Adv Space Res 12:179–189. https://doi.org/10.1016/0273-1177(92)90106-8

11. Withers HR, Hunter N, Barkley HT et al (1974) Radiation survival and regeneration characteristics of spermatogenic stem cells of mouse testis. Radiat Res 57:88–103

12. Ohdaira T, Meguro K, Komatsu K et al (2019) Analysis of radioactive elements in testes of large Japanese field mice using an electron probe micro-analyser after the Fukushima accident. Intech Open 2019:1–9. https://doi.org/10.5772/intechopen.84634

13. Okano T, Ishiniwa H, Onuma M et al (2016) Effects of environmental radiation on testes and spermatogenesis in wild large Japanese field mice (*Apodemus speciosus*) from Fukushima. Sci Rep 6:23601. https://doi.org/10.1038/srep23601

14. Takino S, Yamashiro H, Sugano Y et al (2017) Analysis of the effect of chronic and low-dose radiation exposure on spermatogenic cells of male large Japanese field mice (*Apodemus speciosus*) after the Fukushima Daiichi Nuclear Power Plant accident. Radiat Res 187:161–168. https://doi.org/10.1667/RR14234.1

15. Yamashiro H, Abe Y, Fukuda T et al (2013) Effects of radioactive caesium on bull testes after the Fukushima Nuclear Plant accident. Sci Rep 3:2850. https://doi.org/10.1038/srep02850

16. Yamashiro H, Abe Y, Urushihara Y et al (2015) Electron probe X-ray microanalysis of boar and inobuta testes after the Fukushima accident. J Radiat Res 56(Suppl 1):i42–i47. https://doi.org/10.1093/jrr/rrv070

17. Komatsu K, Iwasaki T, Murata K et al (2021) Morphological reproductive characteristics of testes and fertilization capacity of cryopreserved sperm after the Fukushima accident in raccoon (*Procyon lotor*). Reprod Domest Anim 56:484–497. https://doi.org/10.1111/rda.13887

18. Endo S, Ishii K, Suzuki M et al (2020) Dose estimation of external and internal exposure in Japanese macaques after the Fukushima nuclear power plant accident. In Fukumoto (ed) Low-dose radiation effects on animals and ecosystems. Springer Open, pp 179–191 ISBN 978-981-13-8218-5 (eBook). https://doi.org/10.1007/978-981-13-8218-5

19. Hayama S, Nakiri S, Nakanishi S et al (2013) Concentration of radiocesium in the wild Japanese monkey (*Macaca fuscata*) over the first 15 months after the Fukushima Daiichi Nuclear disaster. PLoS One 8:e68530. https://doi.org/10.1371/journal.pone.0068530

20. Hayama S, Tanaka A, Nakanishi S et al (2022) Time dependence of ^{137}CS contamination in wild Japanese monkeys after the Fukushima Daiichi nuclear accident. Environ Sci Pollut Res 29:88359–88368. https://doi.org/10.1007/s11356-022-23707-0

21. Omi T, Nakiri S, Nakanishi S et al (2020) Concentration of ^{137}Cs radiocaesium in the organs and tissues of low-dose-exposed wild Japanese monkeys. BMC Res Notes 13:121. https://doi.org/10.21203/rs.2.21592/v2

22. Ochiai K, Hayama S, Nakiri S et al (2014) Low blood cell counts in wild Japanese monkeys after the Fukushima Daiichi nuclear disaster. Sci Rep 4:5793. https://doi.org/10.1038/srep05793

23. Urushihara Y, Suzuki T, Shimizu Y et al (2018) Haematological analysis of Japanese macaques (*Macaca fuscata*) in the area affected by the Fukushima Daiichi Nuclear Power Plant accident. Sci Rep 8:16748. https://doi.org/10.1038/s41598-018-35104-0

24. Kurohmaru M, Kanai Y, Hayashi Y (1992) A cytological and cytoskeletal comparison of Sertoli cells without germ cell and those with germ cells using the W/W^v mutant mouse. Tissue Cell 24:895–903. https://doi.org/10.1016/0040-8166(92)90024-2

25. Kopecky M, Semecky V, Nachtigal P (2005) Vimentin expression during altered spermatogenesis in rats. Acta Histochem 107:279–289. https://doi.org/10.1016/j.acthis.2005.06.007

26. Russell LD, Ettlin RA, Sinha Hikim AP et al (1990) Histological and histopathological evaluation of the testis. Cache River Press, Clearwater. (ISBN 0-9627422-0-1-X)

27. Saito H, Yokota S, Kitajima S (2023) Immunohistochemical analysis of the vimentin filaments in Sertoli cells is a powerful tool for the prediction of spermatogenic dysfunction. Acta Histochem 125:152046. https://doi.org/10.1016/j.acthis.2023.152046

28. Fukushima Prefecture (2017) The 4th management plan for Japanese monkeys in Fukushima Prefecture (in Japanese). https://www.pref.fukushima.lg.jp/sec/36021d/kankyou-nougyou-500.html. Accessed 25 Oct 2023. https://www.pref.fukushima.lg.jp/uploaded/life/679784_1914278_misc.pdf; https://www.pref.fukushima.lg.jp/uploaded/life/679784_1914279_misc.pdf; https://www.pref.fukushima.lg.jp/uploaded/attachment/132947.pdf

29. Niigata Prefecture (2017) The 2nd management plan for Japanese monkeys in Niigata Prefecture (in Japanese). https://www.pref.niigata.lg.jp/sec/nosanengei/1341954130416.html. Accessed 25 Oct 2023

30. Primate Research Institute (2015) Kyoto University Guideline for field research for nonhuman primates. http://pri.ehub.kyoto-u.ac.jp/research/Guideline%20for%20field%20research%20of%20non-human%20primates201905.pdf. Accessed 25 Oct 2023

31. Fukushima Prefecture (2023) Radioactivity measurement map in Fukushima revitalization station. https://www.pref.fukushima.lg.jp/site/portal-english/en-m2-3.html. Accessed 25 Oct 2023

32. De Rooij DG, van Alphen MMA, van de Kant HJG (1986) Duration of the cycle of the seminiferous epithelium and its stages in the rhesus macaque (*Macaca mulatta*). Biol Reprod 35:587–591. https://doi.org/10.1095/biolreprod35.3.587

33. Antar M (1971) Duration of the cycle of the seminiferous epithelium and of spermatogenesis in the macaque (*Macaca speciosa*). Anat Rec 169:268–269 (Abstract). https://doi.org/10.1095/biolreprod35.3.587

34. Dreef HC, Esch EV, De Rijk EPCT (2007) Spermatogenesis in the cynomolgus monkey (*Macaca fascicularis*): a practical guide for routine morphological staging. Toxicol Pathol 35:395–404. https://doi.org/10.1080/01926230701230346

35. Fouquet JP, Dadoune JP (1986) Renewal of spermatogonia in the monkey (*Macaca fascicularis*). Biol Reprod 35:199–207. https://doi.org/10.1095/biolreprod35.1.199

36. Zhengwei Y, McLachlan RI, Bremner WI et al (1997) Quantitative (Stereological) study of normal spermatogenesis in the adult monkey (*Macaca fascicularis*). J Androl 18:681–687. https://doi.org/10.1002/j.1939-4640.1997.tb02445.x

37. Chapman DL, Wolgemuth DJ (1994) Expression of proliferating cell nuclear antigen in the mouse germ line and surrounding somatic cells suggests both proliferation-dependent and -independent modes of function. Int J Dev Biol 38:491–497

38. Campion SN, Sandrof MA, Yamasaki Y et al (2010) Suppression of radiation-induced testicular germ cell apoptosis by 2,5-hexanedione pretreatment. III. Candidate gene analysis identifies a role for Fas in the attenuation of X-ray–induced apoptosis. Toxicol Sci 117:466–474. https://doi.org/10.1093/toxsci/kfq205

39. Henriksen K, Kulmala J, Toppari J et al (1996) Stage-specific apoptosis in the rat seminiferous epithelium: quantification of irradiation effects. J Androl 17:394–402. https://doi.org/10.1002/j.1939-4640.1996.tb01805.x

40. Yamasaki H, Sandrof MA, Boekelheide K (2010) Suppression of radiation-induced testicular germ cell apoptosis by 2,5-hexanedione pretreatment. I. Histopathological analysis reveals stage dependence of attenuated apoptosis. Toxicol Sci 117:449–456. https://doi.org/10.1093/toxsci/kfq203

41. Heninger NL, Staub C, Blanchard TL et al (2004) Germ cell apoptosis in the testes of normal stallions. Theriogenology 62:283–297. https://doi.org/10.1016/j.theriogenology.2003.10.022

Chapter 13
Decade-Long Surveys of Morphological Abnormalities of the Pale Grass Blue Butterfly After the Fukushima Daiichi Nuclear Power Plant Accident in the Seven Localities and Iitate Village

Ko Sakauchi, Wataru Taira, Nobuyoshi Ito, and Joji M. Otaki

Abstract Biological impacts of the Fukushima Daiichi Nuclear Power Plant (FNPP) accident have been demonstrated in the pale grass blue butterfly, *Zizeeria maha*, based on field surveys and laboratory experiments that reproduced field conditions. Field surveys have been performed in seven polluted reference localities and in many other localities throughout Japan. Here, we report compiled results of 11-year field surveys, 2011–2021, in the seven reference localities. We also report the results of field surveys, 2013–2024, in Iitate Village. In the reference localities, the morphological abnormality rate peaked in May 2012 and then decreased to the levels of unpolluted localities by 2016. However, Fukushima City had a recurrent peak in August 2014. In Iitate Village, the morphological abnormality rate was relatively high in 2013 and decreased in subsequent years but then increased to the previous level in 2021. These data suggest that adverse biological effects may be recurrent in polluted areas such as Fukushima City and Iitate Village. We speculate that the recurrence may originate from various mechanisms, including synergistic effects of radiation exposure with nonradiation factors, a decrease in genetic diversity in previous years as a result of the initial exposure, and plant stress responses to chronic low-dose radiation exposure in the field.

K. Sakauchi · J. M. Otaki (✉)
Faculty of Science, University of the Ryukyus, Senbaru, Nishihara, Okinawa, Japan
e-mail: otaki@cs.u-ryukyu.ac.jp

W. Taira
Faculty of Science, University of the Ryukyus, Senbaru, Nishihara, Okinawa, Japan

Ryukyu University Museum Fujukan, University of the Ryukyus, Senbaru, Nishihara, Okinawa, Japan

N. Ito
Komiya, Iitate Village, Fukushima, Japan

M. Fukumoto (ed.), *Low-Dose Radiation Effects on Animals and Ecosystems II*,
https://doi.org/10.1007/978-981-95-5559-8_13

Keywords Biological effect · Field survey · Fukushima Daiichi Nuclear Power Plant (FNPP) accident · Low-dose exposure · Pale grass blue butterfly · Radioactive cesium · Recurrence

13.1 Introduction

The Fukushima Daiichi Nuclear Power Plant (FNPP) accident in March 2011 resulted in a massive release of various species of radionuclides to surrounding environments [1]. To understand the biological effects of this accident, the pale grass blue butterfly, *Zizeeria maha*, has been used as an indicator species, which is suitable both for field surveys [2–4] and laboratory experiments [4, 5]. Accumulated results from various field surveys and laboratory experiments have demonstrated that this species of butterfly has been severely affected by the accident [6–11]. One important line of evidence has been provided by long-term field surveys [12]. The morphological abnormality rate was monitored twice a year for 3 years in the period of 2011–2013, corresponding to the 1st–17th generations of this butterfly [12]. It has been reported that the abnormality rate peaked at the second survey in Fall 2011 and then decreased to less than 10% in Fall 2013 [12]. However, based on the field survey in 2016 (5.5 years after the FNPP accident corresponding to the 29th generation), the abnormality rate was still correlated with the ground deposition levels immediately after the accident, implying that the impact of the initial radiation exposure continued [13]. Such an initial exposure may occur through short-lived radionuclides such as iodine-131 (^{131}I) and tellurium-129m (^{129m}Te) or through cesium-134 (^{134}Cs) and ^{137}Cs. In either case, such field studies illustrate the importance of continuous field surveys for many years after the FNPP accident.

Confirmations of these field data have been provided by additional field surveys throughout Japan. The mean value of the abnormality rates in 52 localities in southwestern Japan (summer 2015) has been reported to be 3.8% [14]. Similarly, 44 localities in northeastern Japan have been surveyed [15]. There appeared to be "the gap zone" at approximately 39°N, and the mean abnormality rate south of the gap zone has been reported to be 3.0% [15]. Because Fukushima Prefecture belongs to the southern population of the gap zone, the "normal" abnormality rate there is likely approximately 3%. On the other hand, the populations north of the gap zone showed a mean abnormality rate of 10.6% [15]. This fact indicates that abnormalities are present relatively frequently in the northern populations beyond the gap zone, probably due to low temperatures, but are rare in southern populations, including Fukushima.

In this paper, we present the latest results of the abnormality rates of the pale grass blue butterfly over 11 years after the FNPP accident (May 2011 to September 2021) in seven reference localities, namely, Fukushima City, Motomiya City, Hirono Town, Iwaki City, Takahagi City, Mito City, and Tsukuba City. This species of butterfly requires 1 month for one generation from spring to fall and passes five to six generations per year in the Kanto–Tohoku district. Thus, our surveys cover the period of the 54th–65th generations from the very first generations immediately after the accident. In this study, we present the results of reevaluated abnormalities of all field-caught individuals [16]. We also present the results of the abnormality rates in Iitate Village (2013–2024). Iitate Village is known for its high radioactive pollution. We detected a recurrence of the high abnormality rate of this butterfly in Fukushima City and in Iitate Village. We discuss the present results, considering other recent findings regarding the pale grass blue butterfly in Fukushima Prefecture.

13.2 Materials and Methods

The abnormality rates of the pale grass blue butterfly in 2011–2013 in seven reference localities (Fukushima City, Motomiya City, Hirono Town and Iwaki City in Fukushima Prefecture, and Takahagi City, Mito City, and Tsukuba City in Ibaraki Prefecture) have already been reported in and used here from Hiyama et al. (2015) [12]. Each individual butterfly collected in 2011–2013 in the seven localities was reevaluated and compiled in a public database [16]. The reevaluated data were used in the present study. It should be noted that wing color pattern modifications induced by cold temperatures, which are called temperature-shock-type (TS-type) modifications, can be distinguished visually from abnormalities by researchers [7, 17]. Similarly, unique aberrations of color patterns, called the panda type, are known to occur upon sibling crosses [4, 18], which are also distinguishable visually from other abnormalities by researchers. Therefore, the panda-type aberrations and TS-type modifications were excluded from morphological abnormalities in our system, as in previous studies [6, 7]. We excluded all abnormalities in palpi, considering that abnormalities in palpi are often caused in the field by nongenetic reasons such as physical damage during flight. We also excluded the samples from Watari (Hanamiyama), Fukushima City, because they were not always included in the field surveys.

Adult individuals of the pale grass blue butterfly were newly collected in Iitate Village, Fukushima Prefecture, Japan, in 2020–2024. Adult butterflies were collected using insect nets and individually placed into collection tubes (13 mm in inner diameter and 50 mm in height). These samples were sent to the laboratory at the University of the Ryukyus, Okinawa, Japan, where morphological abnormalities and beak marks were examined. The ground radiation dose rate was measured using the ALOKA pocket survey meter MYRATE PDR-111 (Tokyo, Japan). Data from July 2013 in Iitate Village were obtained from Hiyama et al. (2015) [12]. Data from May–September 2014 in Iitate Village were obtained from Hiyama et al. (2017) [15]. Data from September 2016 in Iitate Village were obtained from Sakauchi et al. (2020) [13]. We did not pay attention to sexual differences in this study.

For new samples from Iitate Village, each adult individual of the pale grass blue butterfly was examined visually under a conventional dissection microscope and a KEYENCE digital microscope VHX-8000 (Osaka, Japan) and by the naked eye for its morphologically abnormal traits and for the presence of beak marks on the wings. The abnormality rate [%] was calculated as the number of individuals with one or more abnormal traits divided by the number of individuals examined. The beak-mark rate [%] was similarly calculated as the number of individuals with one or more beak marks on the wings divided by the number of individuals examined. A beak mark was defined as a physical lack of a region in either the right or left wing or in both wings except for the forewing tip. The capture rate [n/h·person] was obtained as the number of individuals captured in an hour by a single person. To calculate these rates, no distinction was made between sexes.

13.3 Results

13.3.1 Chronological Changes in the Seven Localities

We obtained the abnormality dynamics over 10 years (2011–2021) in the seven reference localities despite the lack of data in some years (Fig. 13.1). We observed the first and largest peak in May 2012 in all localities (mean: 18.0%). Many localities had the second peak in May 2013 (mean: 6.8%). The second peaks were smaller than the first peaks in most localities with the exception of Mito City, in which the second peak was larger than the first peak. In Fukushima City, another peak was observed in August 2014 (7.7%). Overall, the abnormality rates declined to less than 5% in all two or three localities examined in September 2016 and in September 2021.

13.3.2 Chronological Changes in Iitate Village

The abnormality rate was monitored in Iitate Village from July 2013 to October 2024 together with the beak-mark rate, capture rate, and ground radiation dose rate (Fig. 13.2). The abnormality rate was relatively high in July 2013 (17.9%)

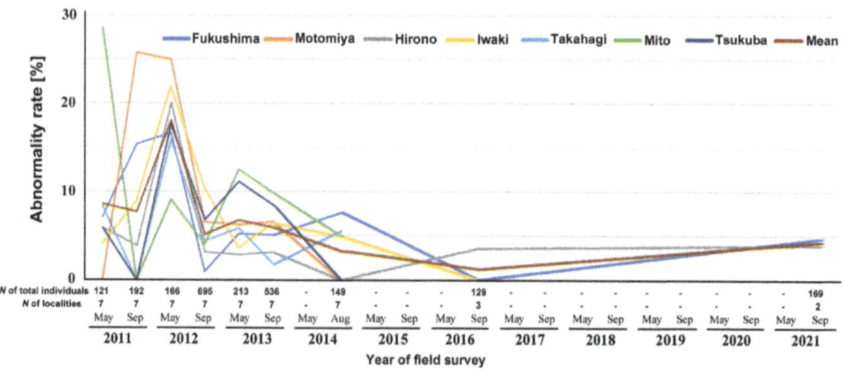

Fig. 13.1 Dynamics of abnormality rate [%] in the period of 2011–2021. Butterflies were sampled at seven reference localities (three in 2016 and two in 2021).

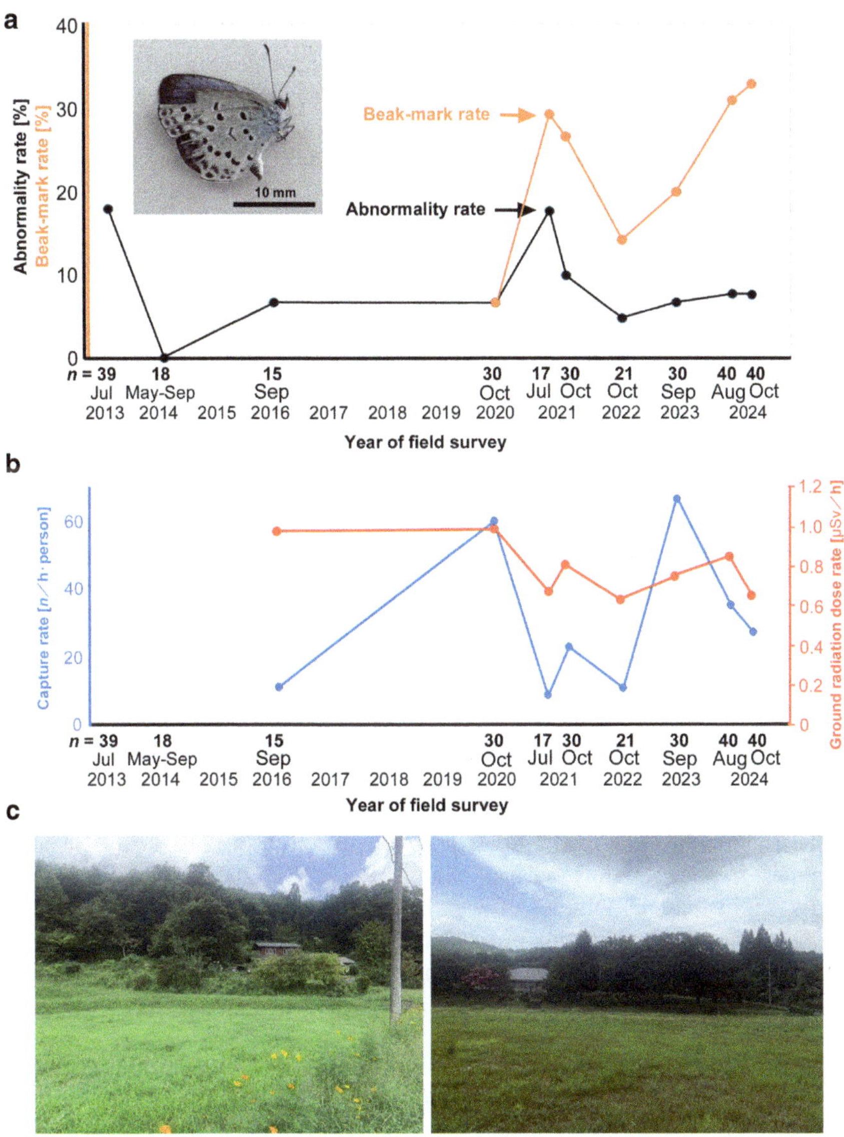

Fig. 13.2 Dynamics of field data in Iitate Village in the period of 2013–2024. (**a**) The abnormality rate [%] (black) and the beak-mark rate [%] (orange). An inset shows an individual with beak marks on the right wings. (**b**) The capture rate [n/h·person] (blue, left vertical axis) and the ground radiation dose rate [μSv/h] (red, right vertical axis). (**c**) Landscape images of Komiya, the sampling site in Iitate Village.

(Fig. 13.2a), which was consistent with the results of the seven reference localities (Fig. 13.1), considering that Iitate Village has been radioactively polluted more than other localities examined. The abnormality rate decreased to 0% in 2014, 6.7% in 2016, and 6.7% in 2020. Unexpectedly, the abnormality rate increased to the previous level in July 2021 (17.6%). This late peak soon declined to 10.0% in October 2021 and then to 4.8% in October 2022. The beak-mark rate showed a sharp peak in July 2021 together with the abnormality rate (Fig. 13.2a). However, beak marks were detected only in the normal individuals (but not in abnormal individuals) throughout these surveys. During this period, the ground radiation dose rate decreased gradually (Fig. 13.2b). On the other hand, the capture rate peaked in October 2020 (Fig. 13.2b).

13.4 Discussion

13.4.1 Changes in the Abnormality Rate in the Seven Localities

Here, we presented the abnormality rate dynamics in the seven reference localities from 2011 to 2021. Although not all years were surveyed, our compiled data covering 11 years in multiple localities are unique and probably second to none in this kind of field surveys after a nuclear pollution event. Although there were some variations among the seven localities, we confirmed that the highest peak was present in May 2012 in most localities. This is an important finding, because the peak was present in September 2011 in the previous study [12]. Another peak was found in some localities in May 2013, but these second peaks were smaller than the first peak in each locality, and they were 6.8% on average. A further decline in the abnormality rate was notable in 2014, 2016, and 2021.

To be sure, there seems to be a tendency that a May population had larger values of the abnormality rate than a September population in 2012 and 2013 in many localities. If we accept this seasonal trend, peaks in May 2013 may not be considered a real increase in pollution effects. The abnormality rate has been recorded as 3.0% in a "normal" population of this butterfly species in northeastern Japan [15]. Therefore, we conclude that the pollution effects on this species of butterflies were no longer detected in the seven localities in 2016 and afterward, at least in terms of the abnormality rates.

Nonetheless, an additional small late peak was found in Fukushima City (and probably also in Takahagi City) in August 2014. This late peak in August 2014 in Fukushima City is not in accordance with the seasonal trend discussed above and thus may be considered important. Interestingly, this late peak is higher than the 2013 peak in Fukushima City. In this sense, the 2014 peak may be considered the recurrence of high abnormalities in this species in Fukushima City if it is caused by radioactive pollution. This possibility is not unrealistic, considering that the adverse effects of radioactive pollution appeared to continue in 2016, 5.5 years after the accident, at least in highly polluted localities [13]. Alternatively, this 2014 peak in Fukushima City may be a "spontaneous" fluctuation irrespective of radioactive pollution in the field, for example, due to climate factors and relationships with predators and the host plant. However, we believe that such a recurrent fluctuation is triggered by radioactive pollution (see below).

13.4.2 Possible Factors for the Recurrent High Abnormality Rate in Iitate Village

As mentioned above, the abnormality rate has been recorded as 3.0% in a "normal" population of this butterfly species in northeastern Japan [15]. On the other hand, the highest abnormality rate in southwestern Japan was 12.5% in Kanazawa and other localities [14]. Considering these points, the abnormality rates in Iitate Village in July 2013 (17.9%) and July 2021 (17.6%) were relatively high. In contrast, in Iitate Village, relatively low levels of abnormality rates were observed in 2014, 2016, and 2020. The 2013 case in Iitate Village is likely caused by the FNPP accident because similar peaks were also seen in the seven localities in 2013. The 2021 case in Iitate Village may be considered the recurrence of biologically adverse effects of radioactive pollution 10 years after the accident, similar to the case of the small recurrence in Fukushima in 2014 discussed above. However, there are other possibilities irrespective of radioactive pollution, considering that the levels of the ground radiation dose rate did not change much from 2016 to 2022.

One possibility is that the 2021 case was caused by low temperatures during winter in Iitate Village irrespective of radioactive pollution. Because Iitate Village is located at a high altitude, abnormal individuals may be relatively frequent there compared to other localities in northeastern Japan. In fact, in the northern border of the "gap zone," a high abnormality rate has been recorded in Oshu City, Iwate Prefecture, showing 16.7% (n = 12) [15]. Another example is found in Nasushiobara City, Tochigi Prefecture, located at a high altitude similar to Iitate Village, showing 17.4% (n = 23), although Nasushiobara City is located at a lower latitude than the gap zone [15]. The annual lowest temperatures of Iitate Village and Fukushima City (note: Fukushima City is located at the highest latitude among the seven reference localities) in 2021 were −14.7 °C and −7.4 °C, respectively [19], showing that Iitate Village is much colder than Fukushima City.

Another possible explanation regarding Iitate's high abnormality rate in 2021 may be related to the high capture rate in October 2020. Such an increase in the population may cause a subsequent increase in predators such as spiders, amphibians, reptiles, and birds. This is supported by the high beak-mark rate in 2021 together with the high abnormality rate in the same year. It is important to recognize that the beak-mark rate and the abnormality rate appear to behave similarly. They peaked immediately after an increase in the capture rate (i.e., an increase in the population size). After the increase in the population size, an increase in the number of predator individuals may result. Predators likely prey on abnormal individuals more frequently than normal individuals because the former are slower in escape behavior, increasing in the beak-mark rate. Immediately after that, a decrease in the abnormality rate will result. This line of discussion suggests that the real abnormality rate in 2021 may be even higher. The beak-mark rate is a new value introduced from 2020. More studies may be necessary to understand its significance.

A population increase in 2020 might have caused sibling crosses in the population because of the low dispersibility of this butterfly species [3], leading to the high abnormality rate the following year. Such a deteriorating effect of sibling crosses on abnormalities has been known in this species [5, 18]. However, sibling crosses often produce unique wing color pattern aberrations known as the panda type [5, 17]. We did not detect any panda-type individuals even when the capture rate was low (i.e., small population size). If predators preyed on these panda-type individuals, which are often small and probably slow to escape, more frequently than the normal and other abnormal individuals, the above scenario of the sibling crosses may not be impossible, but an explanation is not given to the high capture rate in October 2020.

A more likely and simpler explanation is that the previous radiation effect on the high abnormality rate in 2013 and before, possibly because of the high initial exposure in 2011, might have resulted in a general decrease in population size by 2016, leading to a decrease in genetic diversity of this butterfly in Iitate Village (and in many other localities). A population increase in October 2020 may be caused by a different reason, but this increase might have occurred along a general decrease in genetic diversity. This could then cause phenotypic expression of harmful mutations, i.e., an increase in the abnormality rate (but not necessarily an increase in the panda type). We have already obtained such evidence for a decrease in genetic diversity after the FNPP accident [20, 21]. A population increase with low genetic diversity could cause an increase in the abnormality rate as shown in Fig. 13.2. Then, predators indirectly select for genetically robust individuals. In fact, the second peak of the capture rate in Iitate 2023 did not push up the abnormality rate in 2024. This means that natural selection is under way. Repetitive recurrence of the abnormality rate may be a natural selection process in real time. In other words, it seems that we witnessed real-time stabilizing evolution of this butterfly species in Fukushima Prefecture.

An additional viewpoint is the adaptive evolution of the butterfly against radiation exposure or radioactively contaminated leaves. If butterflies have adapted to the polluted environment, the recurrence of the high abnormality rate is not expected. On the other hand, potential adaptive evolution has been demonstrated in butterflies from polluted localities: Resistance against internal and external exposure was correlated with distance from FNPP and with the ground radiation dose rate [22]. By the same token, the pale grass blue butterfly may be expected to have adapted to the high-altitude environments of Iitate Village, but our survey data appear to show that relatively high abnormalities are present at high latitudes and altitudes [15], suggesting that adaptation to high latitudes may still be incomplete. It is possible to speculate that, at high latitudes and altitudes, adaptation to radioactive environments is difficult or delayed in this butterfly. However, this discussion should be reconciled with the results of the generalized linear model (GLM), showing that latitude and altitude were not important factors for the abnormality rate in the localities of lower latitudes than the gap zone [13]. This GLM result might have arisen because the abnormality rate of Iitate Village (6.7%) was not high in 2016 in that study [13].

In 2024, we performed a field survey in August when temperature was more than 32 °C. We confirmed that the August results were similar to the October results in the same year, suggesting that seasonal variation is minimal. Whether or not Iitate's high abnormality rate in 2021 is associated with radioactive pollution is uncertain at this point, but there may be biotic and abiotic factors that are unique to Iitate Village. Thus far, we have discussed a few possible nonradioactive factors of the high abnormality rate in Iitate Village in 2021 (and in Fukushima City in 2014) as if these factors were independent of one another. These potential factors, such as seasonal trends, low temperatures (high altitudes), predator dynamics, sibling crosses, low genetic diversity, and adaptivity, may work synergistically with radioactive pollution. Nonradioactive factors have often been considered "confounding factors" that are assumed to be independent of and unrelated to radioactive pollution. However, such factors may contribute to the high radiation sensitivity of organisms in the field. Such a synergistic effect is one of the important field effects recognized in ecological studies [23] and in Chernobyl (Chornobyl) [24].

In addition to the synergistic field effects, chronic low-dose radiation exposure may often function as a stressor for organisms such as plants. Plant-eating animals, including butterflies and other insects, may be vulnerable to stress-induced metabolites that are produced by plants. Such indirect radiation effects mediated via the food web are called ecological field effects [23].

13.4.3   Possible Ecological Field Effect Through Host Plant Leaves in Iitate Village

Here, we focus on food quality as a potential factor for the recurrent peak in Iitate Village. To do so, we briefly review our experimental results that have been published elsewhere. One of the most important experiments in a series of Fukushima butterfly studies is internal exposure experiments, in which larvae showed deaths or developmental abnormalities after eating host plant leaves collected from polluted sites. The abnormality rate of individuals who ingested the contaminated leaves was dependent on the dose of radioactive cesium (^{134}Cs and ^{137}Cs) in the internal exposure experiments (Fig. 13.3a) [6, 7, 25–27]. Furthermore, larvae that were fed leaves from Iitate Village showed the lowest survival rate among the tested groups (Fig. 13.3b). These results indicate that radioactive contaminants are directly or indirectly responsible for the abnormality rate.

At first glance, these field-oriented studies seemed to indicate that the pale grass blue butterfly is vulnerable to direct radioactive exposure. However, larvae are insensitive to high doses of pure ^{137}CsCl ingested via an artificial diet [28]. The highest dose used in this artificial diet experiment was 4.55×10^7 Bq/kg (diet),

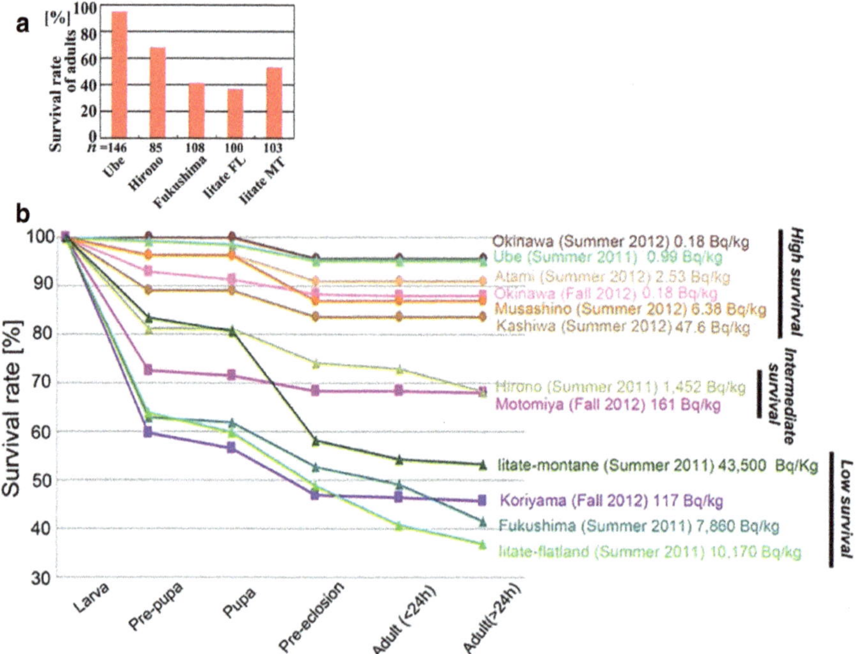

Fig. 13.3 Internal exposure experiments. (**a**) Survival rate of the internal exposure experiment. Butterfly larvae from Okinawa were fed host plant leaves collected from various polluted localities. Samples from Iitate FL (flatland) and Iitate MT (montane) are included. Ube City, Yamaguchi Prefecture is the least polluted among these localities. Reproduced from Hiyama et al. (2013) [7]. (**b**) Survival curves of butterflies that were fed host plant leaves from 12 localities. Two Iitate groups are categorized into the low-survival group. Radioactivity concentrations of the leaves are shown (Reproduced from Nohara et al. (2014) [26]).

which is more than a thousand times higher than the highest dose of the field-collected leaves used in the internal exposure experiments [28]. This result of the laboratory-oriented study is in high contrast to the results of the field-oriented studies: The butterfly is vulnerable to relatively low levels of radioactive pollution in the field but is highly resistant against high levels in laboratory conditions. This is a clear case of the field–laboratory paradox. This paradox can be resolved by considering ecological field effects, in which indirect biological pathways are responsible for the toxicity of pollution [23].

To demonstrate the ecological field effect on the butterfly, chemical constituents of the host plant leaves were analyzed. Nutrients (inorganic ions) in the host plant leaves seem to be important [29]. In addition, metabolomic analyses revealed many upregulated and downregulated chemicals in response to low-dose exposure [30]. It appears that the host plant responds to low-dose radiation by upregulating and downregulating secondary metabolites. Metabolomic profiles of the host plant leaves from polluted areas revealed a unique status of Iitate Village among samples from Fukushima Prefecture in a principal component analysis (PCA) plot

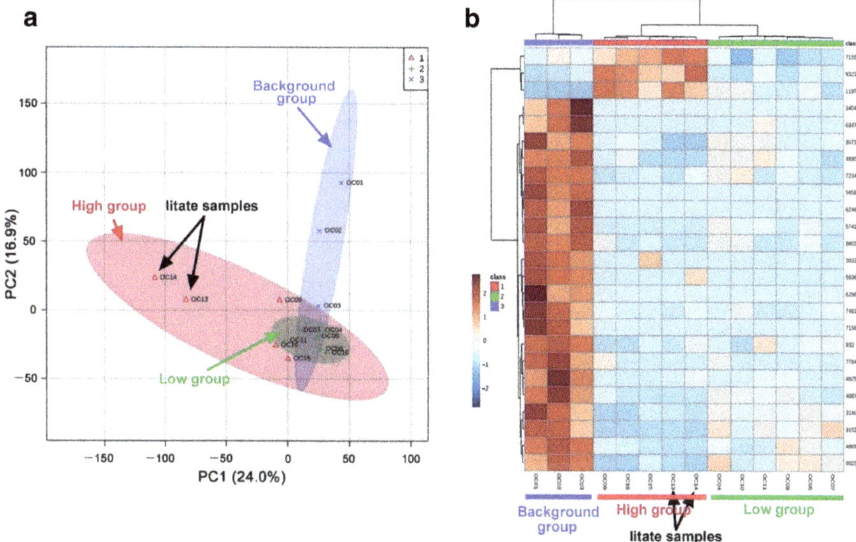

Fig. 13.4 Cluster analyses of liquid chromatography–mass spectrometry (LC–MS) peaks from the host plant leaves collected from 14 localities, including Iitate Village. Two Iitate samples are placed far from other high-group samples and low-group samples. Reproduced with minor modifications from Sakauchi et al. (2022) [30]. (**a**) Principal component analysis (PCA) plot using all detected LC–MS peaks. (**b**) Heatmap using the top 25 LC–MS peaks.

(Fig. 13.4a) [30]. In the plot, the Iitate samples were also very different from Niigata samples (two of the background group, OC01 and OC02) that had negligible radiation exposure from the FNPP accident [30]. This difference in secondary metabolites cannot be attributed to radioactive pollution level alone because other samples from higher levels of pollution did not show this feature. There may be some upregulated secondary metabolites that are specific to Iitate Village. On the other hand, Iitate samples surely share some upregulated metabolites with other localities of the high-dose group in a heatmap (Fig. 13.4b) [30]. The plant might have adapted to the environmental conditions of Iitate Village, which is located at a mountainous high altitude and could have different soil compositions. Interestingly, among the metabolites that were correlated with radiation doses, some were derived from soil microorganisms associated with the plant [30]. Soil microorganisms closely associated with plants might also synthesize stress-induced chemicals in response to radioactive pollution.

Experimentally irradiated leaves from Okinawa (unpolluted locality) using contaminated soil also exhibited upregulation and downregulation of secondary metabolites (Fig. 13.5a–c) [31]. The plant may be sensitive to chronic low-dose radiation exposure to synthesize secondary metabolites that are highly toxic to larvae of this butterfly. One of the upregulated secondary metabolites, lauric acid, has been demonstrated to be toxic to larvae when consumed at high doses (Fig. 13.5d) [32].

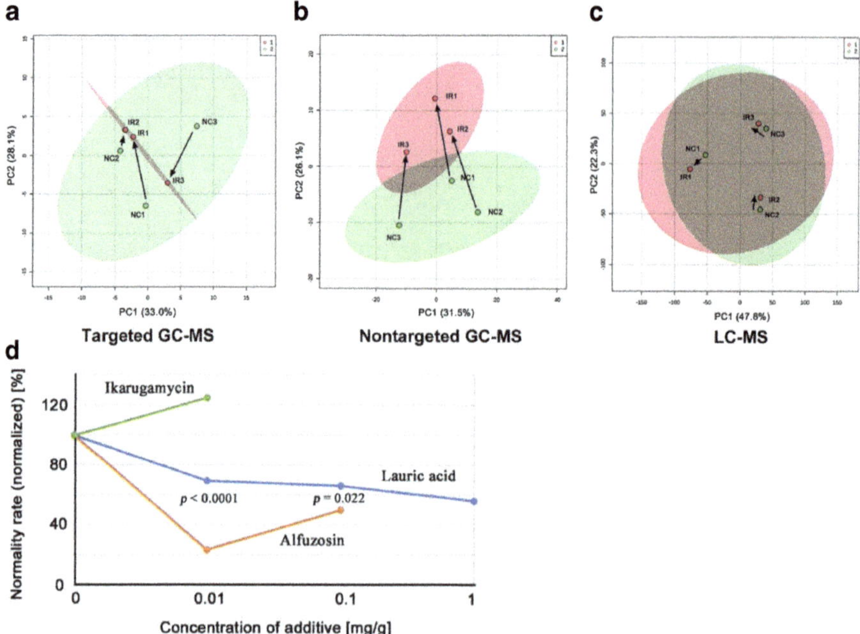

Fig. 13.5 Analyses of metabolites from the host plant leaves from three sites in Okinawa experimentally irradiated with contaminated soil from Fukushima. (**a**) Principal component analysis (PCA) plot of metabolites using targeted gas chromatography–mass spectrometry (GC–MS) peaks. Arrows in **a–c** indicate metabolomic shifts from nonirradiated (NC) to irradiated (IR) states. Reproduced with minor modifications from Sakauchi et al. (2021) [31] (also **b** and **c**). (**b**) PCA plot of metabolites using nontargeted (all detected) GC–MS peaks. (**c**) PCA plot using all detected LC–MS peaks. (**d**) Changes in the normality rate [%] in response to the concentration of an additive in the artificial diet. Three additives tested here (lauric acid, alfuzosin, and ikarugamycin) were chosen based on the results of previous metabolome study [31]. Lauric acid and alfuzosin show significant toxicity to larvae, whereas ikarugamycin shows a beneficial effect (Reproduced from Morita et al. (2022) [32]).

13.4.4 Direct Exposure Effects on Butterflies

Beyond doubt, the direct radiation exposure effect (nonfield effect) is important and should be evaluated quantitatively. This is especially important in the initial exposure event immediately after the FNPP accident because various species of short-lived radionuclides were released [1]. We performed fieldwork to reveal how the pale grass blue butterfly overwintered in Fukushima Prefecture at the time of the FNPP accident in March 2011 [33]. In the seven reference localities, this butterfly was estimated to overwinter as fourth-instar larvae at the time of the FNPP accident. Therefore, the fourth- and fifth-instar larval stages and subsequent prepupal and pupal stages experienced initial exposure in the field. It is important to note that the larval requirement for food consumption drastically increases in these late larval stages, and active cell divisions take place in the subsequent prepupal and pupal stages for metamorphosis. These stages may be a window of vulnerability of butterfly development to radiation exposure due to the high number of cell divisions. Although quantitative estimation of absorbed doses in the butterflies that overwintered in March 2011 and eclosed in May 2011 is expected in the future, the amount of external and internal exposure was probably considerable. The radiation sensitivity of the larvae and the host plant could change under the overwintering dormant conditions in the field, as pointed out in Chernobyl (Chornobyl) research in plants [34]. An imaging plate analysis indicated that radioactive Cs may concentrate on the abdomens of butterflies, suggesting a potential direct exposure effect from concentrated radioactivity, although the accumulation of radioactive Cs over generations has not been detected [35].

13.5 Conclusions

Our field monitoring results of the pale grass blue butterfly in the seven reference localities indicate that the abnormality rate declined to the normal level by 2016. However, possible recurrence was found in 2014 in Fukushima City. Similarly, in Iitate Village, a sudden onset of the abnormality rate was observed in 2021. Considering that such high abnormality rates are relatively rare throughout Japan, these cases may be considered the recurrence of radiation effects *sensu lato*. The recurrence may be repeated at least a few times, and it may be a process of stabilizing evolution of this butterfly species in real time. If so, the recurrence may be caused by the field effects of residual radioactive materials, mostly ^{137}Cs. One example of the field effect is biochemical changes in host plant leaves in response to chronic low-dose-rate radiation exposure. Alternatively, the initial exposure effects that caused a decrease in population size and genetic diversity might have induced recurrent peaks of the abnormality rate as phenotypic expression of harmful genetic mutations. Other possibilities, irrespective of radioactive pollution, including low temperatures, predator dynamics, and sibling crosses, cannot be excluded. However, some nonradiation factors may work synergistically with direct radiation exposure. The present study indicated possible long-term biological impacts of radioactive pollution on organisms potentially through interactions among biotic and abiotic factors in the field.

Acknowledgments The authors are grateful to members of the BCPH Unit of Molecular Physiology for comments. This study was supported by donations from the public who understand the importance of the Fukushima Butterfly Project at the University of the Ryukyus.

References

1. Hirose K (2012) 2011 Fukushima Dai-ichi nuclear power plant accident: summary of regional radioactive deposition monitoring results. J Environ Radioact 111:13–17. https://doi.org/10.1016/j.jenvrad.2011.09.003

2. Hiyama A, Taira W, Sakauchi K et al (2018) Sampling efficiency of the pale grass blue butterfly *Zizeeria maha* (Lepidoptera: Lycaenidae): a versatile indicator species for environmental risk assessment in Japan. J Asia Pac Entomol 21:609–615. https://doi.org/10.1016/j.aspen.2018.03.010

3. Hiyama A, Otaki JM (2020) Dispersibility of the pale grass blue butterfly *Zizeeria maha* (Lepidoptera: Lycaenidae) revealed by one-individual tracking in the field: quantitative comparisons between subspecies and between sexes. Insects 11:122. https://doi.org/10.3390/insects11020122

4. Otaki JM (2020) The pale grass blue butterfly as an indicator for the biological effect of the Fukushima Daiichi Nuclear Power Plant accident. In: Fukumoto M (ed) Low-dose radiation effects on animals and ecosystems, Springer Open, pp 239–247. ISBN 978-981-13-8218-5 (eBook). https://doi.org/10.1007/978-981-13-8218-5

5. Hiyama A, Iwata M, Otaki JM (2010) Rearing the pale grass blue *Zizeeria maha* (Lepidoptera, Lycaenidae): toward the establishment of a lycaenid model system for butterfly physiology and genetics. Entomol Sci 13:239–302. https://doi.org/10.1111/j.1479-8298.2010.00387.x

6. Hiyama A, Nohara C, Kinjo S et al (2012) The biological impacts of the Fukushima nuclear accident on the pale grass blue butterfly. Sci Rep 2:570. https://doi.org/10.1038/srep00570

7. Hiyama A, Nohara C, Taira W et al (2013) The Fukushima nuclear accident and the pale grass blue butterfly: evaluating biological effects of long-term low-dose exposures. BMC Evol Biol 13:168. https://doi.org/10.1186/1471-2148-13-168

8. Taira W, Nohara C, Hiyama A et al (2014) Fukushima's biological impacts: the case of the pale grass blue butterfly. J Hered 105:710–722. https://doi.org/10.1093/jhered/esu013

9. Otaki JM (2016) Fukushima's lessons from the blue butterfly: a risk assessment of the human living environment in the post-Fukushima era. Integr Environ Assess Manag 12:667–672. https://doi.org/10.1002/ieam.1828

10. Otaki JM, Taira W (2018) Current status of the blue butterfly in Fukushima research. J Hered 109:178–187. https://doi.org/10.1093/jhered/esx037

11. Otaki JM, Sakauchi K, Taira W (2022) The second decades of the blue butterfly in Fukushima: untangling the ecological field effects after the Fukushima nuclear accident. Integr Environ Assess Manag 18:1539–1550. https://doi.org/10.1002/ieam.4624

12. Hiyama A, Taira W, Nohara C et al (2015) Spatiotemporal abnormality dynamics of the pale grass blue butterfly: three years of monitoring (2011-2013) after the Fukushima nuclear accident. BMC Evol Biol 15:15. https://doi.org/10.1186/s12862-015-0297-1

13. Sakauchi K, Taira W, Hiyama A et al (2020) The pale grass blue butterfly in ex-evacuation zones 5.5 years after the Fukushima nuclear accident: contributions of initial high-dose exposure to transgenerational effects. J Asia Pac Entomol 23:242–252. https://doi.org/10.1016/j.aspen.2020.01.002

14. Hiyama A, Taira W, Iwasaki M et al (2017) Morphological abnormality rate of the pale grass blue butterfly *Zizeeria maha* (Lepidoptera: Lycaenidae) in southwestern Japan: a reference data set for environmental monitoring. J Asia Pac Entomol 20:1333–1339. https://doi.org/10.1016/j.aspen.2017.09.016

15. Hiyama A, Taira W, Iwasaki M et al (2017) Geographical distribution of morphological abnormalities and wing color pattern modifications of the pale grass blue butterfly in northeastern Japan. Entomol Sci 20:100–110. https://doi.org/10.1111/ens.12233

16. Sakauchi K, Taira W, Otaki JM (2023) Instruction, table, picture sheet, and original pictures: morphological abnormalities in the field samples of the pale grass blue butterfly for three years after the Fukushima nuclear accident. Figshare Collection. https://doi.org/10.6084/m9.figshare.c.6425981.v1

17. Otaki JM, Hiyama A, Iwata M et al (2010) Phenotypic plasticity in the range-margin population of the lycaenid butterfly *Zizeeria maha*. BMC Evol Biol 10:252. https://doi.org/10.118
6/1471-2148-10-252
18. Iwata M, Hiyama A, Otaki JM (2013) System-dependent regulations of colour-pattern development: a mutagenesis study of the pale grass blue butterfly. Sci Rep 3:2379. https://doi.
org/10.1038/srep02379
19. Japan Meteorological Agency. Search for meteorological data in the past. https://www.data.
jma.go.jp/stats/etrn/index.php. Accessed 16 Oct 2023
20. Toki M, Taira W, Sakauchi K, Otaki JM (2025) Mitochondrial genetic mutations in the pale
grass blue butterfly: Possible DNA damage via the Fukushima nuclear accident and real-time
molecular evolution. Diversity 17:275. https://doi.org/10.3390/d17040275
21. Toki M, Taira W, Sakauchi K, Otaki JM (2025) Spatiotemporal dynamics of genetic diversity
in the pale grass blue butterfly after the Fukushima nuclear accident. Diversity 17:668. https://
doi.org/10.3390/d17100668
22. Nohara C, Hiyama A, Taira W et al (2018) Robustness and radiation resistance of the pale
grass blue butterfly from radioactively contaminated areas: a possible case of adaptive evolution. J Hered 109:188–198. https://doi.org/10.1093/jhered/esx012
23. Otaki JM (2018) Understanding low-dose exposure and field effects to resolve the field-
laboratory paradox: multifaceted biological effects from the Fukushima nuclear accident. In:
Awwad NS, AlFaify SA (eds) New trends in nuclear science, IntechOpen, pp 49-71. ISBN
978-1-83881-806-7 (eBook) https://doi.org/10.5772/intechopen.79870
24. Garnier-Laplace J, Geras'kin S, Della-Vedova C et al (2013) Are radiosensitivity data derived
from natural field conditions consistent with data from controlled exposures? A case study
of Chernobyl wildlife chronically exposed to low dose rates. J Environ Radioact 121:12–21.
https://doi.org/10.1016/j.jenvrad.2012.01.013
25. Nohara C, Hiyama A, Taira W et al (2014) The biological impacts of ingested radioactive
materials on the pale grass blue butterfly. Sci Rep 4:4946. https://doi.org/10.1038/srep04946
26. Nohara C, Taira W, Hiyama A et al (2014) Ingestion of radioactively contaminated diets for two
generations in the pale grass blue butterfly. BMC Evol Biol 14:193. https://doi.org/10.1186/
s12862-014-0193-0
27. Taira W, Hiyama A, Nohara C et al (2015) Ingestional and transgenerational effects of the
Fukushima nuclear accident on the pale grass blue butterfly. J Radiat Res 56(Suppl 1):i2–i18.
https://doi.org/10.1093/jrr/rrv068
28. Gurung RD, Taira W, Sakauchi K et al (2019) Tolerance of high oral doses of nonradioactive
and radioactive caesium chloride in the pale grass blue butterfly *Zizeeria maha*. Insects 10:290.
https://doi.org/10.3390/insects10090290
29. Sakauchi K, Taira W, Toki M et al (2021) Nutrient imbalance of the host plant for larvae
of the pale grass blue butterfly may mediate the field effect of low-dose radiation exposure
in Fukushima: dose-dependent changes in the sodium content. Insects 12:149. https://doi.
org/10.3390/insects12020149
30. Sakauchi K, Taira W, Otaki JM (2022) Metabolomic profiles of the creeping wood sorrel *Oxalis
corniculata* in radioactively contaminated fields in Fukushima: dose-dependent changes in key
metabolites. Life 12:115. https://doi.org/10.3390/life12010115
31. Sakauchi K, Taira W, Otaki JM (2021) Metabolomic response of the creeping wood sorrel
Oxalis corniculata to low-dose radiation exposure from Fukushima's contaminated soil. Life
11:990. https://doi.org/10.3390/life11090990
32. Morita A, Sakauchi K, Taira W et al (2022) Ingestional toxicity of radiation-dependent metabolites of the host plant for the pale grass blue butterfly: a mechanism of field effects of radioactive pollution in Fukushima. Life 12:615. https://doi.org/10.3390/life12050615
33. Sakauchi K, Taira W, Toki M et al (2019) Overwintering states of the pale grass blue butterfly
Zizeeria maha (Lepidoptera: Lycaenidae) at the time of the Fukushima nuclear accident in
March 2011. Insects 10:389. https://doi.org/10.3390/insects10110389

34. International Atomic Energy Agency (IAEA) (2006) Environmental consequences of the Chernobyl accident and their remediation: twenty years of experience. Report of the Chernobyl Forum Expert Group 'Environment'. IAEA, Vienna
35. Sakauchi K, Otaki JM (2023) Imaging plate autoradiography for ingested anthropogenic cesium-137 in butterfly bodies: implications for the biological impacts of the Fukushima nuclear accident. Life 13:1211. https://doi.org/10.3390/life13051211

Chapter 14
Dose Estimation and Radiation Effects on Wild Medaka Around Fukushima Daiichi Nuclear Power Plant: A Review

Kouichi Maruyama

Abstract Medaka (*Oryzias latipes*) is a popular small aquarium pet fish in Japan, but it is also an experimental animal established and developed in Japan. Along with zebrafish, it has become an important model animal and is a powerful model vertebrate organism for developmental and molecular studies. Medaka has also been used to study the effects of radiation, and much work has been done using it. The radiosensitivity of medaka is approximately one-fifth that of mammals. The release of radionuclides from the Fukushima Daiichi Nuclear Power Plant (FNPP) accident in 2011 contaminated its surrounding area, and this contamination remains today in 2024. This review focuses on wild medaka living around FNPP and examines the following: (1) ambient dose rate of the habitat, (2) radioactivity concentration of the environmental media (medaka and sediment), (3) estimation of the absorbed dose from the environmental media using the Environmental Risk from Ionising Contaminants: Assessment and Management (ERICA) tool, (4) estimation of the exposure dose using dosimeters placed in the habitats, and (5) radiation effects using the micronucleus assay. Considering the radiosensitivity of medaka, estimated and measured absorbed doses, and actual effects, at present, no detectable radiation effects have been observed in wild medaka around FNPP.

Keywords Medaka · ERICA tool · Micronucleus assay · Radiosensitivity · Fukushima

K. Maruyama (✉)
Institute for Radiological Science, National Institutes for Quantum Science and Technology, Chiba, Japan
e-mail: maruyama.kouichi@qst.go.jp

© The Author(s) 2026

M. Fukumoto (ed.), *Low-Dose Radiation Effects on Animals and Ecosystems II*,
https://doi.org/10.1007/978-981-95-5559-8_14

14.1 Medaka: Characteristics and Basis as an Experimental Animal

Medaka is a small aquarium fish living in freshwater, and its species name is *Oryzias latipes*, which means a fish with a wide pelvic fin living in rice fields. Adult medaka are approximately 3 cm long and live in ponds, rice fields, streams, and reservoirs, forming schools. Wild medaka migrate in relatively shallow waters, feeding on plankton and small insects [1]. Its lifespan is about 2 years under laboratory conditions, while wild medaka have been reported to live for 1 year and a few months [2]. Wild medaka inhabit all parts of Japan except for Hokkaido, the northernmost part of the Japanese archipelago, and are categorized into 67 mitotypes and 15 subclades based on the cytochrome *b* partial sequence [3]. Medaka have been extensively studied in the fields of embryology, biology, behavioral ethology, and evolution, particularly with respect to sex determination and genome analyses [4–6].

14.2 Research on Radiation Effects on Medaka

Research on the effects of radiation on medaka has a long history, and a wide variety of data are available. A large-scale acute irradiation experiment was performed by Egami and Etoh to investigate the relationship between the radiation dose and survival days [7]. When medaka are exposed to 1,280 Gy, they die instantly due to the cessation of central nervous system functions. Exposure to 40–640 Gy causes death within 7–10 days from intestinal failure. Exposure to 20 Gy results in some deaths from anemia within 2 months. Exposure to <20 Gy has no detectable effects. The median lethal radiation dose is estimated to be 20–25 Gy, which is approximately one-fifth the sensitivity of mammals such as humans. A large-scale chronic irradiation experiment on medaka from the embryonic stage to adulthood in a gamma field showed that at 5 Gy/d, the lifespan of fish is shortened and all die before reaching adulthood, while at 1.3–2.4 Gy/d, individuals grow to adulthood but become sterile [8]. In internal exposure experiments, testicular atrophy is observed when adult males are kept in 18.5 GBq/L of tritiated water for 1 month [9]. To date, various studies on the effects of radiation have been conducted on medaka, and a large amount of data have been accumulated, such as age dependency [10], temperature dependency [11], late effects [12], and protective agents [13]. In addition, there are a number of well-known and established systems for detecting radiation effects using medaka: the specific-locus test system, micronucleus assay, brain cell death in embryos, and thymic atrophy [14–17]. Furthermore, radiosensitive mutant and *p53* knockout medaka are available [18, 19]. Radiation sensitivity is approximately one-fifth that of mammals, and the median lethal dose is 20–25 Gy, which is listed along with other experimental animals in the *Handbook of Scientific Tables* [20].

(Note: Old-style units used in cited papers have been unified to Système International d'unités (SI) units. 100 rad = 1 Gy. 1 Ci = 37 GBq.)

14.3   Collection of Wild Medaka

Around 40 years ago, wild populations of medaka were found in rice fields all over Japan and were easy to catch; however, in recent years, numbers have been markedly decreasing due to bank protection construction, pesticides, invasion by alien species, and changes in farming methods. Wild medaka were designated as Vulnerable level (VU) on the Japanese Ministry of the Environment's Red List in 1999 [21]. The area surrounding Fukushima Daiichi Nuclear Power Plant (FNPP) is largely rural with many rivers running through it, and forested areas to the west. We found a wild medaka habitat in two locations (S1 and S2) around FNPP and have been conducting surveys over time [22]. S1 is a stream located 4 km north-northwest of FNPP, and S2 is a reservoir located 7.5 km west-northwest of FNPP (Fig. 14.1).

Wild medaka were collected using scoop nets or four-armed fishing nets. The ambient dose rates at a height of 1 m above the ground at the shore of the sampling sites were measured by a NaI (TI) scintillation detector.

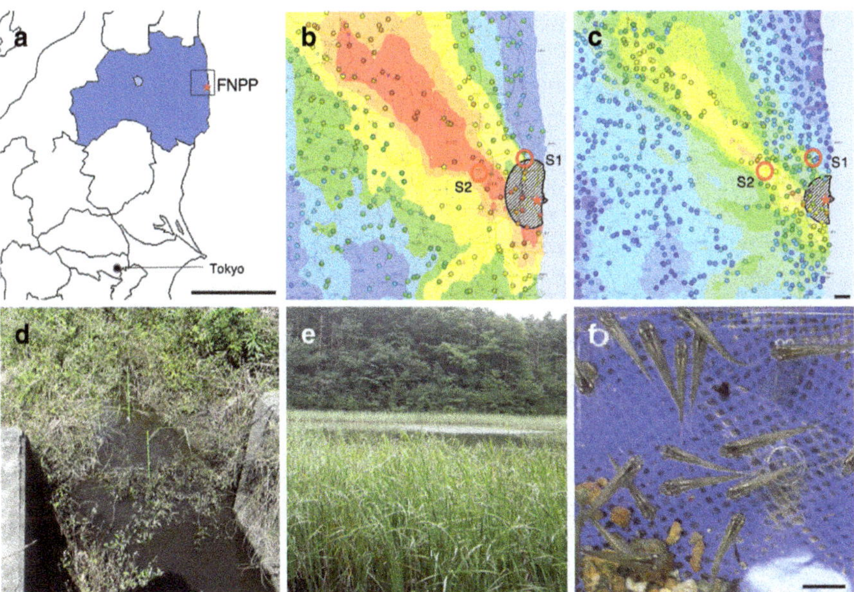

Fig. 14.1 Locations of S1 and S2, the survey sites, and collected medaka. (**a**) Map of Fukushima Prefecture and its surrounding areas. The area in blue represents Fukushima Prefecture. The star symbol indicates the location of FNPP. The symbol ◉ indicates the location of the Japanese capital, Tokyo. Scale bar: 100 km. (**b**) Enlarged map of the area around FNPP (boxed area in **a**). The colored area and spots represent the ambient dose rates: blue, 0–1.0 µSv/h; light blue, 1–1.9 µSv/h; yellowish green, 1.9–3.8 µSv/h; yellow, 3.8–9.5 µSv/h; orange, 9.5–19.0 µSv/h; and red, > 19.0 µSv/h. Shaded area: no survey results available. The small red circles, on the right and left, indicate S1 and S2, respectively. Scale bar: 2 km. This ambient dose rate map was produced using the database for radioactive substance monitoring data [23]. Monitoring was performed on April 29, 2011. (**c**) The same view as shown in **b** on October 29, 2020. (**d**) Scenery image at S1. (**e**) Scenery image at S2. The sight was from shore 3 in Fig. 14.3**b**. (**f**) Collected medaka. Scale bar: 1 cm.

14.3.1 Ambient Dose Rates at the Sampling Sites, S1 and S2

S1 is a narrow and shallow stream along a rice field located in Futaba Town. There are also houses and factories nearby. The stream is about 1 meter wide and about 20 cm deep (Fig. 14.1d). The ambient dose rate was 1.0 μSv/h in 2012. After that, it gradually decreased to 0.09 μSv/h in 2021 (Fig. 14.1b, c). S2 is a reservoir surrounded by hills and forests in Namie Town. It is roughly the same size as a soccer field and is more than 2 m deep. To reach S2, one must go down a 10-meter cliff from the road (Figs. 14.1e and 14.3b). The ambient dose rate was 25 μSv/h in 2012 and subsequently decreased every year, reaching 4.82 μSv/h in 2021, which is approximately one-fifth of the value 10 years ago.

14.3.2 Radioactivity Concentration of Environmental Media

The collected medaka and bottom sediments at S1 and S2 have been measured for radioactive cesium (^{134}Cs + ^{137}Cs) concentration since 2012. Regarding bottom sediment, the surface of the sediment (mud) was collected up to a depth of about 2 cm.

At S1, radioactive Cs concentration in medaka ranged from 19.1 to 90 Bq/kg (wet weight) between 2012 and 2014 (Fig. 14.2). As the value was so low, no further measurement has been performed since then. Radioactive Cs concentration in the sediment ranged from 2,968 to 15,896 Bq/kg between 2012 and 2014, but the value in a sample taken in 2021 had significantly decreased to 1,160 Bq/kg. Since S1 is a stream, there is always a flow, and it is considered that the radioactive Cs on the ground surface has been washed away.

At S2, radioactive Cs concentration of medaka ranged from 201.3 to 3,966.6 Bq/ kg from 2012 to 2014 and gradually decreased to 72.8 Bq/kg in 2021. Radioactive Cs concentration in sediment collected at S2 was extremely high, ranging from 244,169 to 661,520 Bq/kg from 2012 to 2014, but it decreased to 76,690 Bq/kg in 2021 (Fig. 14.2c).

14.3.3 Estimation of Absorbed Dose Rates by the ERICA Assessment Tool

The ERICA assessment tool (ERICA = <u>E</u>nvironmental <u>R</u>isk from <u>I</u>onising <u>C</u>ontaminants: <u>A</u>ssessment and Management) is absorbed dose rate estimation software developed by the European Atomic Energy Community and is freely available to anyone [24]. This software allows estimation of internal and external absorbed dose rates by inputting radioactivity concentrations of sediment, water, environmental media, and several parameters [25]. Table 14.1 shows the estimated absorbed dose rates (sum of internal and external dose rates) obtained by inputting

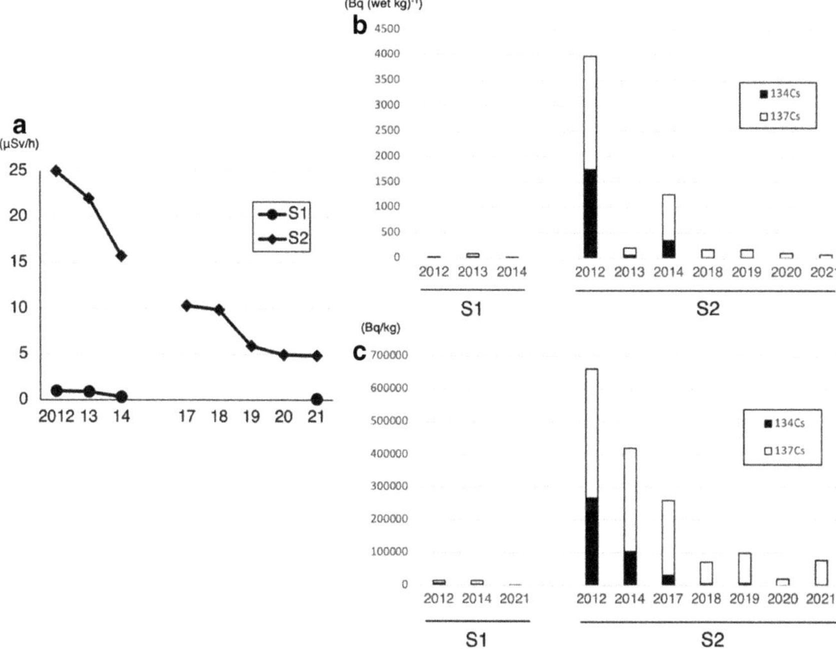

Fig. 14.2 Ambient dose rate and ^{134}Cs and ^{137}Cs concentration in medaka and sediment. (**a**) The transition in ambient dose rate for S1 and S2 from 2012 to 2021. (**b, c**) The transition of ^{134}Cs and ^{137}Cs concentration in medaka and sediment from 2012 to 2021.

radioactivity concentrations of medaka and sediments collected from 2012 to 2021 into the ERICA tool [22].

14.3.4 *In Situ Measurement of External Dose Rate*

Glass dosimeters (GD-302 M, AGC Techno Glass Corporation, Japan) were water-proofed with plastic film and placed with rods overnight to measure external dose rates at locations where wild medaka populations were living [22]. Absorbed dose was obtained by multiplying the calculated air kerma by a factor of 1.103, which is the average ratio of the mass energy absorption coefficients of human muscle to those of air. At S1, glass dosimeters were placed on the water surface and at the stream bottom (approximately 20 cm deep) (Fig. 14.3a). External dose rate measured in 2021 was 0.27 ± 0.02 µGy/h, and no significant difference was observed between the dose rates at the surface and the bottom of the water. At S2, field measurements were performed four times from 2017 to 2021. S2 was a large reservoir with many small plants on the west side, where medaka fry were found (dark gray in Fig. 14.3b). On the north and east sides, the terrain was clay-like and steep, and no individuals were found. On the west and south sides, reeds were abundant and

Table 14.1 Ambient dose rates, estimated absorbed dose rates by ERICA tool, and external dose rates in situ at S1 and S2.

Site	Date	Ambient dose rate (μSv/h)	ERICA estimated absorbed dose rate (μGy/h)	In situ external dose rate[a] (μGy/h) Fry (15–30 cm) Point 1–4	Adult (30–60 cm) Point 1–5	Total (15–60 cm) Point 1	Total (15–60 cm) Point 4	Total (15–60 cm) Point 1–5
S1	2012.05.08	1.0	0.74	–				
	2013.11.06	0.9	0.21	–				
	2014.08.07	0.35	0.63	–				
	2021.10.22	0.09	0.06	0.27 ± 0.02 (n = 8; 0.25–0.3)				
S2	2012.05.08	25.0	48.2					
	2013.11.06	22.0	15.5					
	2014.08.07	15.7	44.3					
	2017.09.05	10.3	16.7	3.81 ± 2.59 (n = 16; 1.9–11.8)	3.07 ± 2.45 (n = 25; 1.2–11.8)	2.66 ± 0.98 (n = 7; 1.3–4.0)	5.79 ± 3.81 (n = 7; 1.4–11.8)	3.21 ± 2.32 (n = 35; 1.2–11.8)
	2018.10.05	9.84	3.62	2.73 ± 1.4 (n = 16; 0.9–6.0)	2.25 ± 1.4 (n = 25; 0.8–7.8)	2.31 ± 0.99 (n = 7; 0.8–3.8)	3.73 ± 2.17 (n = 7; 1.5–7.8)	2.66 ± 1.55 (n = 35; 0.8–7.8)
	2019.10.10	5.87	5.19					
	2020.10.20	4.91	1.39	2.00 ± 1.06 (n = 16; 0.8–4.6)	1.75 ± 1.43 (n = 25; 0.5–7.5)	1.43 ± 0.48 (n = 7; 0.5–1.9)	3.38 ± 2.04 (n = 7; 1.5–7.5)	1.84 ± 1.35 (n = 35; 0.5–7.5)
	2021.10.21	4.82	3.78	2.83 ± 1.74 (n = 16; 1.3–8.2)	1.97 ± 1.24 (n = 25; 0.5–7.0)	1.74 ± 0.48 (n = 7; 0.8–2.6)	3.1 ± 2.15 (n = 7; 1.3–7.0)	2.59 ± 1.89 (n = 35; 0.7–8.2)
				Average		2.04 ± 0.91 (n = 28; 0.5–4.0)	4.0 ± 2.85 (n = 28; 1.3–11.8)	2.58 ± 1.88 (n = 140; 0.5–11.8)

[a]Mean ± SD. Number of measurement points and ranges are shown in parentheses

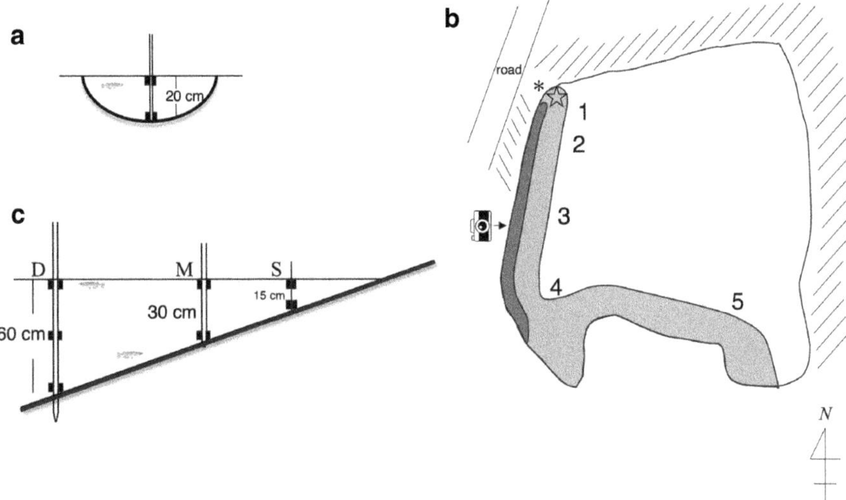

Fig. 14.3 Schematic drawing of the in situ measurement and S2 reservoir. (**a**) Schematic drawing of the in situ measurement at S1. Small black boxes represent glass dosimeters. (**b**) Schematic drawing of the S2 reservoir. The shaded lines indicate cliffs. The eye and arrow indicate the view in Fig. 14.1e. * and ☆ indicate the points where ambient dose rate was measured and sediment was collected, respectively. The numbers represent the points where the glass dosimeters were set. Dark gray color shows where medaka fry were seen. Light gray color indicates where the adult medaka school migrated. (**c**) Schematic drawing of the in situ measurement in S2. A rod with glass dosimeter was installed offshore from the location indicated by the numbers. D, M, and S indicate deep, medium, and shallow, respectively (Modified from Ref. [22]).

many large schools of adult medaka were found migrating (gray in Fig. 14.3b). We selected five points (Points 1–5) inhabited by wild populations and measured the external dose rate at three different depths: deep (D) = 60 cm, median (M) = 30 cm, and shallow (S) = 15 cm below the surface (Fig. 14.3c). The highest dose rate was obtained at Point 4 on the west side of the reservoir, with an average value of 4.0 ± 2.85 μGy/h from 2017 to 2021, which was more than twice as high as that at Point 1 (2.04 ± 0.91 μGy/h) (Table 14.1). The reason for this was likely due to the presence of many shallow areas with abundant mud in the vicinity of Point 4. At the same point, a depth dependency of dose rate was observed, in the order of S (3.37 ± 1.91 μGy/h) > M (2.31 ± 1.7) > D (2.23 ± 1.82) (Table 14.2). Dose rate was higher at the shallow shore and decreased as the position deepened. Regarding the external dose rate at D (Points 1–5), the following order was generally observed: bottom (3.53 ± 2.5 μGy/h) > water surface (2.1 ± 0.62) > middle (1.05 ± 0.42) (Table 14.2). At the bottom, the dose rate was the highest due to γ-irradiation from radioactive Cs in the ground mud. The external dose rate at the water surface was attributed to γ-rays from the surrounding slope soil. The lowest value in the middle of the rod was due to the shielding effect of water. At M and S, external dose rate was higher at the bottom than at the water surface (M: bottom [2.52 ± 2.3

Table 14.2 External dose rates measured in situ from different depths at S2.

Date	in situ external dose rate[a] (μGy/h)									
	D Bottom	D Middle	D Surface	M Bottom	M Surface	S Bottom	S Surface	S Point 1–5	M Point 1–5	D Point 1–5
2017.09.05	4.77 ± 2.65 ($n = 5$; 1.3–9.3)	1.31 ± 0.1 ($n = 5$; 1.2–1.4)	2.23 ± 0.53 ($n = 5$; 1.6–2.9)	4.23 ± 3.81 ($n = 5$; 1.7–11.8)	2.82 ± 0.42 ($n = 5$; 2.1–3.4)	3.39 ± 2.64 ($n = 5$; 1.9–8.7)	3.72 ± 0.61 ($n = 5$; 3.2–4.8)	3.56 ± 1.92 ($n = 10$; 1.9–8.7)	3.52 ± 2.8 ($n = 10$; 1.7–11.8)	2.77 ± 2.14 ($n = 15$; 1.2–9.3)
2018.10.05	3.64 ± 2.24 ($n = 5$; 1.0–7.8)	1.01 ± 0.27 ($n = 5$; 0.8–1.5)	2.7 ± 0.26 ($n = 5$; 2.4–3.1)	1.75 ± 0.68 ($n = 5$; 0.9–2.7)	2.14 ± 0.49 ($n = 5$; 1.7–2.8)	4.21 ± 1.7 ($n = 5$; 1.6–6.0)	3.2 ± 0.73 ($n = 5$; 2.0–4.0)	3.7 ± 1.4 ($n = 10$; 1.6–6.0)	1.95 ± 0.63 ($n = 10$; 0.9–2.8)	2.45 ± 1.7 ($n = 15$; 0.8–7.8)
2020.10.20	3.11 ± 2.33 ($n = 5$; 0.6–7.5)	0.78 ± 0.46 ($n = 5$; 0.5–1.7)	1.61 ± 0.33 ($n = 5$; 1.0–1.9)	1.76 ± 1.23 ($n = 5$; 0.6–4.1)	1.48 ± 0.34 ($n = 5$; 0.8–1.8)	2.19 ± 1.45 ($n = 5$; 0.8–4.6)	1.98 ± 0.4 ($n = 5$; 1.7–2.7)	2.08 ± 1.06 ($n = 10$; 0.8–4.6)	1.62 ± 0.92 ($n = 10$; 0.6–4.1)	1.83 ± 1.69 ($n = 15$; 0.5–7.5)
2021.10.21	2.6 ± 2.24 ($n = 5$; 0.7–7.0)	1.12 ± 0.53 ($n = 5$; 0.5–1.9)	1.84 ± 0.63 ($n = 5$; 0.7–2.6)	2.35 ± 0.79 ($n = 5$; 1.3–3.2)	1.96 ± 0.35 ($n = 5$; 1.3–2.3)	5.41 ± 2.47 ($n = 5$; 1.7–8.2)	2.83 ± 0.75 ($n = 5$; 1.9–4.0)	4.12 ± 2.33 ($n = 10$; 1.7–8.2)	2.16 ± 0.64 ($n = 10$; 1.3–3.2)	1.85 ± 1.5 ($n = 15$; 0.5–7.0)
Average (2017–2021)	3.53 ± 2.5 ($n = 20$; 0.6–9.3)	1.05 ± 0.42 ($n = 20$; 0.5–1.9)	2.1 ± 0.62 ($n = 20$; 0.7–3.1)	2.52 ± 2.3 ($n = 20$; 0.6–11.8)	2.1 ± 0.63 ($n = 20$; 0.8–3.4)	3.8 ± 2.47 ($n = 20$; 0.8–8.7)	2.93 ± 0.9 ($n = 20$; 1.7–4.8)	3.37 ± 1.91 ($n = 40$; 0.8–8.7)	2.31 ± 1.7 ($n = 40$; 0.6–11.8)	2.23 ± 1.82 ($n = 60$; 0.5–9.3)

[a]Mean $\pm$ SD. Number of measurement points and ranges are shown in parentheses

µGy/h] > surface [2.1 ± 0.63]; S: bottom [3.8 ± 2.47 µGy/h] > surface [2.93 ± 0.9]). External dose rates were measured four times over a 5-year period. Most of the values obtained decreased annually, with some exceptions, which could be due to several reasons. The measurement site was selected based on the water level, which changed every year; therefore, the site was not exactly at the same place each year. Furthermore, natural disasters, such as typhoons or heavy rain, generally caused mud mixing and led to changes in the components of mud.

14.3.5   Radiation Effects on Wild Medaka Evaluated by Micronucleus Assay

Wild medaka were collected from S1 and S2, and the effect of radiation was examined by the micronucleus assay in gill cells [26]. As a negative control, we used the micronucleated cells (MNCs) frequency in reared medaka (Hd-rR inbred strain) without irradiation. Furthermore, as a positive control, we analyzed the MNCs frequency of medaka irradiated with X-rays between 0.1 and 2 Gy. At 0.1 Gy, the MNCs frequency was not significantly different from the negative control, whereas at 0.5 Gy or higher doses, significant differences from the control were observed (Fig. 14.4). The MNCs frequency increased dose-dependently between 0.5 and 2 Gy. The MNCs frequency of wild medaka collected from 2013 to 2017 in both S1 and S2 was not different from the non-irradiated medaka.

14.3.6   Estimation of Exposure Dose and Radiation Effects in Fukushima Wild Medaka

Medaka is one of the ideal species for estimating exposed radiation doses relating to the FNPP accident due to the facts that: (1) wild populations inhabit areas around the FNPP, (2) they are similar in size and weight, (3) their behavior and habitat have been clarified, (4) their lifespan is short and stable (1 year and a few months), and (5) experimental data on the effects of radiation on medaka are abundant. In this study, we used three approaches/methods to estimate the exposure dose in wild medaka. The first was the ambient dose rate, which is simple and quick to measure but differs from the actual dose rate that wild populations were exposed to. The second was estimation by the ERICA tool, with dose calculated from environmental media, and this could be used to estimate both internal and external doses. The last was in situ measurement, which measured the dose in the place where individuals were actually present and was considered to be accurate. However, it was not possible to measure internal exposure.

Ambient dose rate at S1 decreased from 1.0 to 0.09 µSv/h from 2012 to 2021. Similarly, the ERICA tool estimate also decreased from 0.74 to 0.06 µGy/h. The in

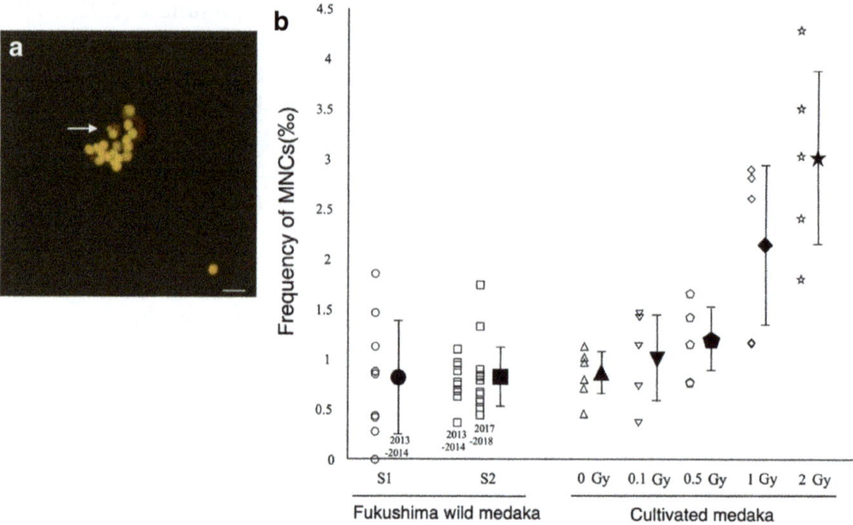

Fig. 14.4 Micronucleus assay. (**a**) Acridine orange-stained gill cells of medaka. The arrow indicates a micronucleus in a cell. The bar represents 10 μm. (**b**) Frequency of micronucleated cells (MNCs) in Fukushima wild and cultivated medaka populations. Wild populations were collected from S1 and S2. The cultivated ones were non-irradiated (0 Gy) or X-ray irradiated (0.1–2 Gy). Each open symbol represents an individual medaka. Closed symbols with vertical bars indicate the average frequency (with standard deviation) of MNCs in each group (Modified from Ref. [26]).

situ dose rate, measured only once in 2021, was 0.27 ± 0.02 μGy/h, which was higher than both the ambient dose rate and the ERICA tool estimate (Table 14.1). This discrepancy was likely due to the fact that the in situ measurement was performed close to the ground and surrounded by concrete revetment walls (Fig. 14.1d). All values were generally low and less than 1 μGy/h. We attempted to calculate the lifetime exposure dose at S1. It is reported that the average lifespan of wild medaka is 1 year and a few months [2]. However, to take considerations about the assurance, the lifetime exposure dose was calculated assuming a lifespan of 2 years. Using the highest ERICA tool value of 0.74 μGy/h at S1, the lifetime cumulative dose was estimated to be 12.96 mGy/life (0.74 [μGy/h] × 24 [hours] × 365 [days] × 2 [years] ÷ 1000 = 12.96 mGy). At S2, from 2012 to 2021, the ambient dose rate decreased from 25.0 to 4.82 μSv/h, and the dose rate estimated using the ERICA tool decreased from 48.2 to 3.78 μGy/h. In situ dose rate decreased from 3.21 ± 2.32 to 2.59 ± 1.89 μGy/h. The ambient dose rate decreased to about one-fifth in 10 years, the ERICA tool value has fluctuated, and the in situ value remained relatively stable for only 5 years after 2017 (Table 14.1).

Furthermore, in order to accurately compare the dose rate values from these three approaches, we focused on Point 1 from in situ data (Table 14.1). Because the ambient dose rate was measured on the shore around Point 1 (* in Fig. 14.3b), and the sediment for measurement in situ was also obtained around Point 1 (star in

Fig. 14.3b). Radioactive Cs concentration of the sediment is the most effective factor for the ERICA tool. As a result, the order of the calculated values of dose rate was as follows: ambient dose rate > ERICA > in situ. The reason for the difference between the ambient dose rate and the dose rate estimated by ERICA was considered to be that estimates by the ERICA tool is highly dependent on radioactive Cs concentration in the sediment.

From 2012 to 2021, radioactive Cs concentration in the sediment decreased by about one-tenth (Fig. 14.2c), and the dose rate estimated by the ERICA tool decreased accordingly. The values calculated by the ERICA tool were higher during 2012–14, and the ambient dose rates were higher after 2018. In addition, the reason why the ambient dose rate was higher than the in situ dose rate is thought to be due to the influence of the surrounding soil, since S2 is surrounded by hills. In fact, radioactive Cs concentration of the surrounding soil was markedly higher than that of the sediment in the reservoir. Of the three approaches for estimating exposure doses, the most reliable was the in situ measurement, which showed lower values. These findings suggest that the use of ambient dose rates and the ERICA tool may overestimate the exposure dose to aquatic organisms. We attempted to calculate the lifetime exposure dose to medaka at S2. Using the highest value of 48.2 µGy/h among the values evaluated by the ERICA tool, the lifetime cumulative external exposure dose to medaka at S2 was estimated to be 844.46 mGy/life (48.2 [µGy/h] × 24 [hours] × 365 [days] × 2 [years] ÷ 1000 = 844.46 mGy). In considering whether there was a possibility of radiation effect on medaka, it was very important to estimate the highest dose rate at S2 after the FNPP accident in March 2011. As the area around FNPP was off-limits, very little research had been done. A study on a pond in Namie, the same town as S2, about 24 km from FNPP and 16 km from S2, reported that the ambient dose rate was 19.6 ± 0.7 µGy/h on May 20, 2011. On March 29, 2012, the dose rate was 16.5 ± 0.9 µGy/h, a decrease of about 15% [27]. Adding 15% to the highest value (48.2 µGy/h) gave an estimated dose rate of 55.4 µGy/h 1 year after the accident, and this value was used to evaluate the possibility of radiation effects. The actual radiation exposure may be much lower than this theoretical value because radiation levels in the S2 reservoir were high in some areas and low in others, and wild medaka always migrate in groups.

A previous study reported that the frequency of abnormal chromosomes in lymphocytes was slightly higher in wild mice near FNPP than in mice in a uncontaminated control area in 2012 and 2014 [28]. The estimated absorbed dose rates at these times were 117.5 and 61.3 µGy/h, respectively. Five years after the FNPP accident, in 2016, the frequency of abnormal chromosomes returned to the non-irradiated control level, and the estimated absorbed dose rate was 33.8 µGy/h [29]. Overall, the dose rate in mice was higher than that in medaka in the present study. Medaka are much less sensitive to radiation than mice (median lethal dose [LD$_{50}$] for medaka: 20–25 Gy; mice: 5–7 Gy) [20]. The value of LD$_{50}$ is generally determined by body temperature and genome size. Medaka is a poikilotherm, and its genome size is about one-third that of a mouse. Furthermore, considering that radiation dose rate in the habitats of medaka was lower than that of mice, it is unlikely that clear effects of radiation can be detected in medaka. We showed that the frequency of MNCs in wild medaka collected at S1 from 2013 to 2014 and further at S2 from 2017 to 2018 did not significantly differ from that of non-irradiated medaka (Fig. 14.4). These findings suggest that wild medaka have not experienced biologically meaningful cytogenetic damage. A proteomics study reported that the protein profile of adult medaka continuously irradiated with a dose of 94 µGy/h for 190 days differs from that of non-irradiated control medaka [30]. The maximum value estimated after the FNPP accident was 55.4 µGy/h, and if wild medaka populations were to continue to be exposed to these levels of radiation, there may be some changes in gene expression levels, but no serious effects were anticipated. Therefore, based on the estimated dose, it is considered that there were no significant radiation-induced effects on wild medaka due to the FNPP accident.

14.4 Future Studies

We recently initiated a new study. In the S2 reservoir, radioactive Cs concentration in medaka remains significantly high, which may be attributed to the bioaccumulation of radioactive Cs through the consumption of plankton and small insects by medaka. To investigate the mechanisms underlying the transfer of radioactive Cs from soil to medaka, we are conducting an experiment by placing radioactive Cs-contaminated soil, zooplankton, phytoplankton, and medaka in a tank and examining the processes by which radioactive Cs is transferred through the ecosystem. The results obtained may provide insights into the mechanisms underlying the transition of radioactive Cs in the future.

Acknowledgments This work was partially supported by the commissioned research fund provided by F-REI (JPFR24050401) and a Grant-in-Aid for Scientific Research (C) from the Japan Society for the Promotion of Science [number: 24K15300].

References

1. Terao O (1985) The habits of wild medaka (in Japanese). Iden 8:47–50
2. Egami N, Terao O, Iwao Y (1988) The life span of wild populations of the fish *Oryzias latipes* under natural conditions. Zool Sci 5:1149–1152
3. Takehana Y, Nagai N, Matsuda M et al (2003) Geographic variation and diversity of the cytochrome b gene in Japanese wild populations of medaka, *Oryzias latipes*. Zool Sci 20:1279–1291. https://doi.org/10.2108/zsj.20.1279
4. Wittbrodt J, Shima A, Schartl M (2002) Medaka—a model organism from the far east. Nat Rev Genet 3:53–64. https://doi.org/10.1038/nrg704
5. Kasahara M, Naruse K, Sasaki S et al (2007) The medaka draft genome and insights into vertebrate genome evolution. Nature 447(7145):714–719. https://doi.org/10.1038/nature05846
6. Matsuda M, Nagahama Y, Shinomiya A et al (2002) DMY is a Y-specific DM-domain gene required for male development in the medaka fish. Nature:559–563. https://doi.org/10.1038/nature751

7. Egami N, Etoh H (1962) Dose-survival time relationship and protective action of reserpine against X-irradiation in the fish. Ann Zool Jpn 35(4):188–198
8. Egami N (1979) Radiation effects on life span of the fish, *Oryzias latipes*. Excerpta Med:431–432
9. Hyodo-Taguchi Y, Egami N (1977) Damage to spermatogenic cells in fish kept in tritiated water. Radiat Res:641–652. https://doi.org/10.2307/3574632
10. Hyodo-Taguchi Y, Egami N (1969) Change in dose-survival time relationship after X-irradiation during embryonic development in the fish, *Oryzias latipes*. J Radiat Res 10:121–125
11. Etoh H, Egami N (1965) Effect of temperature on survival period of the fish, *Oryzias latipes*, following irradiation with different X-ray doses. Ann Zool Jpn 38(3):114–121
12. Egami N, Etoh H (1973) Effect of x-irradiation during embryonic stage in life span in the fish, *Oryzias latipes*. Exp Geron 8(4):219–222
13. Egami N (1969) Temperature effect on protective action by cysteamine against X-rays in the fish, *Oryzias latipes*. Int J Radiat Biol 15(4):393–394
14. Shima A, Shimada A (1991) Development of a possible nonmammalian test system for radiation-induced germ-cell mutagenesis using a fish, the Japanese medaka (*Oryzias latipes*). Proc Natl Acad Sci USA 88:2545–2549. https://doi.org/10.1073/pnas.88.6.2545
15. Takai A, Kagawa N, Fujikawa K (2004) Dose- and time-dependent responses for micronucleus induction by X–rays and fast neutrons in gill cells of medaka (*Oryzias latipes*). Environ Mol Mutagen 44:108–112. https://doi.org/10.1002/em.20042
16. Yasuda T, Yoshimoto M, Maeda K et al (2008) Rapid and simple method for quantitative evaluation of neurocytotoxic effects of radiation on developing medaka brain. J Radiat Res 49(5):533–540. https://doi.org/10.1269/jrr.0617
17. Maruyama K, Iwanami N, Maruyama-Hayakawa T et al (2019) Small fish model for quantitative analysis of radiation effects using visualized thymus responses in GFP transgenic medaka. Int J Radiat Biol 95(8):1144–1149. https://doi.org/10.1080/09553002.2019.1589019
18. Aizawa K, Mitani H, Kogure N et al (2004) Identification of radiation-sensitive mutants in the medaka, *Oryzias latipes*. Mech Dev 121(7–8):895–902. https://doi.org/10.1016/j.mod.2004.04.002
19. Taniguchi Y, Takeda S, Furutani-Seiki M et al (2006) Generation of medaka gene knockout models by target-selected mutagenesis. Genome Biol 7(12):R116. https://doi.org/10.1186/gb-2006-7-12-r116
20. Handbook of scientific tables (2022) National astronomical observatory of Japan. Maruzen Publishing Ltd, Tokyo. ISBN 978-981-3278-51-6
21. Publication of Red List 2020 of the Ministry of the Environment, Japan. https://www.env.go.jp/en/press/107905_00001.html. Accessed 18 Nov 2024
22. Maruyama K, Wang B, Watanabe Y (2023) Dose estimation to wild medaka around Fukushima Dai-ichi nuclear power plant. Radiat Protect Dosi 199(10):1110–1119. https://doi.org/10.1093/rpd/ncad140
23. Japan atomic energy agency database for radioactive substance monitoring data. https://emdb.jaea.go.jp/emdb/. Accessed 18 Nov 2024
24. ERICA HP. https://erica-tool.com. Accessed 18 Nov 2024
25. Brown JE, Alfonso B, Avila R et al (2008) The ERICA tool. J Environ Radioact 99:1371–1383. https://doi.org/10.1016/i.jenvrad.2008.01.008
26. Maruyama K, Wang B, Doi K et al (2021) Radiation effects on wild medaka around Fukushima dai-ichi nuclear power plant assessed by micronucleus assay. J Radiat Res 62:79–78. https://doi.org/10.1093/jrr/rraa116
27. Fuma S, Ihara S, Kawaguchi I et al (2015) Dose-rate estimation of the Tohoku hynobiid salamander, *Hynobius lichenatus*, in Fukushima. J Environ Radioact 143:123–134. https://doi.org/10.1016/j.jenvrad.2015.02.020
28. Kubota Y, Tsuji H, Kawagoshi T et al (2015) Chromosomal aberrations in wild mice captured in areas differentially contaminated by the Fukushima dai-ichi nuclear power plant accident. Environ Sci Technol 49:10074–10083. https://doi.org/10.1021/acs.est.5b01554

29. Shiomi N, Takahashi H, Watanabe Y et al (2022) Chromosomal aberrations in large Japanese field mice (*Apodemus speciosus*) captured in various periods after Fukushima dai-ichi nuclear power plant accident. Radiat Res 198(4):347–356. https://doi.org/10.1667/RADE-21-00162.1
30. Perez-Gelvez YNC, Camus AC, Bridger R et al (2021) Effects of chronic exposure to low levels of IR on medaka (*Oryzias latipes*): proteomic and bioinformatic approach. Int J Radiat Biol 97:1485–1501. https://doi.org/10.1080/09553002.2021.1962570

Chapter 15
Current Status of Long-Term Low-Dose-Rate Radiation Exposure to Masu Salmon (*Oncorhynchus masou*) in Two Rivers Flowing Near Fukushima Daiichi Nuclear Power Plant

Shuhei Naganuma, Gyoh Kawada, Megu Ohtaki, and Masamichi Nakajima

Abstract The Fukushima Daiichi Nuclear Power Plant (FNPP) accident, induced by the Great East Japan Earthquake on March 11, 2011, resulted in extensive contamination of the surrounding environment with radioactive materials. In particular, the forest ecosystem northwest of FNPP in Fukushima Prefecture has been significantly affected, highlighting the need for regular assessment of the status of fish species residing in the rivers running through the contaminated area. This study reports on radioactive cesium-137 (^{137}Cs) concentrations measured in masu salmon in 2014, 2021, 2022, and 2023. Also, the abundance of melanomacrophage centers (MMCs) in the spleen was measured to assess the current status, that is, changes in pollution and its effects on freshwater fish. The results indicate that contamination persists even 12 years after the accident and fish appear to be suffering from the effect of long-term radiation exposure. Correlations between the contamination status of fish at the time of monitoring (2014, 2021, 2023) and the relative area occupied by MMCs in the spleen imply that the increase of MMCs in the spleen was probably caused by long-term low-dose-rate radiation exposure, and therefore MMCs are a candidate biomarker of radiocontamination.

Keywords Masu salmon · Melanomacrophage centers (MMCs) ·
Radioactive cesium

S. Naganuma · M. Nakajima (✉)
Tohoku University Graduate School of Agricultural Science, Aoba-ku, Sendai, Miyagi, Japan
e-mail: masamichi.nakajima.b6@tohoku.ac.jp

G. Kawada
Fukushima Prefectual Inland Water Fisheries Experimental Station, Inawashiro, Yama, Fukushima, Japan

M. Ohtaki
The Center for Peace, Hiroshima University, Hiroshima, Japan

M. Fukumoto (ed.), *Low-Dose Radiation Effects on Animals and Ecosystems II*,
https://doi.org/10.1007/978-981-95-5559-8_15

15.1   Introduction

Following the earthquake and subsequent tsunami that occurred on March 11, 2011, off the Pacific coast of Tohoku, an accident at the Fukushima Daiichi Nuclear Power Plant (FNPP) resulted in the release of large amounts of radioactive materials, which settled on the ground surface in the vicinity of FNPP [1].

Approximately 70% of the area of Fukushima Prefecture is covered by forest. A survey in the Bavarian region of Germany conducted after the Chernobyl (Chornobyl) Nuclear Power Plant accident found that soil inventory of radioactive cesium (^{134}Cs + ^{137}Cs) per unit area was 30% higher in forests than in grasslands [2]. It was shown that ^{137}Cs deposited on the surface of trees in Fukushima migrates over time to the forest floor through defoliation and death, and some of it is absorbed back into the surrounding trees [3]. In the 8 years after the FNPP accident, the amount of ^{137}Cs released from the forest through rivers is estimated to be about 4.8% of the total amount deposited there [4]. These results suggest that the contamination of forests by radioactive materials is likely to be prolonged.

Masu salmon (*Oncorhynchus masou*) is a freshwater salmonid fish widely distributed in Japan. In Fukushima Prefecture, masu salmon and used to be a popular target of mountain stream fishing. They inhabit the upper reaches of rivers that run through forests. Following the FNPP accident, they were widely regulated for human consumption, and restrictions remained in place until 2022 even in Gunma Prefecture, more than 200 km away from FNPP [5]. In a monitoring survey for 16 species of fish in the inland waters of Fukushima Prefecture between 2011 and 2014, a maximum value of 18,700 Bq kg^{-1} wet weight of radioactive cesium was observed in masu salmon in 2012 [6]. It is considered that radioactive Cs in the environment is transferred to stream fish mainly through the insects on which they feed, thereby contaminating them [7]. These findings suggest that masu salmon, in particular, is a species that requires monitoring over a long period.

Since 2014, we have been conducting studies on masu salmon in two water systems, Ukedo and Mano Rivers in Fukushima Prefecture, and, as a control, Hirose River in Miyagi Prefecture away from FNPP (Fig. 15.1). In Ukedo and Mano Rivers, ^{137}Cs concentration in masu salmon muscle was high, accompanied by a positive correlation with the mitochondrial DNA mutation rate [8].

Melanomacrophage centers (MMCs) are aggregates of highly pigmented phagocytes observed in the kidney, spleen, and liver of fish. MMCs are thought to have physiological functions in the immune response, including phagocytosis of unnecessary substances and cells, especially exhausted red blood cells [9]. MMCs are easily identifiable under a microscope and can be quantified using several indices such as area ratio, number per unit and size per unit. MMCs are present in a wide range of fish species and fluctuate in response to environmental stress [10], making them increasingly useful as biomarkers. For example, it has been reported that the number of MMCs per unit area increases with decreasing dissolved oxygen levels [11] and increasing rearing density in fish [12].

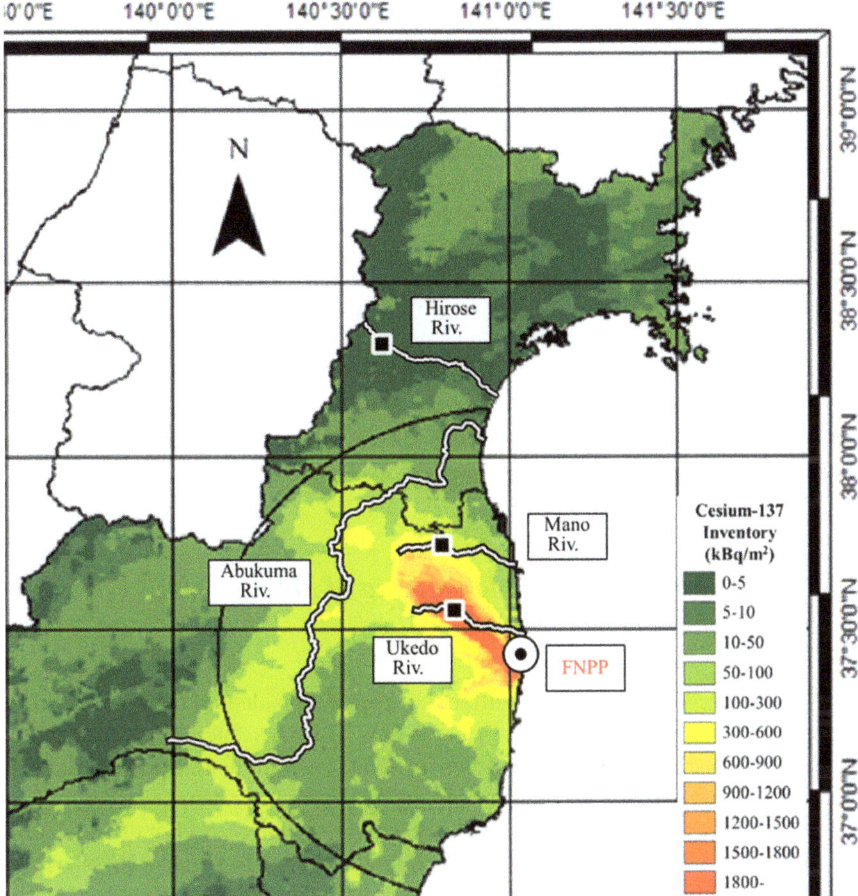

Fig. 15.1 Initial deposition of ^{137}Cs from the FNPP accident in Fukushima Prefecture and surrounding areas and in the rivers where samples were taken. Squares indicate sampling points and the concentric circles indicate FNPP (Modified from Ref [29]). Abukuma River meanders through a number of different areas and was not sampled in the present study.

The purpose of this study is to clarify the current ^{137}Cs contamination status of rivers near FNPP more than 10 years after its accident and its impact on masu salmon that inhabit there. For this purpose, we measured ^{137}Cs concentrations in masu salmon and river sediments and investigated whether long-term low-dose-rate radiation exposure can be monitored by %MMC. Furthermore, by comparing the latest results with those from the 2014 survey, we assessed the change in contamination status over time and the impact of long-term low-dose-rate radiation exposure on fish.

15.2   Materials and Methods

15.2.1   *Materials*

Specimens of *Oncorhynchus masou* (Brevoort, 1856) were sampled using angling and casting nets between June and September of 2014, August and October of 2021, June and October of 2022, and March and October of 2023 in three rivers: Ukedo River and Mano River in Fukushima Prefecture and Hirose River (as unpolluted control) in Miyagi Prefecture. Sampling sites were set up at one fixed point in each river, located 26 km (Ukedo River), 42 km (Mano River), and 106 km (Hirose River) from FNPP, respectively (Fig. 15.1). Spleens of the collected fish were removed, and the spleen-removed fish bodies were frozen for ^{137}Cs measurements. River sediments at each sampling site were collected concurrently, dried overnight at 56 °C and subsequently analyzed for ^{137}Cs concentration. The length of the fish body was measured from the tip of the upper jaw to the base of the caudal fin, which was defined as the standard length (SL).

15.2.2   *Measurement of Relative Area of MMCs in the Spleen (%MMC)*

Half of the spleens were fixed in buffered 4% paraformaldehyde, followed by rinsing and dehydration in ethanol and storage at 4 °C until sectioning. Subsequently, the spleens were embedded in paraffin using conventional methods, and serial sections at 5 μm were prepared and stained with hematoxylin and eosin (H&E).

Ten randomly selected images from the spleen section of each individual were taken at 100× magnification using a DP74 digital camera attached to a BX60 optical microscope (Olympus, Tokyo, Japan). Using the image analysis software ImageJ Fiji (Ver. 1.53t) [13], the average relative area of MMCs (%MMC) of the ten images was calculated, excluding outliers due to measurement error. Samples measured for %MMC in 2014 were remeasured to allow direct comparison between different year groups in the same river.

15.2.3   *Measurement of ^{137}Cs Concentration in Muscle and Sediment*

Frozen fish were thawed, weighed, finely chopped, and then blended using a food processor and placed into polypropylene cylindrical containers (U8 containers, each 55 mm diameter and 64 mm height). For individuals weighing 20 g or more, muscle tissue alone was used, and for smaller individuals, the whole body was used. The minced fish and dried river sediment samples were measured for gamma radiation (662 keV) from ^{137}Cs for 2000 s or (for low concentrations) 5000 s using an ORTEC germanium semiconductor analyzer. Background and attenuation corrections were calculated based on the time difference between the sample collection date and the date of measurement.

15.2.4 Statistical Analysis

Correlations and group differences were analyzed using Python 3.9.0, R 4.2.2, and Excel Toukei Ver. 7.0 (statistical software package; Esumi Co., Ltd., Tokyo). Multiple comparison tests were performed on ^{137}Cs concentration in river sediment and fish muscle, as well as %MMC. These analyses were conducted between groups of different sampling years in the same river and between different river groups in the same sampling year using Kruskal–Wallis and Steel–Dwass tests. Individuals with muscle ^{137}Cs concentration below the limit of measurement were excluded from the correlation analysis. To increase the number of valid individuals, we combined groups that did not show any significant differences in the intergroup test. Consequently, two groups were used: the 2021 and 2023 groups for Mano River; and the 2021, 2022, and 2023 groups for Ukedo River. In the various analyses, ^{137}Cs concentration was converted to base-10 logarithmic form. Also included were unpublished data for the 2014 group obtained previously in our laboratory.

A possible pseudo-correlation was considered: as body length (SL) increases, %MMC also increases. To examine the correlation between ^{137}Cs concentration and %MMC, a multivariate analysis was performed after adjusting for the positive pseudo-correlation with %MMC by SL as shown in the following equation.

$$\log_{10}\left(\%MMC_i\right) = \beta_0 + \beta_1 \mathrm{SL}_i + \beta_2 \, {}^{137}\mathrm{Cs}_i + \varepsilon_i, \quad \left(i = 1,\ldots,99\right),$$

where β_0, β_1, and β_2 are unknown parameters to be estimated, ε_i ($i = 1, \ldots, 99$) denote random error terms subject to a common normal distribution with mean 0 and variance σ^2, which are mutually independent. In order to visually evaluate the impact of ^{137}Cs on %MMC$_i$, an added-variable plot was performed in the above regression analysis, which shows the impact of ^{137}Cs on the objective variable after the impact of other variables has been removed. The added-variable plot helps us understand how specific variables contribute to the model and provides important information for variable selection and model improvement. It is particularly useful for assessing multicollinearity and variable importance in regression analysis [14].

15.3 Results

15.3.1 ^{137}Cs Concentration in River Sediment

The results of the measurement of ^{137}Cs concentration in river sediment are shown in Fig. 15.2 and Table 15.1. Ukedo River has not shown a declining trend since 2014, and high values have been observed every year, significantly exceeding those

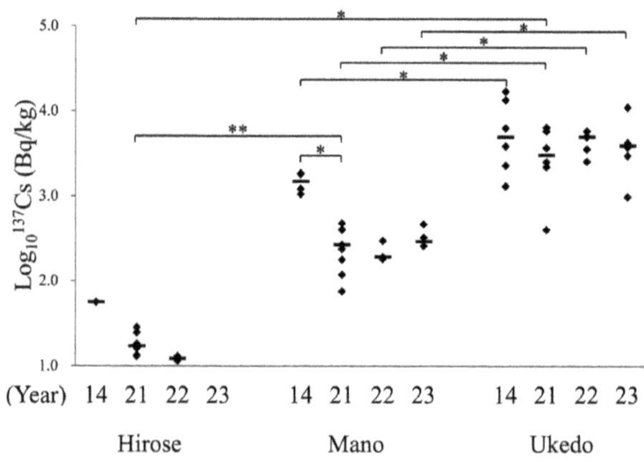

Fig. 15.2 ^{137}Cs concentration in river sediments. ** $p < 0.01$; * $p < 0.05$. Numbers 14, 21, 22, and 23 indicate sampling years: 2014, 2021, 2022, and 2023, respectively.

Table 15.1 ^{137}Cs concentration in river sediments.

River	Year	n	Min (Bq kg⁻¹ dry weight)	Median (Bq kg⁻¹ dry weight)	Max (Bq kg⁻¹ dry weight)
Hirose	2014	1	56	56	56
	2021	6	13	17	28
	2022	9	11	12	13
	2023	0			
Mano	2014	4	1060	1525	1860
	2021	8	75	252	478
	2022	3	182	192	298
	2023	4	9	290	459
Ukedo	2014	6	1320	5535	17,000
	2021	6	403	3114	6403
	2022	5	2554	4973	5854
	2023	6	984	3937	11,124

of Mano River each year. Mano River has shown a significant decline since 2014 but still remained at moderate levels. In the control river (Hirose River), although values were relatively high in 2014, overall values were extremely low.

15.3.2 *^{137}Cs Concentration in Masu Salmon Muscle*

The results of ^{137}Cs concentration in fish muscle are shown in Fig. 15.3 and Table 15.2. In the Ukedo River group, although there were some individuals below the detection limit, most individuals exceeded 1,000 Bq/kg. In the Mano River group, although there were some individuals below the detection limit, most individuals exceeded 100 Bq/kg, and other years revealed slight declines compared to

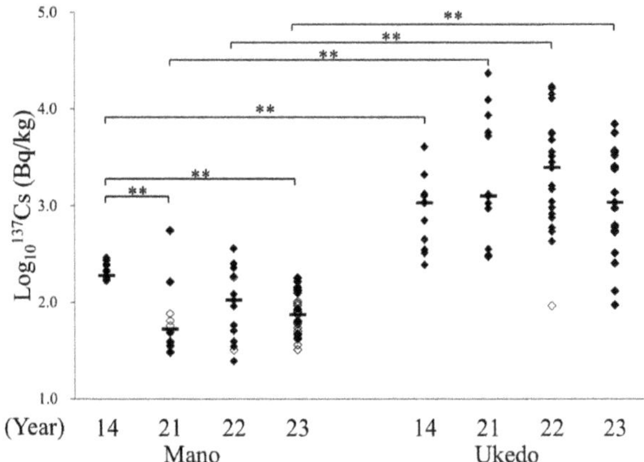

Fig. 15.3 ^{137}Cs concentration in masu salmon muscle (wet weight). ** $p < 0.01$, ** $p < 0.05$. White symbols indicate detection limits for individuals below the detection limit (N.D.). Individuals in the Hirose River are omitted because they are all N.D. The years are expressed in the same way as in Fig. 15.2.

Table 15.2 ^{137}Cs concentration in masu salmon muscle (wet weight).

River	Year	n	Min (Bq kg^{-1} wet weight)	Median (Bq kg^{-1} wet weight)	Max (Bq kg^{-1} wet weight)
Hirose	2014	6	N.D.		N.D.
	2021	5	N.D.		N.D.
	2022	6	N.D.		N.D.
	2023	9	N.D.		N.D.
Mano	2014	16	167	189	290
	2021	10	N.D.	53	551
	2022	15	N.D.	105	360
	2023	26	N.D.	75	179
Ukedo	2014	11	243	1070	4080
	2021	13	296	1267	23,362
	2022	21	N.D.	2487	17,044
	2023	26	94	1089	6996

2014. The Ukedo River samples showed significantly higher values than the Mano River samples in each year.

15.3.3   %MMC Measurements

The results of %MMC are shown in Fig. 15.4 and Table 15.3, and a representative image of spleen histology with MMCs is shown in Fig. 15.5. In 2021, %MMC of the Ukedo River group was significantly higher than that of the Mano and Hirose River groups. In 2022, %MMC was significantly higher than in other years for the Mano and Hirose River groups, respectively. In 2023, %MMC of the Ukedo River group was significantly higher than that of the Mano River group.

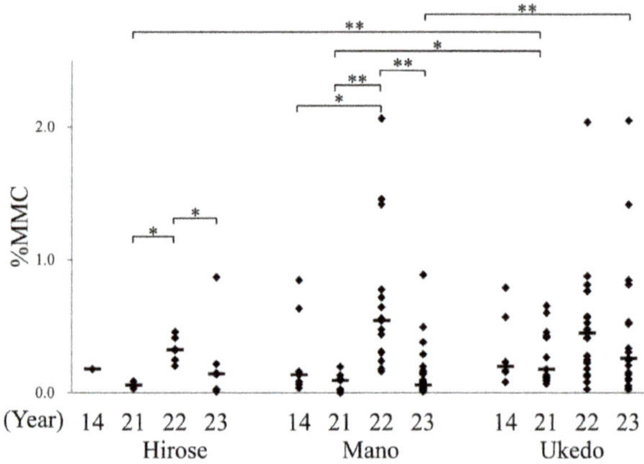

Fig. 15.4 Relative area of MMCs (%MMC) in masu salmon spleen. ** $p < 0.01$; * $p < 0.05$. Numbers on the base line correspond to those in Fig. 15.2.

Table 15.3 Relative area of MMCs in masu salmon spleen.

River	Year	n	Min (%)	Median (%)	Max (%)
Hirose	2014	1	0.18	0.18	0.18
	2021	5	0.03	0.06	0.09
	2022	6	0.20	0.33	0.46
	2023	9	0.01	0.14	0.22
Mano	2014	9	0.04	0.14	0.85
	2021	10	0.00	0.09	0.20
	2022	15	0.17	0.54	2.06
	2023	26	0.01	0.06	0.89
Ukedo	2014	6	0.08	0.20	0.79
	2021	13	0.07	0.18	0.66
	2022	21	0.03	0.45	2.04
	2023	21	0.02	0.26	2.51

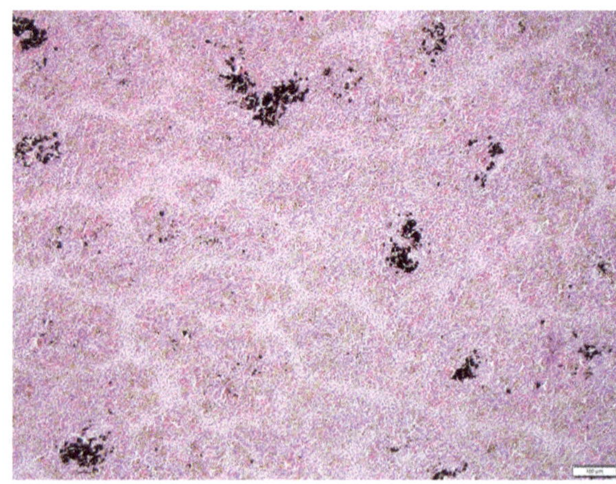

Fig. 15.5 Representative histology of masu salmon spleen containing MMCs (dark deposits). %MMC of this image is 2.0%. Hematoxylin and eosin staining. Scale bar: 100 μm.

15.3.4 Relationship Between ^{137}Cs Concentration in Muscle and %MMC

The relationship between ^{137}Cs concentration in muscle and %MMC for all individuals by year is shown in Fig. 15.6. In 2021, %MMC showed a strong positive correlation with ^{137}Cs concentration ($r = 0.821$, $p < 0.01$), and moderate positive correlations were observed in 2023 ($r = 0.533$, $p < 0.01$) and 2014 ($r = 0.617$, $p < 0.01$), but no significant correlation was found in 2022.

Figure 15.7 is an added-variable plot showing the relationship between the predictor variable ^{137}Cs and the response variable %MMC after controlling for the effect of SL. The estimated correlation coefficient was 0.4139 ($p = 2.08e^{-05}$). The line in the plot represents the fitted values from a linear regression model of the partial residuals of the response variable %MMC against the partial residuals of the predictor variable ^{137}Cs.

15.4 Discussion

15.4.1 Levels of ^{137}Cs

The sampling point for Ukedo River was about 26 km from FNPP, while that for Mano River was about 42 km away. As shown in Fig. 15.1, there has been a large difference in the level of contamination between these two points, and access to the

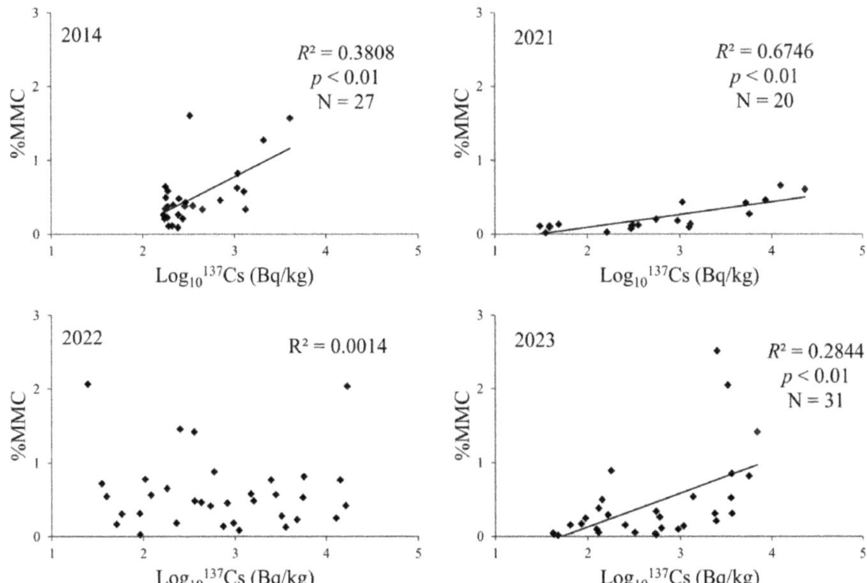

Fig. 15.6 Relationship between ^{137}Cs concentration in muscle and %MMC for each year group.

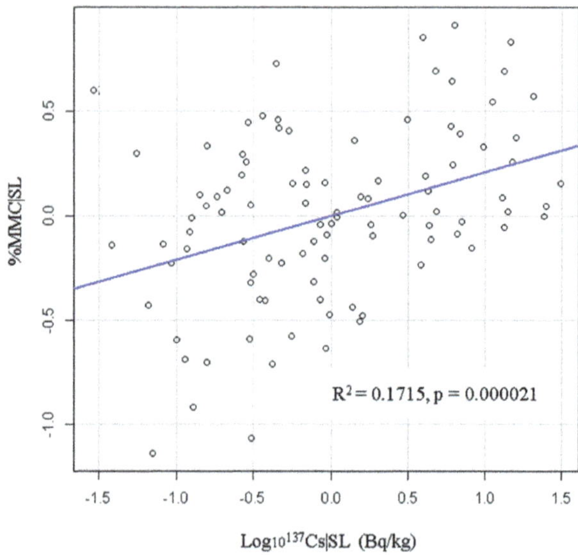

Fig. 15.7 Added-variable plot of the relationship between ^{137}Cs and %MMC, controlling for the effect of SL (standard length).

Ukedo River basin is still restricted in large areas as of 2024. In the control area (Hirose River), ^{137}Cs concentration detected in both sediment and fish muscle samples was extremely low, indicating that radioactive contamination is negligible. Compared to 2014, higher ^{137}Cs concentration was detected in the sediment of Ukedo River in 2021, 2022, and 2023. In each year studied, ^{137}Cs concentration in both fish muscle and river sediment was higher in Ukedo River than in Mano River, indicating that Ukedo River remained at a particularly high level of contamination. Furthermore, there was no significant decrease in contamination levels between years, and values higher than the highest recorded in 2014 were observed in 2021, 2022, and 2023, suggesting that contamination levels in Ukedo River did not decrease even 12 years after the FNPP accident. The ambient dose rate in November 2023 was 5.1 μSv/h at the sampling site on Ukedo River, while compared to 0.35 μSv/h at the sampling site on Mano River [15]. These suggest that ^{137}Cs in the river basin is circulating in the environment and concentrating as well as diluting at the same time.

It is known that ^{137}Cs absorbed by forests in Fukushima Prefecture has been circulating in the environment through a tree-centered cycle and has approached equilibrium dynamics within 5–10 years after the accident [16]. Bioaccumulation of ^{137}Cs in predatory insects in streams has not been observed [17], but insects serving as food for stream fish are reported as the main source of ^{137}Cs [7]. The present study demonstrated that masu salmon in the study area have continued to be exposed to ^{137}Cs, which remained in the environment over 12 years after the accident. In a 2019 survey of masu salmon in Ukedo River, the mean ^{137}Cs concentration was 2670 Bq kg^{-1} wet weight with a maximum of 10,000 Bq kg^{-1} wet weight [18], which is comparable to that found in the present study. Radioactivity monitoring conducted on brown trout living in Norwegian lakes affected by the Chornobyl nuclear accident recorded a peak of 8400 Bq kg^{-1} wet weight in 1984, which then decreased to about 200 Bq kg^{-1} wet weight by 2008 and has remained consistent at this level since then [19]. The situation in Fukushima Prefecture, close to the nuclear power plant where the accident occurred, is different from that in Norway, which is about 1700 km away from Chornobyl. Unless ^{137}Cs is removed from the vast forest areas in Fukushima Prefecture, ^{137}Cs concentration in muscle of masu salmon will likely continue to be similar for a long time.

Higher levels of ^{137}Cs concentration in fish muscle were detected from Ukedo River in 2021 and 2022 compared with 2014. There have been reports from both the Chornobyl [20] and FNPP accidents [6] that ^{137}Cs concentration in fish muscle peaked within 3 years after the accident, so presumably the individuals studied in 2014 were post-peak. The finding that measurements in 2021 and 2022 were higher than those in 2014 in the Ukedo River group suggests that changes in ^{137}Cs concentration in fish are not due to a single cause but rather represent the result of an intricate, ongoing process. Therefore, it is likely that masu salmon will continue to receive ^{137}Cs from the environment, and longer-term, and more detailed studies are needed.

A significant positive correlation was observed between ^{137}Cs concentration in muscle and %MMC in 2014, 2021, and 2023. A relationship between %MMC and body length has been reported, which is considered to be due to aging and increased stress [21]. However, a "size effect" (whereby ^{137}Cs concentration in muscle increases with body length due to factors such as changes in feeding behavior) has also been widely confirmed [22]. In this study, we observed a correlation between ^{137}Cs concentration in muscle and %MMC (Table 15.4), while both ^{137}Cs concentration and %MMC showed a significant positive correlation with body length. Therefore, we considered that body length may be a confounding factor for correlation between ^{137}Cs concentration in muscle and %MMC in the spleen. In this study, multivariate analysis after controlling body length showed a significant positive correlation between ^{137}Cs concentration and %MMC. These results suggest that a spurious correlation via body length is unlikely and that radiation exposure contributes to MMC formation. Low-dose radiation exposure generates reactive oxygen species in vivo [23], while melanin in fish is thought to play a role in absorbing free radicals [24], which may contribute to the association observed between long-term low-dose-rate radiation exposure and %MMC. In contrast, no significant correlation was found between ^{137}Cs concentration in muscle and %MMC in 2022. Notably, %MMC in each river was higher compared to other year groups, presumably because fish

Table 15.4 Single correlations of combinations of two variables among body length, ^{137}Cs, and MMC for each year group.

Year	^{137}Cs-%MMC	^{137}Cs-Body length	%MMC-Body length
2014	0.617**		0.556**
2021	0.821**	0.571**	0.686**
2022			
2023	0.533**		0.427*

Only those correlations that were significant in the no-correlation test are described. ** indicates significant difference at $p < 0.01$; * indicates significant difference at $p < 0.05$

sampled in 2022 were larger than in the other year groups (median SL of 11.7 in 2021 and 19.0 in 2022 in Ukedo River). However, there was no correlation between %MMC and parameters such as body length and muscle ^{137}Cs concentration observed in other years, implying that fish sampled in 2022 were exposed to other forms of stress that had a strong influence on MMC formation, in addition to radiation exposure. Exposure to stress from high temperature is known to decrease liver pigmentation [25]. At the time of sampling in September, the water temperature of Mano River was higher in 2021 than in 2022 (24.4 °C in 2021 vs. 21.7 °C in 2022). Additionally, previous studies have shown that rainbow trout experiencing food deprivation show iron deposition in the spleen [24]. The present study also found variations in ^{137}Cs concentration in the sediment of Mano River, suggesting that ^{137}Cs in the environment is distributed unevenly. Since MMCs are thought to have various functions, multivariate analysis to assess the impact of radiation on %MMC may need to consider variables other than those included in this study.

Yamame refers to a landlocked form of masu salmon that spawn and then die at the age of 3-4 [26]. All sampling sites except for the control area in Hirose River were upstream of the dam, and all individuals were considered to be landlocked Yamame. Although some individuals collected in 2014 were thought to have been in the area immediately after the 2011 FNPP accident, the majority of the fish in this study were likely born after the accident. These suggest that short-lived radionuclides, mainly ^{131}I, which should have been considered immediately after the accident, did not affect %MMC measured in this study.

The present study suggests that long-term exposure to low-dose-rate radiation has caused some stress to the fish and that the effects were observed in the form of an increase in the amount of %MMC in the spleen. It is interesting to know which has a stronger impact on %MMC, dose rate, i.e., ^{137}Cs concentration in muscle, or cumulative dose. Because the biological half-life of ^{137}Cs in captive masu salmon is as short as 56 days [27], ^{137}Cs concentration in the body of an individual may vary over time. However, in this study, ^{137}Cs concentration in the environment and muscle did not vary significantly from year to year, so the cumulative dose of an individual might increase with age, i.e., with body length. %MMC itself is reported to correlate with body length [21]. These findings indicate that %MMC increases more with dose rate than with cumulative dose in this study, which is consistent with the results showing that the effects of radiation are correlated with the internal dose rate of the affected mammals [28].

The results of this study show great potential for %MMC to serve as a biomarker of radiation exposure in fish. However, since %MMC is susceptible to multiple influencing factors, we emphasize that in order to use %MMC as an accurate marker for radiation exposure, it is important to conduct accurate surveys and comprehensive studies, including breeding experiments and measurement of various parameters.

Acknowledgments We are grateful to the staff members of the Fukushima Prefectural Inland Water Fisheries Experimental Station for their help with sample processing and collection. We thank all of the fisheries cooperatives in Fukushima Prefecture who helped us collect masu salmon. This work was partly supported by JSPS KAKENHI Grant (#25252035).

References

1. Yasunari T, Stohl A, Ryugo H et al (2011) Cesium-137 deposition and contamination of Japanese soils due to the Fukushima nuclear accident. Proc Natl Acad Sci 108(49):19530–19534. https://doi.org/10.1073/pnas.1112058108
2. Bunzl K, Schimmack W, Kreutzer K et al (1989) Interception and retention of Chernobyl-derived ^{134}Cs, ^{137}Cs and ^{1064}Ru in a spruce stand. Sci Total Environ 78:77–87. https://doi.org/10.1016/0048-9697(89)90023-5
3. Kuroshima H, Ogata H, Okochi H et al (2014) Distribution and behavior of the atmospherically deposited radioactive cesium in a small forest, *Satoyama* at Namie Town, Fukushima Prefecture. J Japan Soc Atmos Environ 49(2):93–100. https://doi.org/10.11298/taiki.49.93
4. Onda Y, Taniguchi K, Yoshimura K et al (2020) Radionuclides from the Fukushima Daiichi Nuclear Power Plant in terrestrial systems. Nat Rev Earth Environ 1:644–660. https://doi.org/10.1038/s43017-020-0099-x
5. Ministry of Health, Labour and Welfare (MHLW) (2022) https://www.mhlw.go.jp/english/topics/2011eq/dl/(Gunma)press_November_25_2022.pdf
6. Wada T, Tomiya A, Enomoto M et al (2016) Radiological impact of the nuclear power plant accident on freshwater fish in Fukushima: an overview of monitoring results. J Environ Radioact 151(1):144–155. https://doi.org/10.1016/j.jenvrad.2015.09.017
7. Yoshimura M, Yokoduka T (2014) Radioactive contamination of fishes in lake and streams impacted by the Fukushima nuclear power plant accident. Sci Total Environ 482–483(1):184–192. https://doi.org/10.1016/j.scitotenv.2014.02.118
8. Yusof. MFB, Kawada G, Enomoto M et al (2020) Mutations observed in mitochondrial DNA of salmon collected in Mano River, Fukushima Prefecture, Japan. In: Fukumoto M (ed) Low-dose radiation effects on animals and ecosystems, pp 89–98. https://doi.org/10.1007/978-981-13-8218-5_7
9. Natalie C, Steinel, Daniel I et al (2017) Melanomacrophage centers as a histological indicator of immune function in fish and other poikilotherms. Front Immunol 8:827. https://doi.org/10.3389/fimmu.2017.00827
10. Agius C, Roberts RJ (2003) Melano-macrophage centres and their role in fish pathology. J Fish Dis 26(9):499–509. https://doi.org/10.1046/j.1365-2761.2003.00485.x
11. Fournie JW, Summers K, Courtney LA et al (2011) Utility of splenic macrophage aggregates as an indicator of fish exposure to degraded environments. J Aquat Anim Health 13(2):105–116. https://doi.org/10.1577/1548-8667(2001)013<0105:UOSMAA>2.0.CO;2
12. Montero D, Blazer VS, Socorro J et al (1999) Dietary and culture influences on macrophage aggregate parameters in gilthead seabream (*Sparus aurata*) juveniles. Aquaculture 179(1–4):523–534. https://doi.org/10.1016/S0044-8486(99)00185-4
13. Schindelin J, Arganda-Carreras I, Frise E et al (2012) Fiji: an open-source platform for biological-image analysis. Nat Methods 9:676–682. https://doi.org/10.1038/nmeth.2019
14. Hastie T, Tibshirani R, Friedman J (2009) The elements of statistical learning: data mining, inference, and prediction (2nd edn, Springer Series in Statistics). Hardcover
15. Nuclear Regulation Authority. Environmental Raditaion Monitering Data Search Site. https://radioactivity.nra.go.jp/emdb/contents/1/
16. Hashimoto S, Komatsu M, Miura S (2022) Behavior of Radiocesium in the Forest. In: Forest radioecology in Fukushima. Springer, Singapore, pp 21–46. https://doi.org/10.1007/978-981-16-9404-2_3
17. Murakami M, Ohte N, Suzuki T et al (2014) Biological proliferation of cesium-137 through the detrital food chain in a forest ecosystem in Japan. Sci Rep 4:3599. https://doi.org/10.1038/srep03599
18. Teramoto W, Funaki Y, Nakakubo H et al (2021) Relationship between air dose rate and Radiocesium concentrations in mountain stream fish in Fukushima Prefecture. In: Nagao S (ed) Impacts of Fukushima nuclear accident on freshwater environments. Springer, Singapore. https://doi.org/10.1007/978-981-16-3671-4_7

19. Brittain JE, Gjerseth JE (2010) Long-term trends and variation in ^{137}Cs activity concentrations in brown trout (Salmo trutta) from Øvre Heimdalsvatn, a Norwegian subalpine lake. In: Brittain JE, Borgstrøm R (eds) The subalpine lake ecosystem, Øvre Heimdalsvatn, and its catchment: local and global changes over the last 50 years. Hydrobiologia 642:107–113. https://doi.org/10.1007/s10750-010-0155-5
20. Sundbom M, Meili M, Andersson E et al (2003) Long-term dynamics of Chernobyl ^{137}Cs in freshwater fish: quantifying the effect of body size and trophic level. J Appl Ecol 40(2):228–240. https://doi.org/10.1046/j.1365-2664.2003.00795.x
21. Carreras-Colom E, Constenla M, Dallarés S et al (2022) Natural variability and potential use of melanomacrophage centres as indicators of pollution in fish species from the NW Mediterranean Sea. Mar Pollut Bull 176. https://doi.org/10.1016/j.marpolbul.2022.113441
22. Koulikov AO, Ryabov IN (1992) Specific cesium activity in freshwater fish and the size effect. Sci Total Environ 112(1):125–142. https://doi.org/10.1016/0048-9697(92)90243-1
23. Mikkelsen RB, Wardman P (2003) Biological chemistry of reactive oxygen and nitrogen and radiation-induced signal transduction mechanisms. Oncogene 22:5734–5754. https://doi.org/10.1038/sj.onc.1206663
24. Agius C, Agbede SA (1984) An electron microscopical study on the genesis of lipofuscin, melanin and haemosiderin in the haemopoietic tissues of fish. J Fish Biol 24(4):471–488. https://doi.org/10.1111/j.1095-8649.1984.tb04818.x
25. Santos LRDS, Franco-Belussi L, Zieri R et al (2014) Effects of thermal stress on hepatic melanomacrophages of Eupemphix nattereri (Anura). Anat Rec 297(5):864–875. https://doi.org/10.1002/ar.22884
26. Mayama H (1992) Studies on the freshwater life and propagation technology of Masu Salmon, *Oncorhynchus masou* (Brevoort). Sci Report Hokkaido Salmon Hatchery 46:1–156
27. Matsuda K, Yamamoto S, Miyamoto K (2020) Comparison of ^{137}Cs uptake, depuration and continuous uptake, originating from feed, in five salmonid fish species. J Environ Radioact 222:106350. https://doi.org/10.1016/j.jenvrad.2020.106350
28. Urushihara Y, Kawasumi K, Endo S et al (2016) Analysis of plasma protein concentrations and enzyme activities in cattle within the ex-evacuation zone of the Fukushima Daiichi nuclear plant accident. PLoS One 11(5):e0155069. https://doi.org/10.1371/journal.pone.0155069
29. Kato H, Onda Y, Gao. Xiang et al (2019) Reconstruction of a Fukushima accident-derived radiocesium fallout map for environmental transfer studies. J Environ Radioact 210:105996. https://doi.org/10.1016/j.jenvrad.2019.105996

Chapter 16
Assessment of Oxidative DNA Damage in the Affected Cattle After the Fukushima Daiichi Nuclear Power Plant Accident

Kazuaki Kawai, Koichi Fujisawa, Yuko Ootsuyama, Masatoshi Suzuki, Yun-Shan Li, Manabu Fukumoto, and Hiroshi Kasai

Abstract The Fukushima Daiichi Nuclear Power Plant (FNPP) accident has sparked health-related concerns, since a certain amount of radioactive material was released into the environment. To determine the impact of radioactive contamination, many studies have investigated its effects on livestock and wild animals in the ex-evacuation zone. This study aimed to evaluate oxidative DNA damage caused by long-term exposure to low-dose-rate radiation attributed to the FNPP accident by analyzing 8-hydroxy-2′-deoxyguanosine (8-OHdG) levels in the liver, kidney, and skeletal muscle DNA of cattle in the evacuation zone using a high-performance liquid chromatography–electrochemical detector.

The results showed that 8-OHdG levels in the liver and kidney tended to increase in a dose-rate-dependent manner. Further investigation of the mechanism of oxidative DNA damage induced by low-dose-rate irradiation, including organ specificity, is warranted. To our knowledge, this is the first study to evaluate the impact of radioactive contamination by the FNPP accident using 8-OHdG, the most common oxidative DNA damage marker.

Keywords Oxidative DNA damage · 8-hydroxy-2′-deoxyguanosine (8-OHdG) · Low dose-rate radiation · Organ specificity

K. Kawai (✉) · K. Fujisawa · Y. Ootsuyama · Y.-S. Li · H. Kasai
Institute of Industrial Ecological Sciences, University of Occupational and Environmental Health, Japan, Kitakyushu, Japan
e-mail: kkawai@med.uoeh-u.ac.jp

M. Suzuki · M. Fukumoto
International Research Institute of Disaster Science, Tohoku University, Sendai, Japan

© The Author(s) 2026

M. Fukumoto (ed.), *Low-Dose Radiation Effects on Animals and Ecosystems II*,
https://doi.org/10.1007/978-981-95-5559-8_16

16.1 Introduction

Ionizing radiation is known to increase the risk of cancer incidence [1]. Oxidative DNA damage can interfere with normal cellular function and cause abnormalities in processes such as gene expression and the cell cycle [2]. Persistent oxidative DNA damage may lead to a variety of health problems, including cancer, aging, neurodegenerative diseases, and inflammatory diseases [3, 4]. Ionizing radiation may cause oxidative DNA damage through elevated generation of reactive oxygen species [5]. To quantify oxidative damage, 8-hydroxy-2′-deoxyguanosine (8-OHdG) is the most frequently studied due to its mutagenic ability [6]. The levels of 8-OHdG in DNA and biological samples can be accurately detected using a high-performance liquid chromatography–electrochemical detector (HPLC-ECD) system with high sensitivity [7]. The levels of 8-OHdG increase linearly in the range of 20–300 mGy of γ-irradiation in an aqueous deoxyguanosine solution [8]. The formation of 8-OHdG in mouse liver DNA immediately after X-ray irradiation does not significantly increase compared to the nonirradiated group below 0.5 Gy. An increase in urinary 8-OHdG in mice exposed to whole-body X-rays is detectable from 0.2 Gy or higher. In most reports, an increase in 8-OHdG could be detected after irradiation with doses greater than a few Gy. Furthermore, most of the human data were collected from patients undergoing radiotherapy, who usually receive quite high doses of radiation. It is essential to collect lower-dose data to clarify the contribution of oxidative damage to the adverse health effects and to develop protective measures. Recently, several studies have been published on radiation exposure and its effects on wild organisms after the Fukushima Daiichi Nuclear Power Plant (FNPP) accident [9]. To understand the health effects of long-term exposure to low-dose (LD) and low-dose-rate (LDR) radiation, it is necessary to assess the oxidative damage caused in animal organs affected by the FNPP accident. This study aimed to assess oxidative DNA damage resulting from the FNPP accident by measuring 8-OHdG levels in the liver, kidney, and skeletal muscle of cattle obtained in the ex-evacuation zone set within a 20 km radius of FNPP.

16.2 Materials and Methods

16.2.1 Measurement Samples and Estimated Radiation Dose

Frozen liver, kidney, and skeletal muscle stock samples of 11 cattle from the ex-evacuation zone and four cattle from the uncontaminated control area were provided by the Institute of Development, Aging and Cancer, Tohoku University. Samples from radiation-exposed cattle were collected between November 29, 2011 (263 days after the accident) and August 10, 2012 (518 days after the accident) from the ex-evacuation zone of the FNPP accident. The estimated radiation dose for each sample was previously reported [10–12].

This study was approved by the Institutional Animal Care and Use Committee of Tohoku University's Environmental and Safety Committee.

16.2.2 Isolation of Nuclear DNA

Nuclear DNA was isolated from the tissue samples using the sodium iodide method with a DNA Extraction WB Kit (Fujifilm Wako Pure Chemical, Osaka, Japan). To avoid oxidative DNA artifacts, 1 mM deferoxamine mesylate (Sigma Chemical Co., MO, USA) was added to the lysis solution for tissue homogenization and DNA extraction. A 100 mg tissue section was homogenized using a Teflon-glass homogenizer in 1 mL of ice-cold lysis solution. The DNA was isolated according to the manufacturer's instructions.

16.2.3 Analysis of 8-OHdG in DNA

Isolated DNA was digested with 8 units of nuclease P1 (Fujifilm Wako Pure Chemical, Osaka, Japan) in 100 μL of a solution containing 1 mM EDTA and 20 mM sodium acetate (pH 4.5). It was then treated with 2 units of alkaline phosphatase (Roche Diagnostics GmbH, Mannheim, Germany) in 250 mM Tris-HCl buffer (pH 8.0) to obtain a deoxynucleoside mixture. The solution was then filtered through an EKICRODISC filter (LC3CR; Nihon Pall Ltd., Tokyo, Japan). The filtrate was stored at -80 °C until analysis. An aliquot (40 μL) of the filtrate was injected into an HPLC column (Capcell Pak C18 MGII, 3 μm, 4.6 × 250 mm, Shiseido Fine Chemicals, Tokyo, Japan) equipped with ultraviolet (UV-8020, Tosoh Co., Tokyo, Japan) and electrochemical (ECD-300, Eicom Co., Kyoto, Japan, applied voltage: 550 mV) detectors. The mobile phase was 10 mM NaH_2PO_4 containing 8% methanol and 0.13 mM Na_2EDTA, delivered at a flow rate of 0.7 mL/min. The column temperature was set at 32 °C. The amount of 8-OHdG in DNA was determined by comparison with authentic standards. The 8-OHdG value in DNA was calculated as the number of 8-OHdG molecules per 10^6 deoxyguanosine.

16.2.4 Statistical Analyses

The Mann–Whitney U test was used to compare 8-OHdG levels in cattle from the ex-evacuation zone and the control area. Simple linear regression analysis was used to determine the relationship between 8-OHdG levels and radiation dose in each organ.

16.3 Results and Discussion

16.3.1 DNA Levels of 8-OHdG in Cattle from the Ex-evacuation Zone

The levels of 8-OHdG in the liver, kidney, and skeletal muscle DNA tended to be, but not significantly, higher in cattle from the ex-evacuation zone than those from the control area (Fig. 16.1).

In the control group, 8-OHdG levels were highest in the skeletal muscle, followed by those in the liver and kidney. The skeletal muscle parenchyma consists of long-lived postmitotic cells. In contrast, the kidney and liver are composed of relatively short-lived, slow-dividing cells. Oxidative DNA damage is efficiently eliminated in slow-dividing cells [13].

Regarding 8-OHdG levels in cattle DNA of exposed to long-term LDR irradiation, there was a potential association between liver and kidney 8-OHdG (Fig. 16.2a). However, there was no corelation between levels in the skeletal muscle and those in the liver or the kidney (Fig. 16.2b, c). This may be due to differences in the cellular characteristics of the tissues. In addition, cesium-134 (^{134}Cs) (half-life: 2.065 y), ^{137}Cs (half-life: 30.07 y), and silver-110 m (^{110m}Ag) (half-life: 249.8 d) in the liver and tellurium-129 m (^{129m}Te) (half-life: 33.6 d) in the kidney have been detected in cattle from the ex-evacuation zone [10].

Although the half-lives of Ag-110m and Te-129m are relatively short, given the timing of sampling, 263–518 days after the accident, the possibility that these nuclides were involved in oxidative DNA damage in the liver and kidneys cannot be excluded.

The increase in 8-OHdG levels among cattle in the ex-evacuation zone was greater in the liver than in the kidneys. This may be due to the influence of nuclides that accumulate in organs. The accumulation of Ag-110m has been detected in the liver tissues of lambs from Chernobyl fallout [14]. And another thing, exposure to environmental radionuclides has been associated with the upregulation of genes involved in lipid metabolism and fatty acid oxidation in the liver of wild rodents in a study of the Chernobyl Exclusion Zone (CEZ) [15]. Voles inhabiting the CEZ are

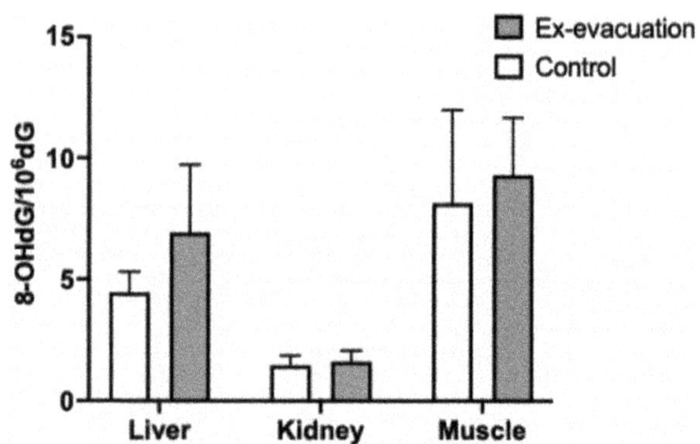

Fig. 16.1 The levels of 8-hydroxy-2′-deoxyguanosine (8-OHdG) in the liver, kidney, and skeletal muscle DNA from the cattle in the ex-evacuation zone and the uncontaminated control area. Values are median ± standard error of mean (SEM).

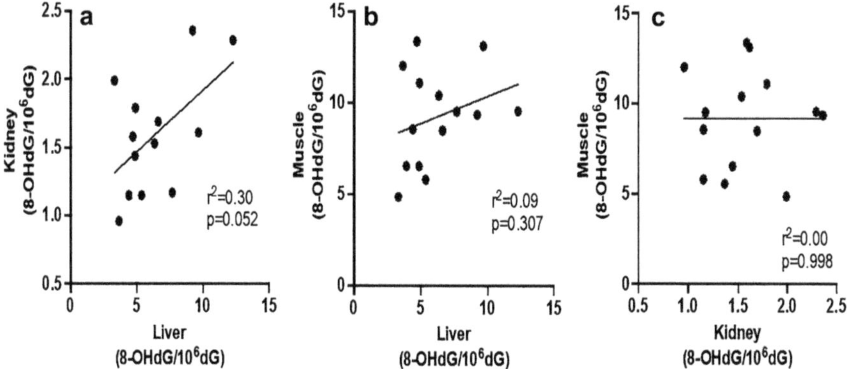

Fig. 16.2 Correlation analysis of 8-OHdG levels in each organ.

characterized by immunosuppression in the liver and spleen, including impaired antigen processing and activation of leukocytes involved in inflammatory responses. Fatty acid oxidation and chronic inflammation are closely related to oxidative stress and DNA damage through the generation of reactive oxygen species [16].

16.3.2 Exposure Dose Rate and DNA 8-OHdG Levels

The levels of 8-OHdG in the liver increased significantly in a dose-rate-dependent manner (Fig. 16.3). This was observed at all internal, external, and total dose rates. In a previous study, significantly higher levels of DNA double-strand breaks have been reported in peripheral lymphocytes of cattle in the ex-evacuation zone than in the uncontaminated control area after the FNPP accident [17]. In addition, several oxidative stress markers have been positively correlated with the radiation exposure dose rate among cattle in the ex-evacuation zone of the FNPP accident [12]. For example, the plasma levels of malondialdehyde and superoxide dismutase activity are positively correlated with the internal dose rate and glutathione peroxidase activity. The 8-OHdG levels in the liver DNA in this study were consistent with these results.

The levels of 8-OHdG in the kidney increased gradually with the external and total dose rates, although the difference was not significant (Fig. 16.3). A single, low-dose subcutaneous administration of ^{137}Cs at 4,000 Bq/kg body weight in mice increases the kidney levels of 8-OHdG [18]. In contrast, 8-OHdG levels in the skeletal muscle tended to decrease (Fig. 16.3). In particular, there was a significant decrease in the internal dose rate. Chronic, very LDR irradiation may enhance antioxidant and DNA repair capacities [19]. We previously reported that radiation-induced urinary 8-OHdG levels increase on administering a nutrient-deficient diet [8]. It is also necessary to investigate factors other than LD radiation that can cause oxidative DNA damage in the evacuation zone. Further research is required to understand why oxidative DNA damage levels vary among different organs.

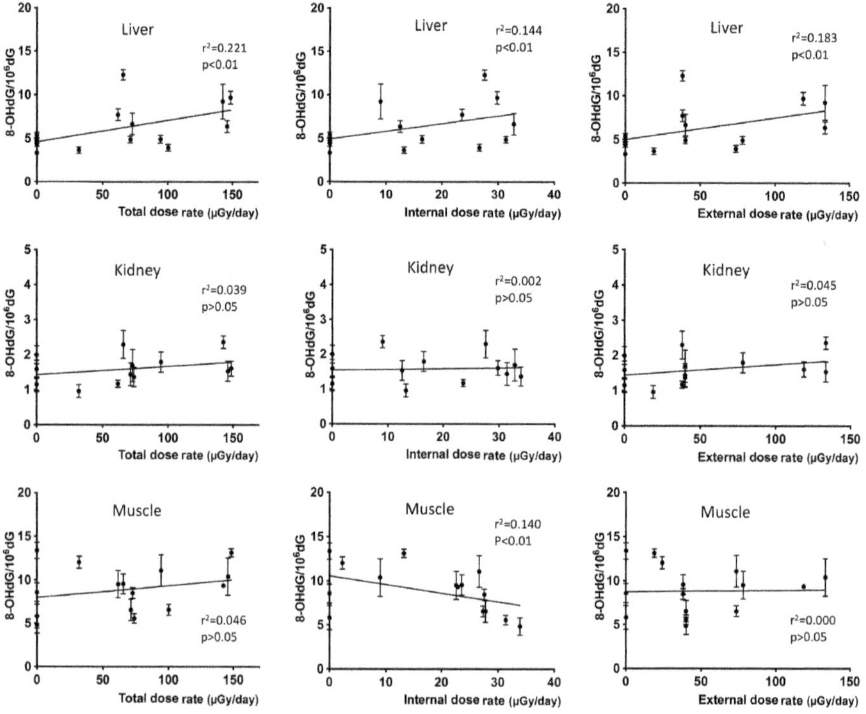

Fig. 16.3 Correlation analysis between estimated exposure dose rate and 8-OHdG levels in each organ. The radiation dose rates were based on the previous study [10, 12]. The data are expressed as the mean ± SEM of three to seven measurements of each sample.

16.4 Conclusions

The levels of 8-OHdG (a key marker of oxidative DNA damage) in the liver tended to increase in a dose-rate-dependent manner among cattle in the ex-evacuation zone of the FNPP accident. The finding in this study that 8-OHdG was elevated in the liver and kidney in relation to dose rate corroborated the results of previous studies that evaluated the effects of the FNPP accidents on animals by analyzing DNA double-strand breaks and other oxidative stress markers. The present study suggests that in skeletal muscle, which is nondividing and accumulates high concentrations of radioactive cesium, long-term LDR radiation exposure may activate mechanisms to repair oxidative DNA damage. Because of the small sample size, this study did not take into account sex and individual age, which are confounding factors known to affect oxidative DNA damage. Further research is required to understand why oxidative DNA damage levels vary among different organs. It is also necessary to investigate factors other than LD radiation that can cause oxidative DNA damage in the cattle in the ex-evacuation zone.

References

1. Land CE (1980) Estimating cancer risks from low doses of ionizing radiation. Science 209(4462):1197–1203
2. Birben E, Sahiner UM, Sackesen C et al (2012) Oxidative stress and antioxidant defense. World Allergy Organ J 5(1):9–19
3. Kasai H, Kawai K (2016) 8-Hydroxyguanine, an oxidative DNA and RNA modification. In: Jurga S, Erdmann (Deceased) V, Barciszewski J (eds) Modified nucleic acids in biology and medicine, Springer International pp 147–185
4. Khansari N, Shakiba Y, Mahmoudi M (2009) Chronic inflammation and oxidative stress as a major cause of age-related diseases and cancer. Recent Patents Inflamm Allergy Drug Discov 3(1):73–80
5. Chatterjee N, Walker GC (2017) Mechanisms of DNA damage, repair, and mutagenesis. Environ Mol Mutagen 58(5):235–263
6. Kasai H (2016) What causes human cancer? Approaches from the chemistry of DNA damage. Genes Environ 38:19
7. Kawai K, Li Y-S, Kasai H (2007) Accurate measurement of 8-OH-dG and 8-OH-Gua in mouse DNA, urine and serum: effects of X-ray irradiation. Genes Environ 29(3):107–114
8. Li Y-S, Song M-F, Kasai H et al (2013) Generation and threshold level of 8-OHdG as oxidative DNA damage elicited by low dose ionizing radiation. Genes Environ 35(3):88–92
9. Fukumoto M(ed) (2020) Low-dose radiation effects on animals and ecosystems long-term study on the Fukushima nuclear accident, Springer Open, pp 43–52. ISBN 978-981-13-8218-5 (eBook). https://doi.org/10.1007/978-981-13-8218-5
10. Fukuda T, Kino Y, Abe Y et al (2013) Distribution of artificial radionuclides in abandoned cattle in the evacuation zone of the Fukushima Daiichi nuclear power plant. PLoS One 8(1):e54312
11. Takahashi S, Inoue K, Suzuki M et al (2015) A comprehensive dose evaluation project concerning animals affected by the Fukushima Daiichi Nuclear Power Plant accident: its set-up and progress. J Radiat Res 56 Suppl 1(Suppl 1):i36–i41
12. Urushihara Y, Kawasumi K, Endo S et al (2016) Analysis of plasma protein concentrations and enzyme activities in cattle within the ex-evacuation zone of the Fukushima Daiichi Nuclear Plant Accident. PLoS One 11(5):e0155069
13. Sohal RS, Agarwal S, Candas M et al (1994) Effect of age and caloric restriction on DNA oxidative damage in different tissues of C57BL/6 mice. Mech Ageing Dev 76(2–3):215–224
14. Martin CJ, Heaton B, Thompson J (1989) Cesium-137, 134Cs and 110mAg in lambs grazing pasture in NE Scotland contaminated by Chernobyl fallout. Health Phys 56(4):459–464
15. Kesaniemi J, Jernfors T, Lavrinienko A et al (2019) Exposure to environmental radionuclides is associated with altered metabolic and immunity pathways in a wild rodent. Mol Ecol 28(20):4620–4635
16. Federico A, Morgillo F, Tuccillo C et al (2007) Chronic inflammation and oxidative stress in human carcinogenesis. Int J Cancer 121(11):2381–2386
17. Nakamura AJ, Suzuki M, Redon CE et al (2017) The causal relationship between DNA damage induction in bovine lymphocytes and the Fukushima nuclear power plant accident. Radiat Res 187(5):630–636
18. Belles M, Gonzalo S, Serra N et al (2017) Environmental exposure to low-doses of ionizing radiation. Effects on early nephrotoxicity in mice. Environ Res 156:291–296
19. Su S, Zhou S, Wen C et al (2018) Evidence for adaptive response in a molecular epidemiological study of the inhabitants of a high background-radiation area of Yangjiang, China. Health Phys 115(2):227–234

Part V
Experimental Approaches to Understanding the Effect of ^{137}Cs on Animals

Chapter 17
Radiation Effects on Lepidopteran Insects: Internal and External Exposure Experiments on the Silkworm, *Bombyx mori*

Sota Tanaka, Tadatoshi Kinouchi, Tsuguru Fujii, Tetsuji Imanaka, Tomoyuki Takahashi, Satoshi Fukutani, Daisuke Maki, Akihiro Nohtomi, and Sentaro Takahashi

Abstract Morphological abnormalities have been reported in insects following the Fukushima Daiichi Nuclear Power Plant (FNPP) accident. Similar abnormalities were also observed during a feeding experiment using contaminated host plants near the FNPP. However, it is unclear whether these morphological abnormalities were directly caused by radiation, as the relationship between the absorbed doses by insects and radiation effects is ambiguous. Therefore, this study aimed to clarify the

---

Sentaro Takahashi passed away before the publication of this book (Deceased 31 July, 2021).

S. Tanaka (✉)
Department of Environmental Science, Faculty of Bioresource Sciences, Akita Prefectural University, Akita, Japan
e-mail: tanaka.sota@akita-pu.ac.jp

T. Kinouchi
Division of Radiation Life Science, Institute for Integrated Radiation and Nuclear Science, Kyoto University, Kumatori, Osaka, Japan

T. Fujii
Laboratory of Silkworm Genetic Resources, Institute of Genetic Resources, Graduate School of Bioresource and Bioenvironmental Sciences, Kyushu University, Fukuoka, Japan

T. Imanaka · T. Takahashi · S. Fukutani
Division of Nuclear Engineering Science, Institute for Integrated Radiation and Nuclear Science, Kyoto University, Kumatori, Osaka, Japan

D. Maki
Oarai Research Center, Chiyoda Technol Corporation, Oarai, Ibaraki, Japan

A. Nohtomi
Quantum Radiation Sciences, Department of Health Sciences, Graduate School of Medical Sciences, Kyushu University, Fukuoka, Japan

S. Takahashi (Deceased)
Professor Emeritus, Kyoto University, Kyoto, Japan

M. Fukumoto (ed.), *Low-Dose Radiation Effects on Animals and Ecosystems II*,
https://doi.org/10.1007/978-981-95-5559-8_17

direct effects of ionizing radiation on lepidopterans by conducting two independent experiments using silkworms: (1) internal exposure using an artificial diet supplemented with cesium-137 (^{137}Cs), and (2) external exposure using γ-ray irradiation. Abnormalities were evaluated by pupal wing-to-whole-body length ratio and somatic mutations via white spots on the larval integument. The results of the internal exposure showed no significant differences in the ratios between the exposed and control groups. A significant difference in the ratio appeared with 80 Gy irradiation in fifth-instar larvae. Additionally, the development of somatic mutations required at least 1 Gy irradiation of eggs. Therefore, it is strongly suggested that low-dose and low-dose-rate exposure to ^{137}Cs radiation is unlikely to cause direct radiation effects in lepidopterans, such as morphological abnormalities and somatic mutations.

Keywords Abnormalities · Mutation · Gamma (γ)-irradiation · Internal exposure · Insects · Silkworm · Cesium-137 (^{137}Cs)

17.1 Introduction

A large amount of radionuclides was released into the environment owing to the Tokyo Electric Power Company's Fukushima Daiichi Nuclear Power Plant (FNPP) accident in March 2011, causing severe radioactive contamination across wide areas in eastern Japan. After the accident, insects, which are generally considered resistant to radiation, showed morphological abnormalities in these areas [1, 2]. In particular, lepidopterans are considered highly tolerant to radiation-induced chromosomal aberrations as they possess holocentric chromosomes [3–5]. Nevertheless, higher-than-expected lethality and morphological abnormalities were observed in the pale grass blue butterfly *Zizeeria maha*, which was exposed to low-dose radiation in contaminated host plants [6–8]. To verify whether the abnormalities observed in butterflies are a consequence of radiation effects, dose–effect relationships based on accurate estimates of absorbed doses should be evaluated, which were lacking in previous studies.

Tanaka et al. (2020) [9] developed a novel internal exposure experimental system using the silkworm, *Bombyx mori*. Given its short generation time (approximately 30 days) and its ability to be reared on an artificial diet under controlled conditions, the silkworm is an ideal model for such studies. Furthermore, many pure lineage variants of silkworms exist, each with different phenotypic characteristics, allowing molecular genetic experiments to be conducted by crossing variants with different genetic backgrounds. In practice, they can be reared from eggs to mature larvae on an artificial diet supplemented with cesium-137 chloride (^{137}CsCl), allowing the absorbed dose required to evaluate the effects of radiation to be estimated.

The purpose of this study was to clarify the effects of low-dose and low-dose-rate radiation exposure on lepidopteran insects using an internal exposure experimental system with silkworms. In addition, this study aimed to determine whether there is a threshold at which direct radiation affects lepidopterans by exposing silkworms to γ-irradiation. The results of this study will help determine the effects of prolonged exposure of insects to low-dose-rate radiation effects following incidents such as the FNPP accident.

17.2   Materials and Methods

17.2.1   Silkworm Strain

The three silkworm strains (l04, p44, and p55) used in this study were provided by the National Bio-Resource Project (NBRP) of the Ministry of Education, Science, Sports, and Culture of Japan. The p55 strain is also referred to as N4. F1 hybrid eggs ($p^S/+^p$ and p^S/p) were obtained by crossing the l04 strain with a p^S mutation and the p44 or p55 strains with the $+^p$ and p alleles. p^S larvae exhibit striped markings, whereas $+^p$ and p larvae exhibit normal and plain markings, respectively. Eggs were used for cobalt-60 (^{60}Co) γ-ray irradiation.

17.2.2   Design of the External and Internal Exposure Experiments

17.2.2.1   External Exposure

The external exposure experiment using γ-ray irradiation was performed at the ^{60}Co γ-ray irradiation facility at the Institute for Integrated Radiation and Nuclear Science, Kyoto University, Japan. Silkworm eggs were irradiated with 0, 0.01, 0.1, 1, 3, and 10 Gy of γ-rays, whereas the fifth-instar larvae were irradiated with 0, 1, 10, 20, 30, 50, 80, 120, and 140 Gy of γ-rays (Fig. 17.1). The irradiation dose rate for both life stages was set to 0.35 Gy/min.

17.2.2.2   Internal Exposure

The internal exposure experiment was performed by adding radioactive cesium chloride (^{137}CsCl) solution, containing 0.05 mg/g CsCl in 0.1 M HCl as a carrier solution, to the silkworm artificial diet (Silkmate 2S; Nosa Co., Yokohama, Japan) (Fig. 17.2). The concentration was set at 1.3×10^3 Bq/g fresh weight (fw), which can be converted to ^{137}Cs ground deposition of approximately 90 MBq/m^2 when ^{137}Cs is distributed within 5 cm of the soil surface and at a soil density of 1.3 g/cm^3. Silkworms were reared on the contaminated diet from the egg stage to the final (fifth

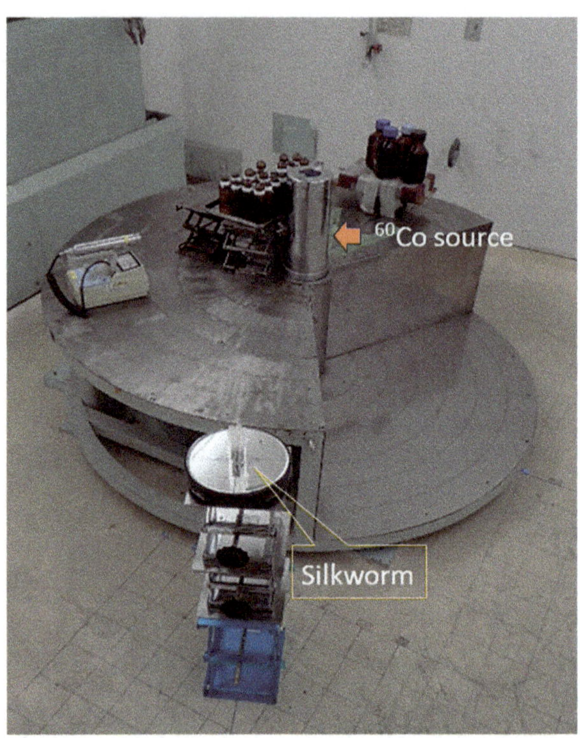

Fig. 17.1 Gamma-ray irradiation of silkworms using a ^{60}Co irradiation facility. Silkworms in vials were placed on a turntable and irradiated while rotating.

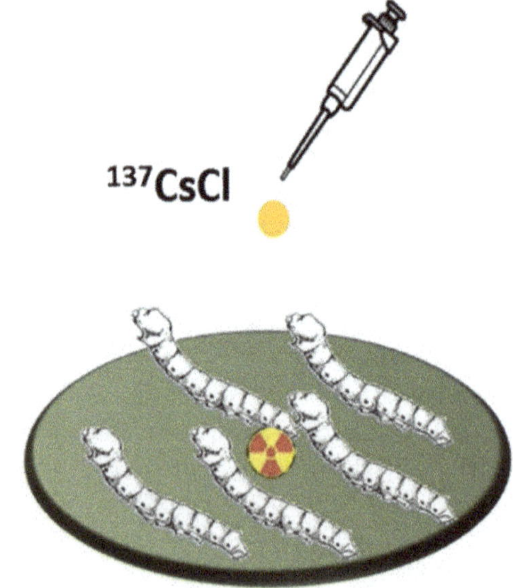

Fig. 17.2 Internal exposure experimental system of silkworms. A ^{137}CsCl solution was uniformly added to the artificial diet to ensure continuous ingestion of the contaminated diet by the silkworms.

instar) larval stage, as described by Tanaka et al. [9]. For the control groups, a non-radioactive CsCl solution containing 0.05 mg/g CsCl in 0.1 M HCl was added to the artificial diet.

17.2.3 Detection of Morphological Abnormalities and Somatic Mutations

Morphological abnormalities were determined by measuring the wing-size-to-whole-body-size ratio of silkworms in the pupal stage (Fig. 17.3). As the shrinkage of the silkworm pupal wings is inversely proportional to increasing irradiation doses [10], this ratio can be used as an effective indicator of radiation sensitivity [11].

An increase in white spots on the black-striped epidermis of fifth-instar larvae hatching from irradiated eggs denotes the occurrence of somatic mutations, as radiation-induced mutations in the p^s allele result in the appearance of white spots on the integument of fifth-instar larvae [12–14].

17.2.4 Estimation of the External and Internal Dose Rates

The external dose rate was estimated using a glass rod dosimeter with a diameter of 1.5 mm × 12 mm (GD-302 M; AGC Techno Glass Corporation, Shizuoka, Japan) equipped with a reader (FGD-1000; AGC Techno Glass Corporation). Beta rays were separated using an approximately 0.6 mm-thick aluminum cover. The ratio of β-to-γ radiation dose was estimated by simple subtraction with and without the aluminum cover. The glass rod dosimeter was placed on the artificial diet (Fig. 17.4) [9]. The internal dose rate was estimated using the Particle and Heavy Ion Transport code System (PHITS) [15], as described by Tanaka et al. [9].

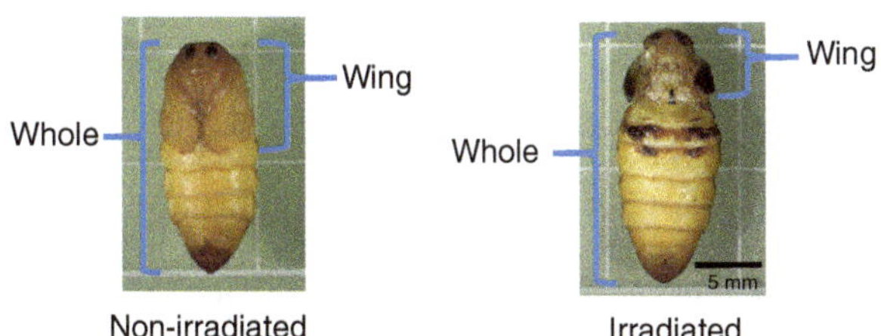

Fig. 17.3 Comparison of wing size and whole-body length of silkworm pupae in nonirradiated and irradiated individuals. Morphological abnormalities were determined by the ratio of wing-to-whole-body length in pupae.

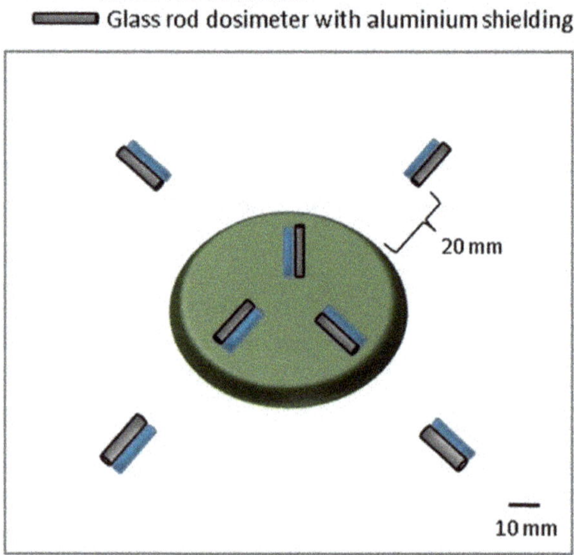

Fig. 17.4 Setting of the glass rod dosimeter on the ^{137}CsCl-supplemented artificial diet.

17.2.5 Statistical Analyses

For changes in the wing-to-whole-body length ratio of silkworm pupae, the lower (Q_1) and upper (Q_3) quartiles and the interquartile range (IQR = $Q_3 - Q_1$) were calculated. Differences in the ratio of control and exposure groups were analyzed using a Student's t-test. One-way analysis of variance (ANOVA), followed by Dunnett's test, was used for multiple comparisons of ratios between the control and irradiated groups. All statistical analyses were performed using R software, version 4.3.0 [16]. Statistical significance is presented as $*P < 0.05$, $**P < 0.01$, and $***P < 0.001$.

17.3 Results

17.3.1 Estimation of Radiation Exposure

The radiation dose was estimated based on a previously published method [9]. The external absorbed dose rates estimated using a glass rod dosimeter are summarized in Table 17.1 [9].

However, the total radiation doses for 3 days, which corresponds to the molting period of silkworm larvae, were measured with glass rod dosimeters placed outside and not on the diet (see Fig. 17.4). The total absorbed dose rates ($\gamma + \beta$ rays) on and beside the diet (20 mm from the edge of the diet pellet) were 0.24 and 0.016 mGy/day, respectively. The total external exposure period was approximately 26 days, of

Table 17.1 Absorbed dose rate from glass rod dosimetry.

mGy/day	γ-ray	β-ray	γ + β	β/γ
On the diet	0.15	0.084	0.24	0.55
Near the diet	0.014	0.0020	0.016	0.14

Table 17.2 Internal dose rate estimated using PHITS.

	Gy/decay	Gy/sec	mGy/day
Electron	1.9E-11	9.1E-09	0.79
Photon	6.6E-13	3.1E-10	0.027

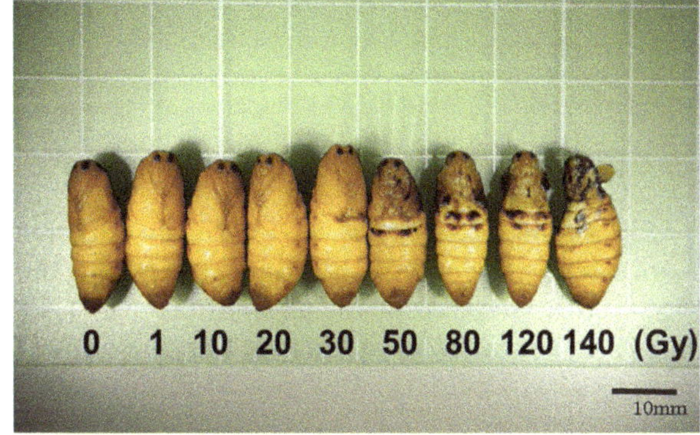

Fig. 17.5 Morphological abnormalities in the pupae after irradiation of fifth-instar larvae. The results of irradiation are within the range of 0–140 Gy.

which the egg period lasted for 6 days. Consequently, the total external absorbed dose of the silkworms was 5.5 mGy, and the average external absorbed dose rate was 0.21 mGy/day.

The internal absorbed dose rates estimated by PHITS are summarized in Table 17.2 [9]. The internal exposure period was 17 days, representing the entire larval stage. The total internal dose was approximately 14 mGy. The average internal absorbed dose rate of the silkworms was 0.82 mGy/day.

Consequently, the average absorbed dose rate for internal and external exposure of the silkworms was approximately 1 mGy/day.

17.3.2 Morphological Abnormalities

Gamma-ray irradiation on fifth-instar larvae revealed that the wings of pupae began to shrink when irradiated with a dose of 50 Gy or more (Fig. 17.5). Consequently, a negative correlation was observed between the wing-to-whole-body length ratio and irradiation dose ($n = 3$–5) (Fig. 17.6).

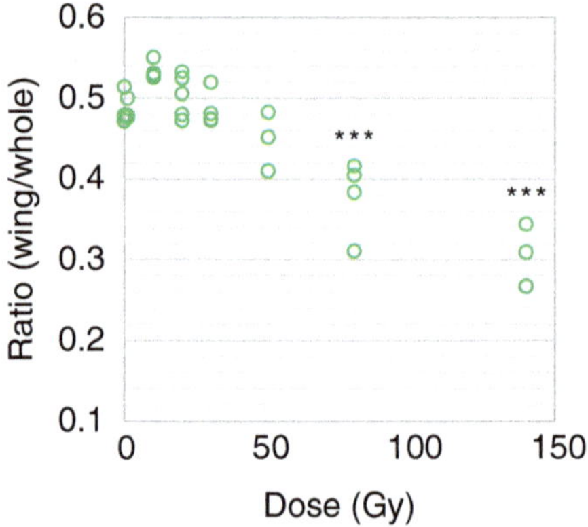

Fig. 17.6 Relationship between wing-to-whole-body length ratio (wing/whole) and irradiation doses (Gy). All results are plotted in the graph (n = 3–5). Asterisks indicate significant differences of control versus all groups by one-way analysis of variance with Dunnett's multiple comparisons test. *P < 0.05; **P < 0.01; ***P < 0.001.

Significant differences in the ratios between the control and exposure groups were observed at external exposure doses of 80 and 140 Gy (Dunnett's test, P < 0.001). However, no significant difference in the ratio between the control (n = 7) and exposure groups (n = 5) was observed in the internal exposure experiment (Student's t-test, P = 0.98; Fig. 17.7).

17.3.3 Somatic Mutations in Silkworms

Gamma-ray irradiation of p^S eggs resulted in the appearance of white spots on the epidermis of fifth-instar larvae at doses of 1 Gy or more (Fig. 17.8), with the frequency of white-spot appearance increasing with irradiation dose. An increase in the number of white spots was observed in more than 46% of the larvae after irradiation at 3 Gy, and in all larvae after irradiation at 10 Gy (Table 17.3).

17.4 Discussion

The ^{137}CsCl concentration used in the internal exposure experiment can be converted to a ^{137}Cs ground deposition of approximately 90 MBq/m^2, which is higher than the initial ^{137}Cs ground deposition in the most highly contaminated area after the FNPP accident. Therefore, in the post-FNPP accident environment, such high levels of ^{137}Cs contamination were unlikely, except at certain hotspots. Furthermore,

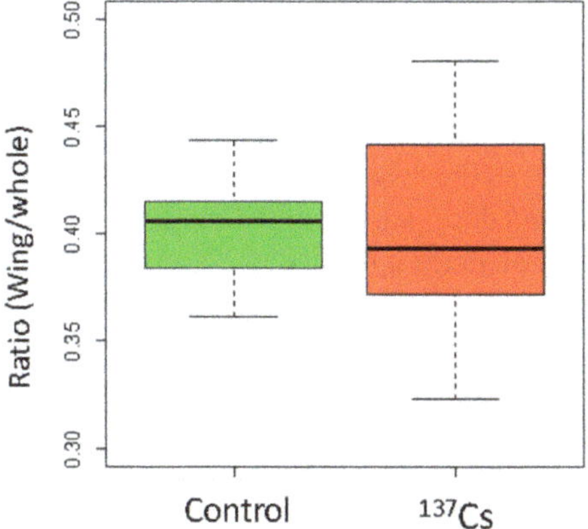

Fig. 17.7 Comparison of the wing-to-whole-body length ratio of silkworm pupae in the internal exposure experiment between the control and exposure groups. The box signifies the upper and lower quartiles, and the median is represented by a horizontal line within the box for the ratio. No significant difference was observed between the control ($n = 7$) and exposure groups ($n = 5$) (Student's t-test, $p = 0.98$).

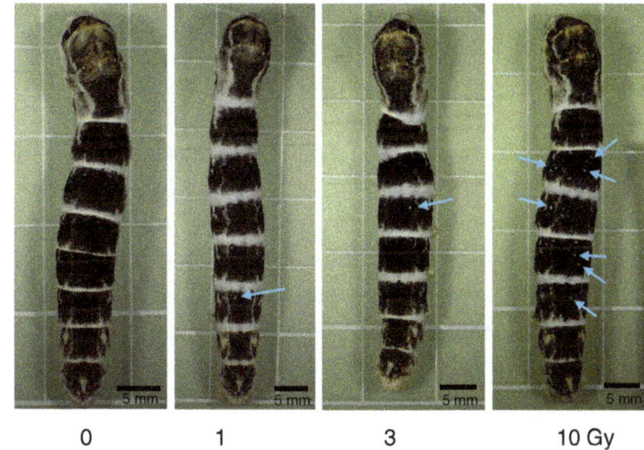

Fig. 17.8 White spots that appeared on p^S fifth-instar larvae after the irradiation of eggs. Arrows indicate the white spots.

Table 17.3 The number of white-spotted and normal *Bombyx mori* individuals recorded at different irradiation doses.

Irradiation dose (Gy)	White spots (No. of individuals)	Normal (No. of individuals)	Appearance rate (%)
0	0	17	0
0.01	0	21	0
0.1	0	20	0
1	4	20	17
3	12	14	46
10	26	0	100

given the low transfer factor of ^{137}Cs from the soil to herbaceous plants [17], it is inconceivable that lepidopterans could directly feed on plants containing such high concentrations of ^{137}Cs for extended periods. Therefore, the present experiment allowed for a conservative assessment of the radiation exposure from ^{137}Cs in the environment. The results of the dose assessment in the internal exposure experiment showed that the estimated dose rate for silkworm larvae was approximately 1 mGy/ day. This value is the dose range specified as "No information" in the International Commission on Radiological Protection (ICRP)'s derived consideration reference levels (DCRL) for insects [18]. Therefore, the data generated in this study are important for estimating the environmental risk of radiation for insects because data on the effects of low-dose-rate exposure are lacking.

The results of the internal exposure experiment showed no morphological abnormalities in silkworms fed an artificial diet containing highly contaminated ^{137}Cs. This suggests that even when directly ingesting concentrations above the postaccident level of ^{137}Cs contamination, there was no obvious impact on the external morphology of lepidopteran insects. In a previous study on the pale grass blue butterfly, *Z. maha*, no morphological abnormalities were observed in experiments involving the addition of ^{137}CsCl to their artificial diet [19]. The results of the present study are therefore consistent with this previous result and support the hypothesis that internal exposure from food sources contaminated with ^{137}Cs does not result in direct radiation effects in Lepidoptera.

The radiation doses required to induce morphological abnormalities in lepidopterans were then assessed. The results of γ-ray irradiation showed morphological abnormalities in fifth-instar larvae exposed to irradiation of 50 Gy and above, and significant differences were observed at 80 Gy. These results are generally consistent with those of previous reports [10], indicating that lepidopterans are radiation-tolerant. In contrast, somatic mutations were detected from 1 Gy after egg irradiation. An increase in the occurrence of somatic mutations in silkworms has been reported from approximately 1 Gy or higher following X-ray irradiation of silkworm eggs [13]. This supports the results of the present study and indicates that exposure to at least 1 Gy of radiation is necessary for somatic mutations to develop.

Irradiation at different growth stages indicated that radiosensitivity varies greatly among lepidopterans at different developmental stages and indicates the importance of evaluating the growth stages of lepidopterans exposed during the initial phase of an accident, including short-half-life radionuclides. However, lepidopterans are generally not expected to be exposed to radiation of 1 Gy, unless they were exposed to short-lived nuclides immediately after the FNPP accident. The total dose from internal and external exposure estimated using conservative values in this study was 1 mGy/day, which is significantly lower than the dose at which morphological changes are clearly induced. Hence, from the perspective of long-term radiation effects, excluding the immediate aftermath of an accident, it is unlikely that these effects will occur in lepidopterans.

17.5   Conclusions

To clarify the direct effects of ionizing radiation on lepidopterans, internal and external radiation exposure experiments were conducted on silkworms. We found no morphological abnormalities in the internal exposure experiments at a dose rate of 1 mGy/day. The effects of radiation on the silkworms were observed as somatic mutations caused by at least 1 Gy of egg irradiation. Therefore, these results suggest that direct radiation exposure to ^{137}Cs after the FNPP accident is unlikely to result in biological effects on Lepidoptera, both now and in the future. To comprehensively clarify the radiation effects of low-dose and low-dose-rate exposure on insects, it is necessary to evaluate both the morphological abnormalities and their effects on reproductive functions to verify the effects of radiation on the next generation.

References

1. Akimoto S (2014) Morphological abnormalities in gall-forming aphids in a radiation-contaminated area near Fukushima Daiichi: selective impact of fallout? Ecol Evol 4:355–369. https://doi.org/10.1002/ece3.949
2. Hiyama A, Nohara C, Kinjo S et al (2012) The biological impacts of the Fukushima nuclear accident on the pale grass blue butterfly. Sci Rep 2:570. https://doi.org/10.1038/srep00570
3. LaChance LE (1967) The induction of dominant lethal mutations in insects by ionizing radiation and chemicals—as related to the sterile-male technique of insect control. In: Wright JW, Pal R (eds) Genetics of insect vectors of disease, pp 617–650
4. Wolf KW, Novák K, Marec F (1997) Kinetic organization of metaphase I bivalents in spermatogenesis of Lepidoptera and Trichoptera species with small chromosome numbers. Heredity 79:135–143. https://doi.org/10.1038/hdy.1997.136
5. Tothová A, Marec F (2001) Chromosomal principle of radiation-induced F1 sterility in *Ephestia kuehniella* (Lepidoptera: Pyralidae). Genome 44:172–184. https://cdnsciencepub.com/doi/10.1139/g00-107
6. Nohara C, Hiyama A, Taira W et al (2014) The biological impacts of ingested radioactive materials on the pale grass blue butterfly. Sci Rep 4:4946. https://doi.org/10.1038/srep04946
7. Nohara C, Taira W, Hiyama A et al (2014) Ingestion of radioactively contaminated diets for two generations in the pale grass blue butterfly. BMC Evol Biol 14:193. https://doi.org/10.1186/s12862-014-0193-0
8. Taira W, Hiyama A, Nohara C et al (2015) Ingestional and transgenerational effects of the Fukushima nuclear accident on the pale grass blue butterfly. J Radiat Res 56:i2–i18. https://doi.org/10.1093/jrr/rrv068
9. Tanaka S, Kinouchi T, Fujii T et al (2020) Observation of morphological abnormalities in silkworm pupae after feeding ^{137}CsCl-supplemented diet to evaluate the effects of low dose-rate exposure. Sci Rep 10:16055. https://doi.org/10.1038/s41598-020-72882-y
10. Takahashi M, Lee JM, Mon H et al (2006) Radiation resistance and its inheritance in the silkworm, *Bombyx mori*. J Fac Agric Kyushu Univ 51:261–264. https://doi.org/10.5109/9239
11. Takada N, Yamauchi E, Fujimoto H et al (2006) A novel indicator for radiation sensitivity using the wing size reduction of *Bombyx mori* pupae caused by γ-ray irradiation. J Insect Biotechnol Sericol 75(3):161–165. https://doi.org/10.11416/jibs.75.161
12. Nakajima M, Takimoto T, Miyakoda T (1972) Radiation effects on silkworm, *Bombyx mori* L., with special reference to the changes in the frequencies of induced somatic mutations

during different stages of larval development. J Sericult Sci Japan 41:359–364. https://doi.org/10.11416/kontyushigen1930.41.359

13. Kotani E, Furusawa T, Nagaoka S et al (2002) Somatic mutation in larvae of the silkworm, *Bombyx mori*, induced by heavy ion irradiation to diapause eggs. J Radiat Res 43:S193–S198. https://doi.org/10.1269/jrr.43.S193

14. Furusawa T, Nojima K, Ichida M et al (2009) Introduction to the proposed Space Experiments Aboard the ISS using the silkworm, *Bombyx mori*. Biol Sci Space 23:61–69. https://doi.org/10.2187/bss.23.61

15. Sato T, Iwamoto Y, Hashimoto S et al (2018) Features of particle and heavy ion transport code system (PHITS) version 3.02. J Nucl Sci Technol 55:684–690. https://doi.org/10.1080/00223131.2017.1419890

16. R Core Team (2023) R: a language and environment for statistical computing. R Foundation for Statistical Computing, Vienna. https://www.R-project.org/

17. Tagami K, Uchida S (2017) Changes of effective half-lives of ^{137}Cs in three herbaceous plants and bioavailable ^{137}Cs fraction in soil after the Fukushima nuclear accident. Appl Geochem 85:162–168. https://doi.org/10.1016/j.apgeochem.2017.01.013

18. International Atomic Energy Agency (IAEA) (2010) Handbook of parameter values for the prediction of radionuclide transfer in terrestrial and freshwater environments. Technical Reports Series No. 472. Vienna. ISBN 978-92-0-113009-9

19. Gurung RD, Taira W, Sakauchi K et al (2019) Tolerance of high oral doses of nonradioactive and radioactive caesium chloride in the pale grass blue butterfly *Zizeeria maha*. Insects 10:290. https://doi.org/10.3390/insects10090290

Chapter 18
What Happens When Mice Are Exposed to Low-Dose Internal Radiation across Generations?: -What we Learned from 40 Generations of Cesium-137 Intake Experiments-

Hiroo Nakajima

Abstract If mice continue to drink water containing cesium-137 (^{137}Cs) for generations, will their offspring be affected? To address this question, this chapter presents the main results of our mouse experiments in which more than 40 generations of mice were fed ^{137}Cs water (100 Bq/mL: 100,000 Bq/L) for 15 years. In addition, I will discuss the possible medical applications of the phenomena that appear to be derived from abscopal effect inducers and radiation-induced gene expression observed in this series of experiments.

Keywords Cesium-137 (^{137}Cs) · Generation · Genetic effect · Abscopal effect

18.1 Introduction

A nuclear and radiation accident is defined by the International Atomic Energy Agency (IAEA) as "an event that has led to significant consequences to people, the environment or the facility." The International Nuclear and Radiological Event Scale (INES) was developed in 1990 by international experts convened by the IAEA and the Organisation for Economic Co-operation and Development/Nuclear Energy Agency (OECD/NEA) with the aim of communicating the safety significance of events at nuclear installations [1].

The scale has seven levels, with each higher level increasing the severity of the event by approximately one order of magnitude. The highest level, level 7, is a "major accident." The 2011 Fukushima Daiichi nuclear plant (FNPP) accident was deemed a level 7 accident, and has been only the second time since the 1986 Chernobyl disaster that a nuclear reactor core was damaged and large amounts of

H. Nakajima (✉)
Research Center for Nuclear Physics, Osaka University, Osaka, Japan
e-mail: nakajima@irs.osaka-u.ac.jp

© The Author(s) 2026

M. Fukumoto (ed.), *Low-Dose Radiation Effects on Animals and Ecosystems II*,
https://doi.org/10.1007/978-981-95-5559-8_18

radioactive isotopes were released [2]. However, the total amount of fallout is estimated to be approximately one-sixth of that of Chornobyl (FNPP: 900Peta Bq, Chornobyl: 5,200Peta Bq) [3]. The FNPP accident was triggered by the tsunami due to the Great Tohoku Earthquake (magnitude 9).

In a nuclear accident, many kinds of radioactive materials are produced as a result of nuclear fission and released. However, the one that is of greatest concern in terms of its impact on living organisms and the human body is cesium-137 (^{137}Cs), which has a long half-life and is deposited in soil over a wide area.

It is certainly true that a large amount of ^{137}Cs has been dispersed over a wide area, increasing radiation levels in addition to existing natural levels [4]. However, we need to be cautious about assuming that all of the ^{137}Cs added to the natural radiation dose due to the accident poses any health effects. In fact, ^{137}Cs released from the atmospheric nuclear tests (528 times) conducted by the United States, USSR, United Kingdom, France, and China from 1945 to 1998 fell on land around the world and were added to the pre-1945 natural radiation levels [5]. No clear evidence has been determined that these additional doses have caused a clear increase in human health effects outside of the nuclear test sites. This indicates that even if there are human health effects due to soil deposition of ^{137}Cs, they may not be detectable (excluding highly contaminated areas near nuclear test sites such as Semipalatinsk and Rongelap Island). It can be affirmed that external and internal exposure to large amounts of ^{137}Cs clearly causes significant radiation damage to the human body and is extremely dangerous. However, as mentioned above, it can also be said that there is a certain amount of radiation that clearly has no detectable effect on the human body. Then, how much is that?

To address this question, we have conducted a series of experiments on chronic exposure to ^{137}Cs using mice. The following is a summary of what we have learned so far through our experiments.

The reasons for using mice in these experimenst are as follows:

1. The ultimate effects of low-dose radiation of concern are carcinogenesis and genetic effects. Mice are experimental animals that provide a large amount of data to simultaneously assess carcinogenicity and genetic effects.
2. Because mice belong to the same class, Mammalia, as humans, it is likely that results obtained in mice can be extended to humans.
3. Because they have a shorter lifespan and generation than humans, it is possible to examine carcinogenic effects and effects on offspring in a shorter period of time than is required for observation in humans.
4. It is possible to examine not only effects on the next generation but also effects on offspring through multigenerational exposure experiments.
5. The spontaneous germline mutation rate in the next generation of mice is almost the same as that of humans (humans: 3.6×10^{-6}, mice: 6.1×10^{-6}) [6].
6. Based on previous studies, the effects of radiation on the next generation of mice can be quantitatively detected.
7. Lung tumors in mice develop like countable bacterial colonies in the lungs, making them excellent for quantifying tumor incidence and growth rate. A/J mice,

one of the strains with a high incidence of lung tumors, can be used to quantitatively detect spontaneous lung tumor incidence, chemical-induced lung tumor incidence, and their lung tumor growth rates.

8. Mutation and carcinogenesis rates can be quantitatively compared using inbred mouse strains (A/J, C57BL/6) and a radiation–hypersensitive mouse strain (*Msh2* transgenic mice).

18.2 Experimental Methods and Results

Two pairs of littermates of A/J mice were selected; one pair was kept as a low-dose internal exposure group with free access to ^{137}Cs water (100 Bq/mL), and the other was kept as a control group with drinking water without ^{137}Cs. The offspring of both pairs were sibling-mated for more than 40 generations (equivalent to about 800 years in humans), and the following analyses (1–9) were conducted at any given generation.

1. Distribution of ^{137}Cs in mice.

   When drinking ^{137}Cs water (100 Bq/mL) daily, ^{137}Cs gradually accumulated in each organ. After 3–4 weeks, however, the ^{137}Cs concentrations in the organs reached equilibrium, with concentrations in muscle about 1.6 times that of drinking water (160 Bq/g organ weight) and about half that of muscle in other organs. Replacement with ^{137}Cs-free water caused a slight decrease in muscle ^{137}Cs concentration, but a rapid decrease in other organs [7].

2. Effects on litter size and sex ratio in each generation:

   Drinking ^{137}Cs water (100 Bq/mL) throughout 1–18 generations had no effect on the birth sex ratio or litter size of mice [7].

3. Induction of DNA double-strand breaks:

   Radiation exposure causes DNA double-strand breaks, and the amount of which can be measured by the γ-H2AX focus count. In the ^{137}Cs water group, internal exposure of approximately 37 mGy (2313 Bq per mouse, average 93.54 Bq/g body weight, 59.5 Bq per liver) was observed per generation (108 days). A significant increase in the number of γ-H2AX foci was observed in hepatocytes in the ^{137}Cs water group compared to the control group [8].

4. Chromosome aberration and the micronucleus test:

   Chromosome aberration analysis using multicolor fluorescence in situ hybridization (FISH) and the micronucleus test was performed in the tenth-generation mice. No common chromosomal aberration was found in bone marrow cells of the ^{137}Cs water group. Although the frequency of DNA double-strand breaks increased as described in the above-mentioned Section 3, no common chromosomal changes that could be passed on to the next generation were observed even after ten generations of mice. No significant increase in micronuclei was also observed in the ^{137}Cs water group [8].

5. Analysis of DNA sequence variation by whole genome sequencing in liver cells:

   Base mutations in noncoding regions of DNA (introns, intergenic sequences) are expected to be more likely to accumulate across generations because they have less impact on the maintenance of life than mutations in coding regions. Therefore, we attempted whole genome analysis in the 1st, 2nd, 5th, 18th, and 25th generations of mice. The results showed that the number of single-nucleotide variant (SNV) mutations in any region (exons, introns, and intergenic regions) tended to increase progressively with each successive generation in both the ^{137}Cs water group and the control group. However, there was no significant difference in the frequency of sequence variations between the ^{137}Cs water group and the control group. Similarly, there was no difference in insertion/deletion (InDel) mutation frequency between the two groups. Furthermore, there was no distinctive pattern of base deletions in each group [8].

6. Interaction between low-dose radiation and chemical carcinogens:

   The incidence of lung tumors and mean tumor volume were quantified at 10 months of age in A/J mice; there was no difference in the incidence of spontaneous and chemically induced (Urethane-induced) lung tumors between the ^{137}Cs water and control groups.

   This indicates that trace doses of radiation are not additive or synergistic factors in chemical carcinogenesis. But surprisingly, the mean tumor volume in the ^{137}Cs water group was significantly smaller than in the control group. Thus, chronic low-dose internal exposure with ^{137}Cs does not affect tumor incidence, but may significantly inhibit tumor growth [8].

7. Analysis of cytokine levels in blood plasma:

   As described in item 6 above, tumor growth was significantly suppressed in the ^{137}Cs water group compared to the control group. A possible reason for this could be the difference in immunocompetence between the two groups. Therefore, we measured the amount of cytokines in the blood between the ^{137}Cs water group and the control group. The cytokines examined were interleukin (IL)-1α, -1β, -2, -3, -4, -5, -6, -9, -10, -12p40, -12p70, -13 and IL-17, eotaxin, granulocyte colony-stimulating factor (G-CSF), granulocyte-macrophage colony-stimulating factor (GM-CSF), interferon-gamma (IFN-γ), keratinocyte chemoattractant (KC/CXCL1), monocyte chemotactic protein-1 (MCP-1), macrophage inflammatory protein-1α (MIP-1α), MIP-1β, regulated on activation normal T cell expressed and secreted (RANTES), and TNF-α. Interestingly, blood levels of the Th1-type cytokines (IL-2, IFN-γ, and TNF-α, as well as IL-9, -13, and GM-CSF were significantly higher in the ^{137}Cs water group than in the control group [8].

   These results suggest that low-dose radiation activates antitumor immunity in mice. These also may be related to the abscopal effect, in which tumors in the radiation field shrink at the same time as distant tumors outside the radiation field shrink due to radiation therapy [8].

8. Gene expression analysis in the small intestine:

   It was shown that Cd226 gene expression, which induces the cytotoxic activity of NK cells, was approximately two-fold higher in the ^{137}Cs water group, and

IL-2 inducible T cell kinase (ITK) gene expression, which is involved in the proliferation and differentiation of T cells, was 1.8-fold higher compared to the control group. These results may be consistent with the Th1-type cytokine predominance observed in the previous cytokine assay results of item 7. The expression of these two genes was also increased by external ^{137}Cs γ-ray irradiation (1 Gy). This suggests that a certain dose of radiation has an immunostimulatory effect.

9. Oxidative stress and antioxidant stress capacity in plasma:

    Metabolome analysis showed that the glycolytic system was suppressed in the ^{137}Cs water group, and the antioxidants glutathione (GSH) and cysteine were decreased. Therefore, the state of balance between oxidative stress and antioxidant stress capacity in the body, which is thought to be affected by internal radiation exposure, was examined. In the ^{137}Cs water group, there was a significant increase in plasma 8-oxodihydroguanine, an indicator of oxidative stress. However, there was no significant difference in antioxidant stress capacity compared to the control group. It was considered that the oxidative stress occurring was within the tolerable range of the organism [8]. Similar findings were observed in analyses of plasma protein concentrations and enzyme activities in cattle within the evacuation zones following the Fukushima Daiichi nuclear power plant accident [9].

18.3 Discussion and Conclusion

Radiation-induced genetic effects, including carcinogenesis and transgenerational effects, have been observed in mice. The mutation induction rate per genome has been shown to be surprisingly lower than would have been expected from previous results with specific locus tests in the mice [10]. It has also been predicted that the same may be true for humans belonging to the same class, Mammalia, as mice. However, studies conducted over the past 70 years on the effects of radiation exposure on second-generation of A-bomb survivors [11, 12], the effects of radiation therapy on the children of childhood cancer patients [13, 14] and whole genome analysis of the children of Chornobyl decontaminators [15] have not yet demonstrated any genetic effects in the dose range that would result in the birth of future generations, even if exposed.

The effects of low-dose exposure to ^{137}Cs, including internal exposure, have become a major social issue, as the FNPP accident has raised concerns about genetic effects and carcinogenicity. In this context, efforts to present risk assessments based on quantitative scientific evidence are important, and this series of studies was undertaken to contribute to these efforts.

Despite the fact that humans have a much larger number of somatic cells and a longer life span than mice, the spontaneous mutation rate to the next generation is almost the same, 3.6×10^{-6} per gene per generation in humans and 6.1×10^{-6} in mice [6]. However, while mice develop cancer within 2 years, the average age at which humans develop cancers is about 50 years (lifetime cancer mortality rate is 11 ~ 30%), and considering that the total cell number is about 2,000 times that of mice, humans have by far a lower cancer rate than mice. Therefore, it is difficult to extrapolate the mouse experiment directly to humans. However, even if the mice are more susceptible to cancer than humans, if we can show a radiation dose that does not increase cancer or the effects on future generations of mice, the effect on the human body at that dose level is considered to be even lower. In other words, if we can experimentally demonstrate a dose range that does not affect the next generation in mice, we will be able to present a safety range for humans.

In this series of experiments, assuming that equilibrium has been reached because of continuous drinking, the body fluids of the ^{137}Cs-drinking mice have been completely replaced with water containing ^{137}Cs. In other words, each mouse weighing 30 g would have more than 2820 Bq of ^{137}Cs (equivalent to more than 4,700,000 Bq in a whole human body weighing 50 kg). Whole genome sequencing after 25 generations of mice in this condition showed no significant differences from the control group. Based on this experiment, it is believed that even if A/J mice were given water containing 100,000 Bq/L of ^{137}Cs, this would be a dose that would have no effect on future generations. Therefore, the Codex Alimentarius Commission's food regulatory limit of 1,000 Bq/kg, which is set at 1/100 of the present study, is considered to be within a safe range, even if taking into account the existence of humans who are highly sensitive to radiation. As an aside, the standard in Japan has been set at 100 Bq/kg for food and 10 Bq/kg for drinking water, which are extremely strict and one-tenth of the international standards.

18.4 Derivative Findings from Our Study and Their Applications

1. Abscopal effect.

The abscopal effect was first suggested by Mole. He irradiated only one of the tumors implanted bilaterally in mice and found that the unirradiated tumor on the opposite side also regressed. Mole proposed the term "abscopal" ("ab"—away from, "scopus"—target) to refer to this effect of ionizing radiation [16]. Since the abscopal effect was a rare phenomenon in radiotherapy, it was skeptical from the beginning and was not the subject of much research. However, with the increase in opportunities for particle therapy in recent years, the abscopal effect has been observed in many cases. This effect is thought to be the result of the unknown immunostimulatory effect that occurs in the process of killing tumors in the irradiated field, causing simultaneous regression of distant tumors [17].

It is reported that administration of a programmed death-ligand 1 (PD-L1) inhibitor after chemoradiotherapy led to long-term progression-free and overall survival benefits in patients with stage III lung cancer [18]. Radiation therapy can be considered as a trigger of systemic antitumor immune responses and used as a curative and systemic treatment, which may be added to the current standard treatment plan for patients with metastatic cancer. Clinical trials are underway to identify the optimal schedule of radioimmunotherapy to induce the abscopal effect. In addition, it is thought that the "radscopal effect," which uses low-dose radiation to reprogram the tumor microenvironment, may amplify the occurrence of the abscopal effect and overcome treatment resistance [19]. In this study, sustained low-dose-rate whole-body internal exposure caused significant fluctuations in the levels of antitumor cytokines. It is likely that some signals from the exposed tumor cells are required for the development of the abscopal effect. The results of lung tumor growth inhibition in the ^{137}Cs water group may be related to the abscopal effect. However, the ^{137}Cs water group may have an unknown response mechanism that is not necessarily limited to a specific tumor by radiation stimulation, since the anti-tumor cellular immune system is stimulated in the ^{137}Cs water group despite the absence of tumors. In fact, the relationship between standardized mortality ratios for aircraft pilots and exposure to cosmic radiation revealed that the higher the lifetime radiation dose, the lower the cancer mortality rate [20]. It is well known that radiation is carcinogenic, but this series of studies has revealed that very long-term low-dose radiation exposure also has the opposite effect. It is thought that radiation causes inflammation [21] and increases oxidative stress [22], which may be the background to carcinogenesis. In the future, it will be necessary to identify conditions that will eliminate these adverse effects and enhance immune function [23].

In addition, a comparison of cancer mortality rates between British radiologists and general practitioners based on 100 years of medical records showed that radiologists with higher lifetime radiation doses have a higher cancer mortality rate than general practitioners. However, the cancer mortality rate of radiologists with lifetime exposure doses of 100 mGy or less is significantly lower than that of general practitioners [24]. Therefore, the possibility that low-dose radiation exposure may have a cancer prevention effect cannot be denied, but the optimal dose needs to be considered.

2. Induction of organ-specific enzymes in the body by radiation and their application to medicine.

Figure 18.1 is a heat map showing the increase/decrease in gene expression in the liver of mice in the group exposed to 1 Gy external acute irradiation, the group subcutaneously administered urethane (1.0 mg/body weight) as a carcinogen, and the third-generation group continuously fed with ^{137}Cs water. The red bars indicate genes that increased compared to the untreated group, and the green bars indicate those that decreased. The two-colored arrows indicate the gene groups that significantly increased (red↑) and decreased (green↑) in the third-generation mice that continuously ingested ^{137}Cs water. The number and magnitude of the increased or decreased genes are shown below the heat map. Among these genes with increased expression, several genes showed enzyme expression (data not shown).

If these enzymes are expressed in an organ-specific manner by radiation, they can be used to treat cancer and other diseases. For example, enzymes induced in an organ-specific manner by radiation exposure could be used to activate an inactive

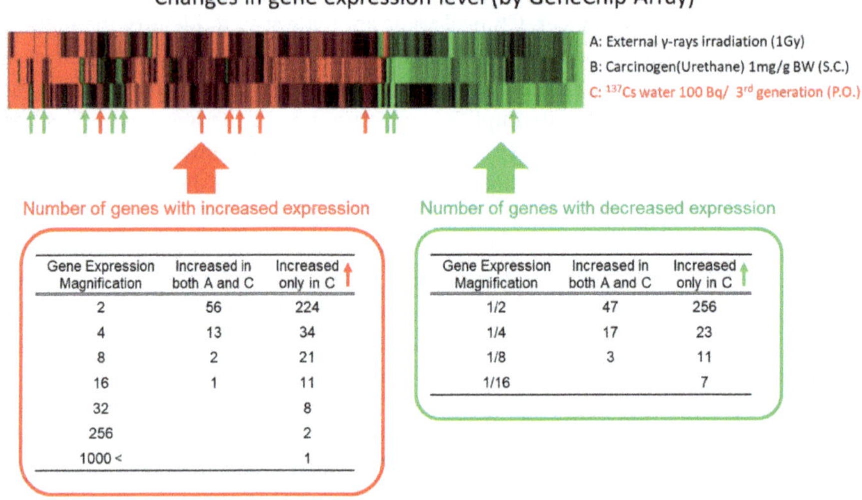

Fig. 18.1 Changes in gene expression level (by GeneChip Array).

drug (prodrug) that has been systemically administered in advance to produce a drug effect at the target organ.

Chemotherapy with systemic administration of anticancer drugs is burdensome to the bodies of patients. The key issue is how to selectively and effectively deliver the drug only to cancer tissues. The advantage of radiation in cancer treatment is that it can be administered noninvasively from outside the body, and the dose distribution (site-specific doses) within the body can be controlled. Depending on the location of the cancer, radiation therapy is also generally less physically demanding than surgery.

To date, the use of radiation in cancer therapy has been based on its cell-killing effect at high doses. The idea of this chapter, however, is a completely new approach: using low-dose-rate radiation as a switch on metabolic activity in the body.

18.5 Summary

Currently, the hereditary effects and carcinogenicity of radiation are evaluated based on the linear no-threshold (LNT) hypothesis. Therefore, concerns about carcinogenicity and hereditary effects remain even at low doses of radiation. To quantitatively evaluate the low-dose radiation effects of this concern, we conducted a series of experiments in which mice were fed 100,000 Bq/L of ^{137}Cs water as drinking water while undergoing repeated generation cycles (approximately 37 mGy per generation). And then, quantitative analysis of genetic effects using DNA sequence mutations as an indicator in the 25th generation of mice revealed no significant differences compared to the control group. In addition, no significant cancer-promoting effect was observed in the ^{137}Cs group.

This demonstrated that even in mice, which are more sensitive to mutations and carcinogenesis than humans, there exists a radiation dose at which the effects of radiation exposure cannot be significantly detected. Considering that the regulatory limits for food (Codex: 1000 Bq/kg or less for food; Japan's standard values: 100 Bq/kg or less for food, 10 Bq/g or less for drinking water) are less than one-hundredth of the conditions used in this experiment, levels below the current regulatory limits are considered to be within a range that is sufficiently safe for humans.

In addition, in carcinogenicity experiments in groups that ingested ^{137}Cs, an unexpected inhibitory effect on tumor growth was observed. Analysis of plasma cytokines for the purpose of studying immunocompetence showed that low-dose radiation stimulated anti-tumor immunity.

The series of studies presented in this chapter suggest the existence of biological phenomena that are different from the negative image of damage caused by low-dose radiation exposure from atomic bombs and nuclear accidents. We hope that more researchers will become interested in this new research field, the effects of low-dose radiation.

Acknowledgments I would like to thank my coresearchers, Mizuki Ohno (Kyushu Univ.), Kazuko Uno (Louis Pasteur Center for Medical Research), Satoru Endo (Hiroshima Univ.), Masatoshi Suzuki (Tohoku Univ.), and Hiroshi Toki and Tadashi Saito (Osaka Univ.).

I would like to thank Yamaguchi, Y., Tanigawa, H., Oda, S., and Ginama, H. (Osaka Univ.) for their excellent technical assistance.

This work was supported by Research project on the Health Effects of Radiation Organized by the Ministry of the Environment, Japan (2015, 2016, 2017, 2019, 2020, 2021, and 2022 to H.N.) and JSPS KAKENHI (Grant-in-Aid for Challenging Exploratory Research [JP26550039], Grant-in-Aid for Scientific Research (C)[JP20510052], and Grant-in-Aid for Scientific Research (B) [JP23310037] to H.N.).

The views of the author do not necessarily reflect those of the two sponsoring governments.

Competing Interests The author has no competing interests to declare.

References

1. The Use of the International Nuclear and Radiological Event Scale (INES) for Event Communication. IAEA Safety Standards and Related Publications. https://www-pub.iaea.org/MTCD/Publications/PDF/INES_web.pdf
2. The International Nuclear and Radiological Event Scale. User's Manual 2008 Edition. IAEA. https://www-pub.iaea.org/MTCD/Publications/PDF/INES2013web.pdf
3. The official report of The Fukushima Nuclear Accident Independent Investigation Commission. The National Diet of Japan. National Diet Library, archived October 25, 2012. https://warp.da.ndl.go.jp/info:ndljp/pid/3856371/naiic.go.jp/en/report/
4. Uchiyama M, Nakamura Y, Kobayashi S (1996) Analysis of body-burden measurements of ^{137}Cs and ^{40}K in a Japanese group over a period of 5 years following the Chernobyl acci-

dent. Health Phys 71:320–325. https://doi.org/10.1097/00004032-199609000-00008. Pubmed:8698573

5. Norris RS, Arkin WM (1998) Known nuclear tests worldwide, 1945–98. Bull At Sci 54(6):65–67. https://doi.org/10.1080/00963402.1998.11456906

6. Drost JB, Lee WR (1995) Biological basis of germline mutation: comparisons of spontaneous germline mutation rates among drosophila, mouse, and human. Environ Mol Mutagen 25(Suppl 26):48–64. https://doi.org/10.1002/em.2850250609. Pubmed:7789362

7. Nakajima H, Yamaguchi Y, Yoshimura T et al (2015) Fukushima simulation experiment: assessing the effects of chronic low-dose-rate internal ^{137}Cs radiation exposure on litter size, sex ratio, and biokinetics in mice. J Radiat Res 56(Suppl 1):i29–i35. https://doi.org/10.1093/jrr/rrv079. Pubmed:26825299

8. Nakajima H, Ohno M, Uno K et al (2024) Effects of generational low dose-rate ^{137}Cs internal exposure in descendant mice. Int J Radiat Biol 100(11):1560–1578. https://doi.org/10.1080/09553002.2024.2400521. Pubmed: 39302823

9. Urushihara Y, Kawasumi K, Endo S et al (2016) Analysis of plasma protein concentrations and enzyme activities in cattle within the ex-evacuation zone of the Fukushima Daiichi Nuclear Plant accident. PLoS One 11(8):e0159282. https://doi.org/10.1371/journal.pone.0159282

10. Nakamura N (2017) Why genetic effects of radiation are observed in mice but not in humans. Radiat Res 189(2):117–127. https://doi.org/10.1667/RR14947.1

11. Neel JV, Schull WJ, Awa AA et al (1990) The children of parents exposed to atomic bombs: estimates of the genetic doubling dose of radiation for humans. Am J Hum Genet 46:1053–1072. https://www.ncbi.nlm.nih.gov/pubmed/2339701. Pubmed: 2339701

12. Izumi S, Suyama A, Koyama K (2003) Radiation-related mortality among offspring of atomic bomb survivors: a half-century of follow-up. Int J Cancer 107:292–297. https://doi.org/10.1002/ijc.11400. Pubmed: 12949810

13. Green DM, Kawashima T, Stovall M et al (2009) Fertility of female survivors of childhood cancer: a report from the childhood cancer survivor study. J Clin Oncol 27:2677–2685. https://doi.org/10.1200/JCO.2008.20.1541. Pubmed: 19364965

14. Winther JF, Olsen JH, Wu H et al (2012) Genetic disease in the children of Danish survivors of childhood and adolescent cancer. J Clin Oncol 30:27–33. https://doi.org/10.1200/JCO.2011.35.0504. Pubmed: 22124106

15. Yeager M, Machiela MJ, Kothiyal P et al (2021) Lack of transgenerational effects of ionizing radiation exposure from the Chernobyl accident. Science 372:725–729. https://doi.org/10.1126/science.abg2365. Pubmed:33888597

16. Mole RH (1953) Whole body irradiation; radiobiology or medicine? Br J Radiol 26:234–241. https://doi.org/10.1259/0007-1285-26-305-234. Pubmed:13042090

17. Demaria S, Ng B, Devitt ML et al (2004) Ionizing radiation inhibition of distant untreated tumors (abscopal effect) is immune mediated. Int J Radiat Oncol Biol Phys 58:862–870. https://doi.org/10.1016/j.ijrobp.2003.09.012. Pubmed:14967443

18. Pujol JL (2022) Durvalumab induces sustained survival benefit after concurrent Chemoradiotherapy in stage III non–small-cell lung cancer. J Clin Oncol 40:1301–1311. https://doi.org/10.1200/JCO.22.00204

19. Barsoumian HB, Hsu J, Nanez S et al (2023) Technique as an immune adjuvant to treat cancer. Ther Immunol 3(1):74–85. https://doi.org/10.3390/immuno3010006

20. Langner I, Blettner M, Gundestrup M et al (2004) Cosmic radiation and cancer mortality among airline pilots: results from a European cohort study (ESCAPE). Radiat Environ Biophys 42:247–256. https://doi.org/10.1007/s00411-003-0214-7

21. Schaue D, Micewicz ED, Ratikan JA et al (2015) Radiation and inflammation. Semin Radiat Oncol 25(1):4–10. https://doi.org/10.1016/j.semradonc.2014.07.007

22. Meng QM, Zaharieva EK, Sasatani M et al (2021) Possible relationship between mitochondrial changes and oxidative stress under low dose-rate irradiation. Redox Rep 26:160–169. https://doi.org/10.1080/13510002.2021.1971363. Pubmed:34435550

23. Zhang Z, Liu X, Chen D et al (2022) Radiotherapy combined with immunotherapy: the dawn of cancer treatment. Signal Transduct Target Ther 7(1):258. https://doi.org/10.1038/s41392-022-01102-y
24. Berrington A, Darby SC, Weiss HA et al (2001) 100 years of observation on British radiologists: mortality from cancer and other causes 1897–1997. Br J Radiol 74(882):507–519. https://doi.org/10.1259/bjr.74.882.740507

Part VI
Key Issues Emerging from the FNPP Accident

Chapter 19
Differentially Expressed Genes in Normal Human Epithelial Cells Exposed to Type B Radioactive Cesium-Bearing Microparticles (CsMPs)

Masatoshi Suzuki, Satoru Endo, Kazuhiko Ninomiya, Koichi Chida, and Manabu Fukumoto

Abstract Following the Fukushima Daiichi Nuclear Power Plant (FNPP) accident, water-insoluble silicon dioxide microparticles adsorbing radioactive cesium (CsMPs) were found in the environment. CsMPs are classified into two categories, designated as type A and type B, based on their size and radioactivity. Inhalation of CsMPs is thought to affect surrounding cells at the deposition sites, both through exposure to ionizing radiation and contact with silica particles.

In this study, to understand the cellular effects of CsMPs, we performed a comparative analysis of gene expression changes in epithelial cells co-incubated with a type B CsMP or with a control nonradioactive (mock) particle using DNA microarray analysis. Gene expression was defined as upregulated when it increased by 1.5-fold or more, and downregulated when it decreased by 1.5-fold or lower after

M. Suzuki (✉)
International Research Institute of Disaster Science, Tohoku University, Sendai, Japan

Graduate School of Medicine, Tohoku University, Sendai, Japan

Fukushima Institute for Research, Education and Innovation, Sendai, Japan
e-mail: masatoshi.suzuki.c7@tohoku.ac.jp

S. Endo
Graduate School of Advanced Science and Engineering, Hiroshima University, Higashi-Hiroshima, Japan

K. Ninomiya
Natural Science Center for Basic Research and Development, Hiroshima University, Higashi-Hiroshima, Japan

K. Chida
International Research Institute of Disaster Science, Tohoku University, Sendai, Japan

Graduate School of Medicine, Tohoku University, Sendai, Japan

M. Fukumoto
International Research Institute of Disaster Science, Tohoku University, Sendai, Japan

© The Author(s) 2026

M. Fukumoto (ed.), *Low-Dose Radiation Effects on Animals and Ecosystems II*,
https://doi.org/10.1007/978-981-95-5559-8_19

co-incubation with the particle. Confluent normal human retinal epithelial hTERT-RPE1 cells were co-incubated with either of the particles in a 6.4 mm diameter well for 24 h. Co-incubation with the CsMP revealed that the number of upregulated genes was greater than that of downregulated genes. Gene Ontology Biological Process (GO-BP) analysis revealed that five pathways were enriched for the upregulated gene set. Three of these were related to viral infection, while the other two were related to interferon. The CsMP upregulated several interferon-stimulated genes (ISGs), whose basal expression is reported to protect cells from stress. STAT1 is known to up-regulate the expression of its downstream ISGs. These suggest that type B CsMP, which has high radioactivity and is not phagocytosed by cells, activates the STAT1-ISG pathway in cells surrounding its deposition. As a result, it is surprising that the particle nature of CsMPs cannot be ruled out as a factor that may mitigate the biological effects on normal cells.

Keywords Radioactive cesium-bearing microparticle (CsMP) · Insoluble radioactive microparticle · Fukushima Daiichi Nuclear Power Plant accident · Differentially expressed genes

19.1 Introduction

Following nuclear disasters, insoluble radioactive particles have been found in the environment, the nature of which varies depending on each nuclear event. The atomic bombings of Hiroshima and Nagasaki activated manganese oxides (MnO_2) in the soil, forming radioactive particles, $^{56}MnO_2$ [1]. The radioactive particles produced in the Chernobyl (Chornobyl) nuclear accident were uranium oxides, a component of nuclear fuel material [2]. Following the Fukushima Daiichi Nuclear Power Plant (FNPP) accident, water-insoluble radioactive cesium-bearing microparticles (CsMPs) formed by the adhesion of radioactive cesium ($^{134}Cs + ^{137}Cs$) to fine particles mainly composed of silicon dioxide were found in the environment [3]. The activity ratio of $^{134}Cs/^{137}Cs$ released into the environment was found to be 1.1 from Unit 1 and 0.92 from Units 2 and 3 [4, 5]. CsMPs from Units 2 and 3 are classified as type A with particle sizes in the range of 0.1–10 μm and radioactivity of 10^{-2}–10^2 Bq. Type B CsMPs, which are larger than type A particles with radioactivity of 10–10^4 Bq, have also been discovered. The radioactivity of ^{90}Sr and $^{238+239}Pu$ measured in type B particles is extremely small, 10^{-4}–10^{-6} relative to ^{137}Cs activity, and the main radiation emitted from CsMPs is β-particles and γ-rays derived from radioactive Cs [6, 7].

CsMPs are poorly soluble in water, and inhalation of highly radioactive type B particles in particular is of concern as a cause of localized internal exposure in humans. The site of deposition of particles in the respiratory tract after inhalation depends on particle size [8]. The International Commission on Radiological Protection (ICRP) has shown, using a human respiratory airway model, the half-life of particle clearance for each deposition site [9]. Type B particles are deposited mainly in the upper respiratory tract and are excreted from the body with a half-life of about 18 h. Type A particles penetrate deep into the lung and have a slow excretion half-life exceeding 1,000 days. It is generally recognized that the induction of DNA double-strand breaks is important in the manifestation of the biological effects of radiation [10]. In our study, type B particles but not type A induce DNA double-strand breaks, determined by immunohistochemistry for 53BP1. In this study, we therefore analyzed the cellular effects of type B particles. Cells exposed to radiation are known to induce inflammatory reactions in surrounding cells through the production of inflammatory cytokines [11]. To understand the effects of CsMPs on cells, it is necessary to consider not only radiation but also physical factors of contact with insoluble particles. In this study, we co-incubated immortalized human 2n epithelial cells with a type B CsMP and analyzed changes in gene expression in cells within a 3 mm radius of the particle.

19.2 Material and Methods

19.2.1 CsMPs and Cell Culture

CsMPs, kindly provided by Drs. Sueki and Satou (Tsukuba University, Japan) were isolated from soil collected in the ex-evacuation zone, which is within the 20-km radius of FNPP [5]. Radioactivity of CsMPs was measured in a germanium semiconductor spectrometer (ORTEC Co., Oak Ridge, TN). The CsMP used in this study was a type B particle with a diameter of 500 μm, in which 234 Bq of ^{134}Cs and 1,677 Bq of ^{137}Cs were contained. Human telomerase reverse transcriptase–immortalized retinal pigment epithelial (hTERT-RPE1) cells [12], kindly provided by Dr. Hara (Osaka University, Japan), were cultured in Dulbecco's Modified Eagle Medium (DMEM; Nissui, Tokyo, Japan) supplemented with 10% fetal bovine serum (FBS; ThermoFisher Scientific, NY) and maintained in the logarithmic growth phase. Non-radioactive (mock) particles were prepared by mixing silica particles into non-radioactive CsOH melted at approximately 300 °C in a crucible, followed by the application of an air jet to generate droplets [13].

19.2.2 Gene Expression Analysis

The calculated dose decreases rapidly with distance from the CsMP. In this experiment, we analyzed the effect of a single type B CsMP on cells in an entire well with a radius of 3.2 mm (96-well microplate, TPP, Trasadingen, Switzerland) (Fig. 19.1a). Cells (50,000 cells/well) were seeded into a well, the CsMP was placed on confluent cells for 24 h (CsMP group), and total RNA was extracted (Fig. 19.1a, b). To analyze the effect of radiation exposure, gene expression profiles were compared

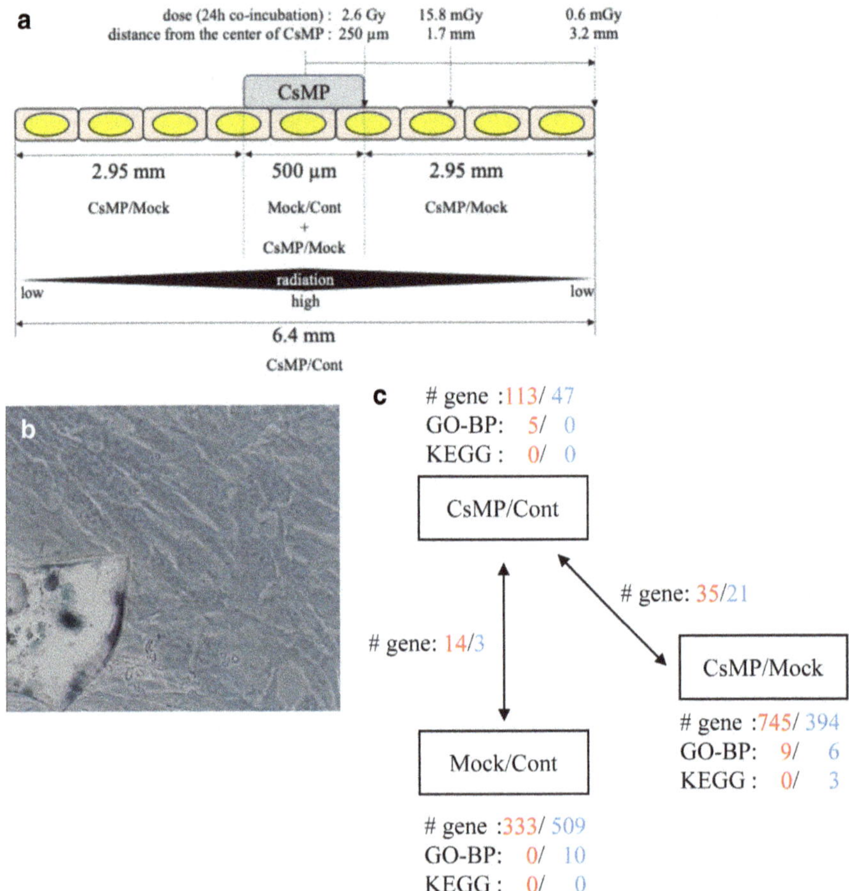

Fig. 19.1 Overview of the co-incubation experiment and microarray analysis. (**a**) Schematic diagram of the co-incubation of hTERT-RPE1 cells with a CsMP in a 96-well plate. (**b**) Co-incubation of hTERT-RPE1 cells with the CsMP. (**c**) Microarray analysis results. The "# gene" numbers indicate the number of upregulated genes (red) and downregulated genes (blue), respectively. The GO-BP and KEGG numbers indicate the number of enriched pathways in the upregulated gene set (red) and downregulated gene set (blue), respectively.

among the CsMP group, the Mock group and the negative control (Cont) group without any particles. Each comparison was performed independently in duplicate using the same extracted RNA. Genes exhibiting a fold-change of ≥ 1.5 or ≤ 0.67 (1/1.5) across two independent experiments, relative to Cont or Mock groups, were defined as significantly upregulated or downregulated. Human Oligo chip 25 k (TORAY, Kanagawa, Japan) was used for microarray analysis. Gene Ontology-Biological Process (GO-BP) analysis was performed on the upregulated or downregulated gene groups using Database for Annotation and Visualization and Integrated Discovery v2025_1 (DAVID, https://davidbioinformatics.nih.gov/summary.jsp) [14, 15].

Table 19.1 qRT-PCR primer sequences.

Gene	Forward	Reverse
BST2	ACGCGTCTGCAGAGGTGGAG	GCAGCGGAGCTGGAGTCCT
ISG15	CGCAGATCACCCAGAAGATCG	TTCGTCGCATTTGTCCACCA
OAS1	TGAGGTCCAGGCTCCACGCT	GCAGGTCGGTGCACTCCTCG
STAT1	GGCACGCACACAAAAGTGAT	AGAGGTCGTCTCGAGGTCAA

Changes in gene expression extracted from microarray analysis were confirmed by quantitative reverse transcription polymerase chain reaction (qRT-PCR) using TB Green Premix Ex Taq II (Takara, Tokyo, Japan). The primer sequences used in qRT-PCR are shown in Table 19.1. Confluent hTERT-RPE1 cells cultured in a T25 flask (ThermoFisher Scientific, NY) were exposed to 2, 4, 6, 8, or 10 Gy of X-rays (M150-WE, SOFTEX, Kanagawa, Japan), and 24 and 72 h after irradiation, total RNA was extracted.

19.3 Result

19.3.1 *Differentially Expressed Genes (DEGs) in Cells After Co-Incubation with a Single Type B CsMP*

Compared to Cont, 113 genes were upregulated, and 47 genes were downregulated in the CsMP group (the CsMP/Cont comparison in Fig. 19.1c). Compared to Cont, 333 genes were upregulated, and 509 genes were downregulated in the Mock group (the Mock/Cont comparison in Fig. 19.1c). In the CsMP/Cont comparison and the Mock/Cont comparison, 14 genes were commonly upregulated, and 3 genes were commonly downregulated. The expression of these genes is thought to be fluctuated by physical contact regardless of whether the particle was radioactive or not. Compared to the Mock group, 745 genes were upregulated, and 394 genes were downregulated in the CsMP group (the CsMP/Mock comparison in Fig. 19.1c). In both the CsMP/Cont and CsMP/Mock comparisons, 35 genes were commonly upregulated and 21 genes were downregulated. The expression of these genes is thought to be affected by radiation exposure.

Figure 19.2 is the heat map showing genes that were up- or downregulated in the CsMP/Cont comparison and were also up- or downregulated in the Mock/Cont or the CsMP/Mock comparison. Three genes, *DACT1* and *SLC14A1*, and *ADM* exhibited opposite regulation between the Mock/Cont and the CsMP/Mock comparisons. *DACT1* and *SLC14A1* were downregulated by particle contact (the Mock/Cont comparison), but were upregulated in both the CsMP/Cont and CsMP/Mock comparisons, indicating that their upregulation was induced by radiation *per se* (Fig. 19.2a). *ADM* was upregulated by radiation exposure (the CsMP/Mock comparison), but was downregulated by the particle contact, resulting in overall downregulation in the CsMP/Cont comparison.

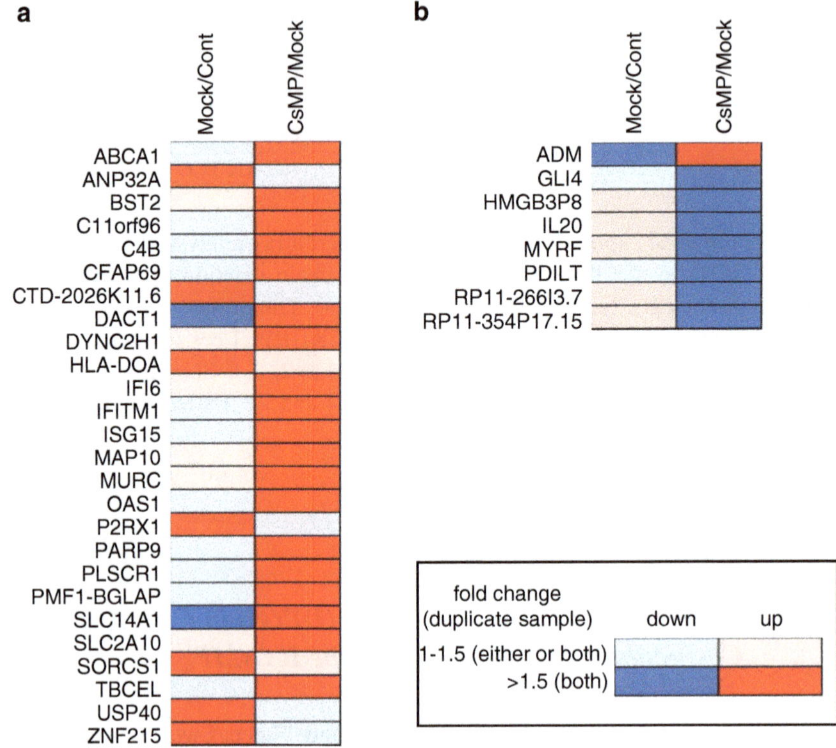

Fig. 19.2 Heatmap of genes differentially expressed after co-incubation with or a mock particle. Genes whose expression was upregulated (**a**) or downregulated (**b**) by exposure to the CsMP (the CsMP/Cont comparison) were extracted, and comparative analysis of each gene expression was conducted with the data of the Mock/Cont and the CsMP/Mock comparisons. Changes in gene expression are visualized by the color scale.

19.3.2 Functions of Genes with Altered Expression

Enrichment analyses reveal biological insights by detecting overrepresented pathways or functions within a gene set. Gene ontology- biological process (GO-BP) enrichment classifies genes by their functions, cellular locations, and biological roles. Kyoto Encyclopedia of Genes and Genomes (KEGG) enrichment analysis maps genes to specific metabolic or signaling pathways, revealing how these genes work together in biological systems. The GO-BP analysis identified five pathways enriched for the upregulated gene set in the CsMP/Cont comparison (Fig. 19.1c). Among these five pathways, three were related to viral infection and the other two to interferon (Table 19.2). GO-BP analysis identified 9 pathways enriched for the upregulated gene set in the CsMP/Mock comparison (Fig. 19.1c). Among these pathways, "defense response to viruses" was common to the result of the CsMP/ Cont comparison (Table 19.2). These suggest that the "defense response against

Table 19.2 GO-BP analysis of up-regulated genes.

	Term	# Genes (%)[a]	FDR
CsMP/Cont (5)	Defense response to virus	12 (11.4)	1.8×10^{-5}
	Negative regulation of viral genome replication	7(6.7)	2.5×10^{-5}
	Response to virus	8(7.6)	3.0×10^{-4}
	Type I interferon-mediated signaling pathway	6(5.7)	8.0×10^{-4}
	Response to interferon-beta	4(3.8)	2.7×10^{-3}
CsMP/Mock (9)	Negative regulation of transcription by RNA polymerase II	69(9.8)	3.9×10^{-6}
	Negative regulation of DNA-templated transcription	49(7.0)	3.9×10^{-6}
	Apoptotic process	43(6.1)	2.5×10^{-3}
	Positive regulation of DNA-templated transcription	48(6.8)	3.5×10^{-3}
	Regulation of DNA-templated transcription	57(8.1)	2.2×10^{-2}
	Negative regulation of cell population proliferation	32(4.5)	2.2×10^{-2}
	Positive regulation of apoptotic process	26(3.7)	3.8×10^{-2}
	Regulation of autophagy	11(1.6)	4.6×10^{-2}
	Defense response to virus	21(3.0)	4.9×10^{-2}

[a]Genes involved in the term (percentage involved gene/total gene)

viruses" pathway is activated by radiation *per se* rather than by the particle nature of the CsMP. In this pathway, the commonly upregulated genes in both comparisons were *BST2, IFI44L, IFI6, IFIH1, IFITM1, ISG15, OSAL, PARP9, PLSCR1,* and *STAT1* (Table 19.3).

The genes, except for *STAT1*, are known to be transcriptionally activated by STAT1. Although these genes are classified as interferon-stimulated genes (ISGs), gene expression levels of interferon were unchanged in the CsMP/Cont comparison (data not shown). These results suggest that radiation derived from CsMPs, but not the particle nature, induces increased expression of STAT1, resulting in activation of interferon-related pathways. The GO-BP and KEGG analyses revealed that pathways related to the cell cycle, DNA replication, and metabolism were enriched in the downregulated gene set in the CsMP/Mock comparison (Fig. 19.1c, Tables 19.4 and 19.5). However, these pathways were different from those enriched for the downregulated gene set in the CsMP/Cont comparison.

19.3.3 Radiation Effects on Gene Expression

In both the CsMP/Cont and CsMP/Mock comparisons, 35 genes were commonly upregulated. Among them, *BST2, ISG15, OAS1,* and *STAT1* were involved in multiple pathways enriched for the upregulated gene set found by GO-BP analysis.

Table 19.3 Genes involved in the pathways enriched for the up-regulated gene set in the CsMP/Cont comparison.

Genes	Terms					
	defense response to virus		negative regulation of viral genome replication	response to virus	type I interferon-mediated signaling pathway	response to interferon-beta
	CsMP/Cont	CsMP/Mock				
ADARB1		○				
BST2	○	○	○	○		○
DDX60	○			○		
EIF2AK2		○				
HERC5		○				
IFI16		○				
IFI44				○		
IFI44L	○	○				
IFI6	○	○				
IFIH1	○	○	○	○	○	
IFIT3		○				
IFITM1	○	○	○	○	○	○
IFNG		○				
IRF9		○				
ISG15	○	○	○	○		
ITCH		○				
LSM14A		○				
OSA1	○		○	○	○	
OSAL	○	○	○	○	○	
PARP9	○	○				
PLSCR1	○	○	○			○
PMAIP1		○				
POLR3E		○				
SIN3A					○	
STAT1	○	○			○	○

Table 19.4 GO-BP analysis of down-regulated genes.

	Term	# Genes (%)[a]	FDR
Mock/Cont (10)	Negative regulation of transcription by RNA polymerase II	63 (13.0)	5.1×10^{-11}
	Positive regulation of transcription by RNA polymerase II	60 (12.4)	3.0×10^{-5}
	Negative regulation of DNA-templated transcription	36(7.4)	4.4×10^{-5}
	Positive regulation of apoptotic process	23(4.8)	1.8×10^{-3}
	Positive regulation of DNA-templated transcription	36(7.4)	4.1×10^{-3}
	Regulation of autophagy	10(2.1)	7.6×10^{-3}
	Apoptotic process	31(6.4)	7.6×10^{-3}
	Transforming growth factor beta receptor signaling pathway	11(2.3)	2.2×10^{-2}
	Positive regulation of autophagy	10(2.1)	3.2×10^{-2}
	Negative regulation of apoptotic process	26(5.4)	3.8×10^{-2}
CsMP/Mock (6)	Cell division	27(7.4)	1.3×10^{-6}
	Chromosome segregation	14(3.8)	9.6×10^{-6}
	Mitotic cell cycle	13(3.6)	2.6×10^{-3}
	Mitotic sister chromatid segregation	7(1.9)	6.9×10^{-3}
	Mitotic spindle assembly checkpoint signaling	6(1.6)	3.8×10^{-2}
	DNA replication	9(2.5)	4.7×10^{-2}

[a]Genes involved in the term (percentage involved gene/total gene)

Table 19.5   KEGG pathway analysis of down-regulated genes.

	Term	# Genes (%)[a]	FDR
CsMP/Mock (3)	DNA replication	8(2.2)	1.3×10^{-3}
	Cell cycle	12(3.3)	2.9×10^{-2}
	Retinol metabolism	8(2.2)	2.9×10^{-2}

[a]Genes involved in the term (percentage involved gene/total gene)

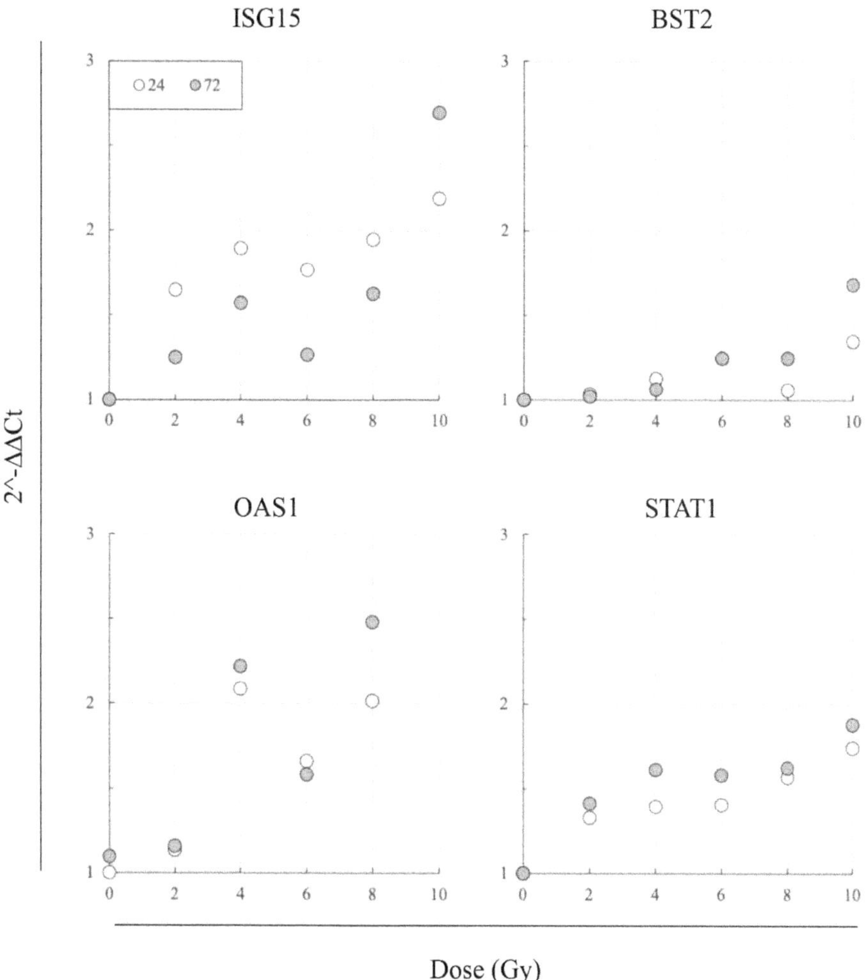

Fig. 19.3 Verification of gene expression in response to ionizing radiation exposure. The expression of *ISG15*, *BST2*, *OAS1*, and *STAT1* was examined by qRT-PCR. Total RNA was extracted from hTERT-RPE1 24 (white) and 72 h (gray) after irradiation.

The expression of these four genes increased in a dose-dependent manner, particularly at doses of 2 Gy or more, and persisted for up to 72 h after irradiation (Fig. 19.3).

19.4 Discussion

Type B CsMPs are larger than the cell body and cannot be taken up into the cell. Therefore, once type B CsMPs are deposited, cells are affected by both the physical effect of contact with the silica particle and radiation exposure. In this study, to understand the characteristics of biological response to type B CsMPs, we compared genes whose expression was altered by CsMP treatment (the CsMP/Cont comparison) with genes whose expression was altered by contact with particles (the Mock/Cont comparison) and radiation exposure (the CsMP/Mock comparison). Radiation exposure to cells surrounding a CsMP is nonuniform, and dose-rate decreases proportionally to the square of distance from the CsMP. The type B CsMP used in this study demonstrated to induce DNA double-strand breaks in cells located within a 1 cm radius (*manuscript submitted*). Therefore, all cells co-incubated with the CsMP in this study were affected by radiation.

DACT1 and *SLC14A1* were upregulated following radiation exposure (the CsMP/ Mock comparison) but downregulated by particle-contact (the Mock/Cont comparison) (Fig. 19.2). *DACT1* overexpression is reportedly enhanced apoptosis [16], and overexpression of *SLC14A1* causes mitochondrial dysfunction, leading to the generation of mitochondrial reactive oxygen species [17]. *ADM* mRNA levels and secretion are upregulated by γ-irradiation [18] and induce IL-6 secretion [19]. In this study, *ADM* was upregulated by radiation exposure (the CsMP/Mock comparison); however, it was downregulated in the CsMP/Cont and the Mock/Cont comparisons. These support the need to consider particle contact when analyzing the biological effects of CsMPs, including their potential to mitigate radiation effects by particle contact. The GO-BP analysis enriched three virus-infection-related pathways and two interferon-related pathways for the gene set upregulated in the CsMP/ Cont comparison (Table 19.2). Of these five pathways, the "defense response to viruses" was the pathway with the highest number of upregulated genes (Table 19.3). Among the upregulated genes in the CsMP/Cont comparison, *BST2*, *IFI44L*, *IFI6*, *IFIH1*, *IFITM1*, *ISG15*, *OASL*, *PARP9*, *PLSCR1*, and *STAT1* were also upregulated in the CsMP/Mock comparison, suggesting that the "defense response to viruses" pathway is activated by radiation exposure per se. Genes whose expression is upregulated by virus infection via interferon, such as *IFI44L*, *IFITM1*, *OAS1*, and *OASL*, are called interferon-stimulated genes (ISGs) [20–22]. It is known that overexpression of STAT1 increases expression of ISGs in human fibroblasts [22, 23]. In this study, we did not detect upregulation of interferon genes in the CsMP/Cont comparison, but nine ISGs genes (*IFITM1*, *OAS1*, *OASL*, *PLSCR1*, *IFI44*, *BST2*, *IFIH1*, *IFI44L*, and *IFI35*) were upregulated. These suggest that the exposure of cells to CsMPs induces STAT1-mediated but interferon-independent expression of ISGs, which is induced by radiation exposure *per se*. Sustained low level of interferon causes a steady-state expression of ISGs and resistance to DNA damage [24, 25]. In this study, we found upregulation of ISGs genes in the CsMP/Cont comparison. Therefore, the pathways related to viral infection, which were enriched for the upregulated gene set in the CsMP/Cont comparison, may induce stress tolerance in the cells affected by CsMPs. It is surprising that CsMPs may have radiation-protective effects on normal cells even though the range of the cells with which they directly come into contact is extremely limited. A detailed investigation is required into the effects of non-uniform radiation doses relative to the distance from CsMPs and the so-called bystander effects.

Acknowledgments This work was supported by the Research Project on the Health Effects of Radiation, organized by the Ministry of the Environment, Japan, and the Research Project for Reconstruction from Nuclear Disaster, organized by Tohoku University Fund. This work was partly supported by JSPS KAKENHI (grant number: 23K28227, 23K11429, 24K03080) and Network-type Joint Usage/Research Center for Radiation Disaster Medical Science. This work is an activity of the Disaster Resilience Co-creation Center and Core-Research Cluster of Disaster Science, IRIDeS, Tohoku University.

References

1. Tanaka K, Endo S, Imanaka T et al (2008) Skin dose from neutron-activated soil for early entrants following the A-bomb detonation in Hiroshima: contribution from beta and gamma rays. Radiat Environ Biophys 47:323–330. https://doi.org/10.1007/s00411-008-0172-1
2. Zheltonozhsky V, Mück K, Bondarkov M (2001) Classification of hot particles from the Chernobyl accident and nuclear weapons detonations by non-destructive methods. J Environ Radioact 57:151–166. https://doi.org/10.1016/s0265-931x(01)00013-3
3. Adachi K, Kajino M, Zaizen Y et al (2013) Emission of spherical cesium-bearing particles from an early stage of the Fukushima nuclear accident. Sci Rep 3:2554. https://doi.org/10.1038/srep02554
4. Miura H, Kurihara Y, Yamamoto M et al (2020) Characterization of two types of cesium-bearing microparticles emitted from the Fukushima accident via multiple synchrotron radiation analyses. Sci Rep 10:11421. https://doi.org/10.1038/s41598-020-68318-2
5. Satou Y, Sueki K, Sasa K et al (2018) Analysis of two forms of radioactive particles emitted during the early stages of the Fukushima Dai-ichi nuclear Power Station accident. Geochem J 52:137–143. https://doi.org/10.2343/geochemj.2.0514
6. Igarashi J, Zheng J, Zhang Z et al (2019) First determination of Pu isotopes (^{239}Pu, ^{240}Pu and ^{241}Pu) in radioactive particles derived from Fukushima Daiichi Nuclear Power Plant accident. Sci Rep 9:11807. https://doi.org/10.1038/s41598-019-48210-4
7. Igarashi J, Ninomiya K, Zheng J et al (2024) Fukushima Daiichi nuclear power plant accident: understanding formation mechanism of radioactive particles through Sr and Pu quantities. Environ Sci Technol 58:14823–14830. https://doi.org/10.1021/acs.est.4c03428
8. Rostami AA (2009) Computational modeling of aerosol deposition in respiratory tract: a review. Inhal Toxicol 21:262–290. https://doi.org/10.1080/08958370802448987
9. International Commission on Radiological Protection (ICRP) (2015) Occupational intakes of radionuclides: part 1. ICRP Publication 130. Ann ICRP 44(2). https://doi.org/10.1177/0146645315577539
10. El-Nachef L, Al-Choboq J, Restier-Verlet J et al (2021) Human Radiosensitivity and Radiosusceptibility: what are the differences? Int J Mol Sci 22:7158. https://doi.org/10.3390/ijms22137158
11. Schaue D, Kachikwu EL, McBride WH (2012) Cytokines in radiobiological responses: a review. Radiat Res 178:505–523. https://doi.org/10.1667/RR3031.1
12. Bonder AG, Ouellette M, Frolkis M et al (1998) Extension of Life-Span by Introduction of Telomerase into Normal Human Cells. Science 279:15729. https://doi.org/10.1126/science.279.5349.349

13. Ninomiya K (2020) Properties of radioactive Cs-bearing particles released by the Fukushima Daiichi Nuclear Power Plant accident and trace element analysis. Fukumoto M (ed) Low-Dose Radiation Effects on Animals and Ecosystems. 195–204

14. Sherman BT, Hao M, Qiu J et al (2022) DAVID: a web server for functional enrichment analysis and functional annotation of gene lists (2021 update). Nucl Acids Res 50(W1):W216–W221. https://doi.org/10.1093/nar/gkac194

15. da Huang W, Sherman BT, Lempicki RA (2009) Systematic and integrative analysis of large gene lists using DAVID bioinformatics resources. Nat Protoc 4(1):44–57. https://doi.org/10.1038/nprot.2008.211

16. Zhu K, Jiang B, Yang Y et al (2017) DACT1 overexpression inhibits proliferation, enhances apoptosis, and increases daunorubicin chemosensitivity in KG-1α cells. Tumour Biol 39(10):1010428317711089. https://doi.org/10.1177/1010428317711089

17. Shi J, Sha R, Yang X (2023) Role of the human solute carrier family 14 member 1 gene in hypoxia-induced renal cell carcinoma occurrence and its enlightenment to cancer nursing. BMC Mol Cell Biol 24:10. https://doi.org/10.1186/s12860-023-00473-6

18. Zhong G, Chen F, Bu D et al (2003) Effects of cobalt-60 gamma-radiation on the synthesis of adrenomedullin and endothelin in rat vascular smooth muscle cells. Heart Vessel 18:207–212. https://doi.org/10.1007/s00380-003-0709-9

19. Isumi Y, Minamino N, Kubo A et al (1998) Adrenomedullin stimulates interleukin-6 production in Swiss 3T3 cells. Biochem Biophys Res Commun 244:325–331. https://doi.org/10.1006/bbrc.1998.8261

20. Wang W, Yin Y, Xu L et al (2017) Unphosphorylated ISGF3 drives constitutive expression of interferon-stimulated genes to protect against viral infections. Sci Signal 10:eaah4248. https://doi.org/10.1126/scisignal.aah4248

21. Tanaka Y, Chen ZJ (2012) STING specifies IRF3 phosphorylation by TBK1 in the cytosolic DNA signaling pathway. Sci Signal 5:ra20. https://doi.org/10.1126/scisignal.2002521

22. Nan Y, Wu C, Zhang YJ (2018) Interferon independent non-canonical STAT activation and virus induced inflammation. Viruses 10:196. https://doi.org/10.3390/v10040196

23. Cheon H, Stark GR (2009) Unphosphorylated STAT1 prolongs the expression of interferon-induced immune regulatory genes. Proc Natl Acad Sci U S A 106:9373–9378. https://doi.org/10.1073/pnas.0903487106

24. Wilkins C, Woodward J, Lau DT et al (2013) IFITM1 is a tight junction protein that inhibits hepatitis C virus entry. Hepatology 57:461–469. https://doi.org/10.1002/hep.26066

25. Cheon H, Borden EC, Stark GR (2014) Interferons and their stimulated genes in the tumor microenvironment. Semin Oncol 41:156–173. https://doi.org/10.1053/j.seminoncol.2014.02.002

Chapter 20
Highly Efficient Uptake of Radioactive Cesium by Intestinal and Probiotic Bacteria

Kazuki Saito, Kengo Kuroda, Rie Mukozono, Yasushi Kino, Junko Nishimura, Manabu Fukumoto, and Emiko Isogai

Abstract After the Fukushima Daiichi Nuclear Power Plant (FNPP), biological and chemical methods have been developed to reduce radioactive contamination. We hope to know efficient technology to remove radioactive cesium (Cs) from animal and human bodies to avoid internal exposure to contaminated water and foods. It was shown that common enteric bacteria, such as genus *Bacteroides* and *Clostridium*, were able to trap cesium-137 (^{137}Cs) in BHI medium (the uptake ratio 45.0–81.2% in vitro). When potassium ion (K^+) increased in the medium, % uptake decreased (21.0–24.5%). Viable bacteria are essential because heat-killed bacteria cannot act adsorptive agent.

Bifidobacterium longum (intestinal and probiotic bacterium) could grow in BHI (K ion: 2×10^2 ppm) but not in lactobacilli medium. The uptake ratio of *B. longum* was 37.8% in BHI medium. Lactobacilli, as probiotic bacteria, strongly require K+ ion and can grow in MRS medium with high K^+ concentration (1.5×10^3 ppm). It was suspected that K^+ inhibits the uptake of ^{137}Cs in MRS medium. Lactobacilli could grow in skim milk medium (5% skim milk, K ion: 7×10^2 ppm), and the uptake of ^{137}Cs increased from 28.7% to 35.7% in *Lactobacillus gasseri*, from 35.3% to 51.3% in *Lactobacillus delbrueckii* subsp. *bulgaricus* and from 33.0% to 82.9% in *Lacticaseibacillus casei*. Thus, ^{137}Cs uptake may depend on the concentration of K^+ in the media under suitable bacterial growth.

It was considered that intestinal bacteria are important to remove radioactive Cs from human and animal bodies, although intestinal flora itself can change with

K. Saito · K. Kuroda · R. Mukozono · E. Isogai (✉)
Graduate School of Agricultural Science, Tohoku University, Sendai, Japan
e-mail: emiko.isogai.a7@tohoku.ac.jp

Y. Kino
Faculty of Science and Graduate School of Science, Tohoku University, Sendai, Japan

J. Nishimura
Faculty of Food and Agricultural Sciences, Fukushima University, Fukushima, Japan

M. Fukumoto
International Rersearch Institute of Disaster Science, Tohoku University, Sendai, Japan

M. Fukumoto (ed.), *Low-Dose Radiation Effects on Animals and Ecosystems II*,
https://doi.org/10.1007/978-981-95-5559-8_20

aging, diet, and various factors. We also described the possibility of probiotic bacteria for the elimination of radioactive Cs.

Keywords Radioactive cesium (Cs) · ^{137}Cs · Intestinal flora · Probiotic bacteria · Elimination · Fukushima Daiichi Nuclear Power Plant (FNPP)

20.1 Introduction

Following the Fukushima Daiichi Nuclear Power Plant (FNPP) accident in March 2011, large amounts of radionuclides were released into the environment, and radioactive cesium (^{134}Cs + ^{137}Cs) in food became a serious problem in Japan [1]. Radioactive contamination caused by the FNPP accident was detected in water, vegetables, fruits, milk, and beef [2, 3]. Fukuda et al. reported the distribution of radioactive substances in abandoned cattle within a 20-km radius of FNPP, revealing that the highest distribution of radioactive Cs was in the skeletal muscle [4]. Organ distribution and egestion of radioactive Cs are important for the assessing food safety and for human/animal health. Because Cs$^+$ is chemically similar to K$^+$, it can enter mammalian cells via potassium channels and transporters. In humans, radioactive Cs is thought to be excreted mainly in urine (85%), followed by feces (13%) and sweat (2%) [5]. In addition, dairy cows excrete radioactive Cs via their milk [2]. Figure 20.1 shows the dynamics of radioactive Cs in the body of cattle.

Recently, we reported that cattle feces contained high concentrations of ^{137}Cs, and that intestinal bacteria trapped ^{137}Cs [6]. Based on these findings, we speculated that intestinal flora plays an important role in the elimination of radioactive Cs in domestic animals. In almost all examined animals, including cattle and inobuta (a boar–pig hybrid), the concentration of ^{137}Cs in feces was higher than that in urine, which is generally considered a major route for egestion of radioactive Cs. Furthermore, the ^{137}Cs concentration in feces was higher than that in skeletal muscle, where the highest concentration of radioactive Cs shows among organs. These observations suggest that abundant bacteria in the intestinal flora contribute to the elimination of radioactive Cs from the body. Therefore, we examined the contribution of intestinal bacteria to ^{137}Cs excretion. Radioactive Cs encounters up to 10^{14} bacteria in the mammalian intestine [7]. It is considered that radioactive Cs uptake is mediated through the metabolic system of the intestinal bacteria.

Food microbes can modify the normal flora of the human body, and the replacement of harmful microbes with beneficial microbes is possible. The most widely used bacteria as probiotics are *Bifidobacterium* and *Lactobacilli*. These bacteria are so-called lactic acid-producing bacteria and are very important probiotics that are used for the treatment of many disorders [8, 9]. Probiotics are beneficial microorganisms that are consumed in foods or dietary supplements and can survive in the intestine [10]. In this chapter, we discuss how probiotic bacteria interact to absorb radioactive Cs. Here, we introduce Cs uptake by intestinal bacteria and probiotic bacteria.

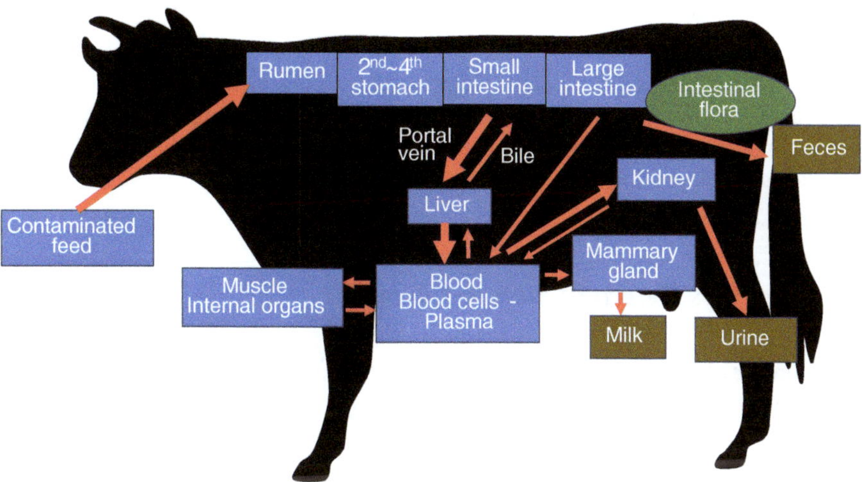

Fig. 20.1 The dynamics of radioactive cesium in the body of cattle.

20.2 Materials and Methods

20.2.1 Bacterial Strains, Media and Cultures

Bacteroides fragilis RIMD 0230001, *Bacteroides vulgatus* JCM 5826, *Clostridium perfringens* JCM 1290, *Clostridium ramosum* JCM 1298, and *Bifidobacterium longum* subsp. *longum* JCM 1217 were used as the major intestinal bacteria. These bacterial strains were propagated in 10 mL of Brain–Heart Infusion (BHI) broth (Difco Laboratories, Detroit, MI, USA) in Anaero-Pack systems (Mitsubishi Gas Chemical, Tokyo, Japan) at 37 °C for 24 h, as previously described [6].

Bifidobacterium breve ATCC 15700, *Lacticaseibacillus casei* (*L. casei*) ATCC 393, *Lactobacillus gasseri* JCM 1131^T (*L. gasseri*), and *Lactobacillus delbrueckii* subsp. *bulgaricus* JCM 1002^T (*L. bulgaricus*) were used as probiotic bacteria. These bacterial strains were propagated in 10 ml of de Man, Rogosa, and Sharpe (MRS) medium (Difco Laboratories, Detroit, MI, USA) or reconstituted skim milk (RSM; Morinaga Milk Industry Co., Tokyo, Japan) supplemented with 0.5% (w/v) Proteose peptone No.3 and 0.5% (w/v) Yeast extract (Nissui Pharmaceutical Co., Tokyo, Japan) using a 1% (v/v) inoculum. All indigenous bacteria were incubated anaerobically with an Anaero-Pack (Mitsubishi Gas Chemical, Tokyo, Japan) at 37 °C for 24 h. MRS medium was sterilized at 121 °C for 15 min. RSM was sterilized at 115 °C for 15 min. MRS or RSM was used because probiotic bacteria cannot grow in BHI medium.

20.2.2 ^{137}Cs-Containing Muscle Samples for Medium

Muscles were sampled from cattle living within a 20-km radius of the FNPP, and muscle extract was prepared by boiling. BHI agar containing 10% (v/v) of the ^{137}Cs-containing extract was used as the incubation medium for the bacterial ^{137}Cs uptake assay, as previously described [6].

20.2.3 ^{137}Cs Determination in Bacteria

The number of viable bacteria was adjusted to 10^8 colony-forming units (CFUs)/ml, and 100 µl of each bacterial strain was inoculated onto the medium and incubated at 37 °C for 48 h under anaerobic conditions [6]. After incubation, the medium was washed three times with 1 ml of sterile Dulbecco's phosphate-buffered saline (PBS) (Nissui Pharmaceutical Co., Tokyo, Japan). The bacterial suspension was recovered and poured into U8 (100 mL) polypropylene containers (Yamayu, Osaka, Japan). The agar medium was also melted and poured into a separate U8 polypropylene container. The agar medium from three petri dishes was poured into U8 containers. Heat-killed bacteria were also used for the assay. The concentration of radioactive ^{137}Cs in the bacteria and the medium was determined using a germanium γ-ray spectrometer.

20.2.4 Inhibition of ^{137}Cs Uptake by K^+ Ion

To examine the ^{137}Cs uptake inhibition caused by K^+ in the medium, K_2HPO_4 was added to BHI or RSM at a final concentration of 1,500 ppm, which is a similar level to that of MRS medium. After cultivation under anaerobic conditions, the concentration of ^{137}Cs was measured in both bacterial cells and the media, as described above. To confirm the K concentration in the medium used, a LAQUA Twin Compact Water Quality Meter (HORIBA Ltd., Kyoto, Japan) was used according to the provided protocols.

20.2.5 Statistical Analysis

Data were expressed as mean ± standard deviation. Differences in the uptake ratio of ^{137}Cs in media with or without K^+ were analyzed with the two-way analysis of variance (ANOVA). Furthermore, for significance tests, the Turkey-Kramer test was used among strains, and the Student's t test was used between media with and without K^+ addition. If $p < 0.05$, the difference was considered significant.

20.3   Results and Discussion

20.3.1   Absorption or Uptake of Radioactive Cesium

Recently, many papers evaluating the excretion of ^{137}Cs have been published. Table 20.1 lists intestinal, probiotic and environmental bacteria that have been reported to be able to active uptake radioactive Cs [6, 11–14]. In Table 20.2, some chemical absorbents are listed [15–20].

We tried to examine the possibility of improving ^{137}Cs excretion from farm animals and humans using intestinal bacteria [6]. Bacteria take up radioactive Cs through their metabolic system. Althogh their capacity for uptake of radioactive Cs differs depending on genera and species, bacteria are well suited to promoting excretion of radioactive Cs because they activate their metabolic systems.

Candidate chemical adsorbents of radioactive Cs were ammonium–ferric ferro-cyanide (AFCF), zeolite, Prussian blue (PB), activated charcoal (AC), and others (Table 20.2). These chemical adsorbents, such as AFCF, have been used for broiler chicks [15] and farm animals [16–19]. PB is one of the Cs adsorbents used for radioactive Cs decontamination, and it has been reported to be useful for cows [19, 20]. We tried to measure the absorption percentage using the same process applied

Table 20.1   Potential bacterial biosorbents for radioactive Cs.

Material	Function	Target for	Effects	Reference
Intestinal bacteria	Uptake	Farm animals and humans	Accumulation of ^{137}Cs in the bacterial body	[6] This review
Probiotic bacteria	Uptake	Farm animals and humans	Accumulation of ^{137}Cs in the bacterial body	This review
Environmental bacteria	Uptake	Environment	Accumulation of radioactive Cs in the bacterial body	[11, 12]
Environmental and intestinal bacteria	Absorption	Environment and human	Reduction of radioactive Cs in the environment	[13]
Probiotic bacteria	Absorption	Human	Use of non-radioactive Cs. Possibility of reduction of radioactive Cs in the body	[14]

Table 20.2   Potential chemical adsorbents for radioactive Cs.

Material	Function	Usage for	Effects	Reference
AFCF and clinoptilolite	Absorption	Broiler chicks	Reduction of ^{137}Cs	[15]
Boli with AFCF	Absorption	Farm animals	Reduction of ^{137}Cs	[16]
AFCF, other ferric ferrocyanide	Absorption	Farm animals	Reduction and inhibition of the incorporation of ^{137}Cs	[17, 18]
PB, AFCF, others	Absorption	Cow	Reduction of radioactive Cs	[19, 20]

AFCF Ammonium–ferric ferrocyanide, *PB* Prussian blue

to bacteria by using BHI medium. Instead of bacteria, PB or activated charcoal (200 mg) was spread on the agar medium with various concentrations of K^+. PB absorption percentages were 8, 16, 13 and 15% in BHI medium with K^+ concentrations of 200, 500, 1,000 and 1,500 ppm, respectively. AC absorption percentages were 7.7, 8.2, 8.5, and 7.2% in medium with K^+ concentrations of 200, 500, 1,000 and 1,500 ppm, respectively.

20.3.2 Uptake of ^{137}Cs by Intestinal Bacteria

The uptake rate was defined as the radioactivity in the bacterial suspension divided by the total radioactivity (bacterial suspension plus medium) expressed as a percentage (uptake %). Analysis revealed that the bacterial suspension had a higher ^{137}Cs concentration than the medium. While ^{137}Cs uptake was observed across all tested strains, the uptake ratio varied significantly by species, with *B. vulgatus* exhibiting the highest accumulation efficiency. Statistically significant differences between the species are summarized in Table 20.3.

In the blank control, the amount of ^{137}Cs extracted by water was less compared to the bacterial uptake. The uptake % ranged from 45.0 to 81.2 when BHI medium was used for the assay, supporting that intestinal bacteria take up ^{137}Cs. Given the high density of viable bacteria typically present in feces, it is possible that the uptake of ^{137}Cs by intestinal bacteria is related to its high distribution in feces. It has been demonstrated that the concentration of ^{137}Cs in feces is higher than in ruminal contents [6]. This result is likely due to the intestinal bacteria taking up ^{137}Cs and subsequently secreting it into the intestinal tract, and then excreting it through the feces. Therefore, these findings emphasize that feces is the major route of ^{137}Cs excretion in bovine physiology.

Table 20.3 Uptake of ^{137}Cs in intestinal bacteria grown on BHI medium with low and high concentrations of K^+.

Bacteria used	K^+ ion content[a]	Bacteria (Bq/kg)	BHI medium (Bq/kg)	Uptake %[b]
B. fragilis	Low	9 ± 1	4 ± 2	70.9 ± 1.2
	High	33 ± 2	101 ± 3	24.5 ± 0.6[c]
B. vulgates	Low	11 ± 1	3 ± 2	81.2 ± 1.2
	High	30 ± 2	103 ± 3	22.3 ± 0.4[c]
C. perfringens	Low	10 ± 2	12 ± 4	45.0 ± 2.8
	High	27 ± 2	103 ± 4	21.0 ± 0.6[c]
C. ramosum	Low	9 ± 1	3 ± 2	74.8 ± 1.1
	High	29 ± 1	102 ± 4	22.0 ± 0.5[c]

[a]Low: 2×10^2 ppm (non-supplement BHI); High 1.5×10^3 ppm (BHI added K_2HPO_4)
[b]The main effect for both strains and concentration, and the interaction are significant [Strains $F_{(4, 20)} = 37.10$, $p < 0.01$, Concentration $F_{(1, 20)} = 1094.37$, $p < 0.01$, Interaction $F_{(4, 20)} = 243.10$, $p < 0.01$]
[c]Significant differences compared with the group of media without added K^+ ($p < 0.01$)

We thought that intestinal bacteria are able to trap ^{137}Cs and the uptake ratio differs among the bacterial species depending on the balance between intake and excretion. Due to their nature as alkali metal congeners, uptake of ^{137}Cs and K$^+$ occurs through the Na$^+$/K$^+$ pump located on the cell membrane [5, 21]. *Bacteroides* species and *C. ramosum* showed high uptake ratios. Uptake ratio of radioactive Cs in *C. perfringens* was significantly lower than that of others ($p < 0.01$). This could be related to the structure of the bacterial surface layers and metabolic system.

In addition, it was reported by Kato et al. [9] that *Bacteroidetes* and *Flavobacterium* spp. appear to have significant tolerance to high concentrations of Cs$^+$. Therefore, it is thought that *B. fragilis* and *B. vulgatus* are able to accumulate ^{137}Cs actively. We demonstrated that intestinal bacteria contribute to ^{137}Cs excretion in the host. K$^+$ transporter can help to excrete ^{137}Cs.

20.3.3   Inhibition of ^{137}Cs$^+$ Uptake by K$^+$ Ion in Intestinal Bacteria

^{137}Cs uptake rate of the intestinal bacteria was lower in the supplemented medium (high concentration of K$^+$, final concentration the same as MRS medium) than in the non-supplemented BHI (low concentration of K$^+$) ($P < 0.01$). The addition of K$^+$ to the medium significantly inhibited ^{137}Cs$^+$ uptake, decreasing it from 45.0–81.2% to 21.0–24.5% (Table 20.3). These results indicated that the uptake of ^{137}Cs could be inhibited by an increase of the K$^+$ concentration in the medium.

This further suggests that the uptake of ^{137}Cs$^+$ is mediated by a K$^+$ transporter system. It has been reported that ^{137}Cs uptake in soil bacteria is inhibited by K$^+$ in soil in a dose-dependent manner [22]. In the intestine, Cs uptake can be inhibited in a K$^+$ concentration-dependent manner.

20.3.4   Uptake of Radioactive Cs by B. longum

B. longum, an excellent colonizer, is one of the most common bifidobacteria present in the gastrointestinal tracts. The significance of *Bifidobacterium* to human health can be appreciated from its early colonization of the neonatal gut [23]. Several *B. longum* strains have thus been developed as probiotics [23, 24]. *B. longum* is a unique bacterium because it is not only an intestinal bacterium but also a probiotic bacterium.

As shown in Fig. 20.2, radioactive ^{134}Cs and ^{137}Cs were detected in *B. longum*. Natural ^{208}Tl and ^{214}Bi were also detected in the bacteria and the medium. The uptake ratio is 37.8 ± 1%. The total volume of the medium was 20 ml, while the bacterial cell mass was 30–100 mg on the agar plate. This means that the bacteria have a strong ability to take up radioactive Cs. *B. longum* showed a significant increase of Cs uptake from 37.8 ± 1.3 to 59.5 ± 1.4% after the addition of K$^+$ (final

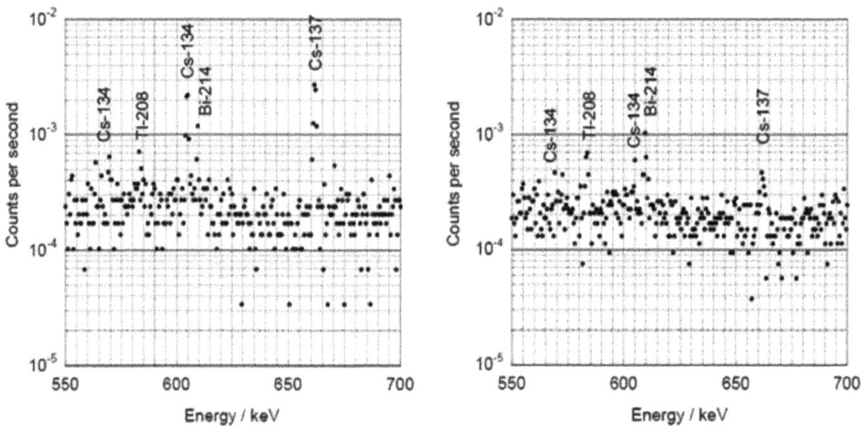

Fig. 20.2 Detection of radioactive Cs in *B. longum* after cultivation. Left: agar medium without bacteria. Right: bacterial cells. Tl-208 (^{208}Tl) and Bi-214 (^{214}Bi) are naturally occurring radioactive nuclides.

concentration 1.5×10^3 ppm) ($P < 0.01$). It is thought that K^+ is an essential element for bacteria. In various bacteria, K^+ is required for the activity of the ribosome and a lot of enzymes [25].

No detection of radioactive Cs was recognized in the heat-killed bacteria, indicating that the bacteria should be alive.

20.3.5   Uptake of Radioactive Cs by Probiotic Bacteria

Common probiotic bacteria could not grow in BHI medium. When MRS medium was used for their growth, Cs uptake was observed in the probiotic bacteria such as *B. longum* (68.7%), *B. breve* (34.5%), *L. casei* (33.0%), *L. bulgaricus* (35.3%), and *L. gasseri* (28.7%) (Table 20.4). The concentration of K^+ in BHI, MRS, and RSM was about 2×10^2 ppm, 1.5×10^3 ppm and 7×10^2 ppm, respectively. It was considered that the uptake of radioactive Cs was inhibited by K^+. We tried to show high uptake using a low K^+ concentration medium (RSM, similar K ion concentration to BHI medium) for probiotic bacteria. The uptake percentage was 34.0 in *B. longum*, 41.3 in *B. breve*, 82.9 in *L. casei*, 51.3 in *L. bulgaricus*, and 35.7 in *L. gasseri*. In some strains, the uptake was clearly increased by using RSM ($p < 0.01$). Furthermore, the uptake was decreased to 27.7% in *B. longum*, 31.5% in *B. breve*, 33.0% in *L. casei*, and 29.8% in *L. bulgaricus* when RSM supplemented with K (K+ ion: 1.5×10^3 ppm) was used compared with RSM. On the other hand, the uptake was increased to 75.9% in *L. gasseri* compared with RSM.

Table 20.4 Uptake of ^{137}Cs in probiotic bacteria grown on MRS or RSM.

Strain	Medium[a]	Bacteria (Bq/kg)	Medium (Bq/kg)	Uptake %[b]
B. longum	MRS	110 ± 4.1	50 ± 3.9	68.7 ± 0.9
	RSM	97 ± 3.7	188 ± 4.2	34.0 ± 0.4*
	RSM + K	69 ± 3.3	180 ± 5.2	27.7 ± 0.4*
B. breve	MRS	140 ± 5.2	266 ± 4.1	34.5 ± 0.5
	RSM	140 ± 3.6	199 ± 3.2	41.3 ± 0.2*
	RSM + K	86 ± 4.0	187 ± 4.4	31.5 ± 0.5*
L. casei	MRS	101 ± 2.1	205 ± 3.0	33.0 ± 0.1
	RSM	890 ± 4.5	184 ± 4.1	82.9 ± 0.3*
	RSM + K	127 ± 3.5	258 ± 5.9	33.0 ± 0.1
L. bulgaricus	MRS	128 ± 3.6	234 ± 5.0	35.3 ± 0.6
	RSM	250 ± 2.9	237 ± 3.8	51.3 ± 0.1*
	RSM + K	95 ± 4.2	223 ± 4.5	29.8 ± 0.5*
L. gasseri	MRS	109 ± 4.3	272 ± 8.3	28.7 ± 0.2
	RSM	151 ± 6.3	273 ± 5.6	35.7 ± 0.5*
	RSM + K	150 ± 5.3	48 ± 3.2	75.9 ± 0.6*

[a]K^+ concentration: MRS; 1.5×10^3 ppm, Skim milk 7×10^2 ppm, RSM 1.5×10^3 ppm
[b]*indicates significant differences compared to growth in MRS medium at $P < 0.01$, as calculated by Dunnett's test
Abbreviations: *RSM + K* supplemented RSM with K ions

In conclusion, we demonstrated that intestinal bacteria contribute to elimination of ^{137}Cs from the body. During the digestive process, ^{137}Cs is not only absorbed into the blood but also taken up by intestinal bacteria and subsequently discharged via the fecal route. Uptake of radioactive Cs by probiotic bactera is useful for elmination of the materials.

References

1. Yasunari TJ, Andreas S, Ryugo SH et al (2011) Cesium-137 deposition and contamination of Japanese soils due the Fukushima nuclear accident. Proc Natl Acad Sci USA 108:19530–19534. https://doi.org/10.1073/pnas.1112058108
2. Manabe N, Takahashi T, Li J et al (2013) Changes in the transfer of fallout radiocaesium from pasture harvested in Ibaraki prefecture, Japan, to cow milk two months after the Fukushima Daiichi nuclear power plant accident. In: Nakanisi TM, Tanoi K (eds) Agricultural implications of the Fukushima nuclear accident. Springer, Tokyo, pp 87–95. https://doi.org/10.1007/978-4-431-54328-2_9
3. Hosono H, Kumagai Y, Sekizaki T (2013) Development of an information package of radiation risk of beef after the Fukushima Daiichi nuclear power plant accident. In: Nakanisi TM, Tanoi K (eds) Agricultural implications of the Fukushima nuclear accident. Springer, Tokyo, pp 187–204. https://doi.org/10.1007/978-4-431-54328-2_17
4. Fukuda T, Kino Y, Abe Y et al (2013) Distribution of artificial radionuclides in abandoned cattle in the evacuation zone of the Fukushima Daiichi Nuclear Power Plant. PLoS One 8:e54312. https://doi.org/10.1371/journal.pone.0054312

5. Leggett RW, Williams LR, Melo DR et al (2003) A physiologically based biokinetic model for cesium in the human body. Sci Total Environ 317:235–255. https://doi.org/10.1016/S0048-9697(03)00333-4

6. Saito K, Kuroda K, Suzuki R et al (2019) Intestinal bacteria as powerful trapping lifeforms for the elimination of radioactive cesium. Front Vet Sci 12(6):70. https://doi.org/10.3389/fvets.2019.00070

7. Garrett WS, Gordon JI, Glimcher LH (2010) Homeostasis and inflammation in the intestine. Cell 140:859–870. https://doi.org/10.1016/j.cell.2010.01.023

8. Lebeer S, Vanderleyden J, de Keersmaecker SC (2008) Genes and molecules of lactobacilli supporting probiotic action. Microbiol Mol Biol Rev 72:728–764. https://doi.org/10.1128/MMBR.00017-08

9. Mazziotta C, Tognon M, Martini F et al (2023) Probiotics mechanism of action on immune cells and beneficial effects on human health. Cells 12:184. https://doi.org/10.3390/cells12010184

10. Hill C, Guarner F, Reid G et al (2014) The International Scientific Association for Probiotics and Prebiotics consensus statement on the scope and appropriate use of the term probiotic. Nat Rev Gastroenterol Hepatol 11:506–514. https://doi.org/10.1038/nrgastro.2014.66

11. Avery SV (1995) Caesium accumulation by microorganisms: uptake mechanisms, cation competition, compartmentalization and toxicity. J Ind Microbiol 14:76–84. https://doi.org/10.1007/BF01569888

12. Gadd GM (1996) Influence of microorganisms on the environmental fate of radionuclides. Endeavour 20:150–156. https://doi.org/10.1016/s0160-9327(96)10021-1

13. Kato S, Goya E, Tanaka M et al (2016) Enrichment and isolation of *Flavobacterium* strains with tolerance to high concentrations of cesium ion. Sci Rep 6:20041. https://doi.org/10.1038/srep20041

14. Kinoshita H, Sato Y, Ohtake F et al (2015) In vitro mass-screening of lactic acid bacteria as potential biosorbents of cesium and strontium. J Microbiol Biotechnol Food Sci 4:383–386. https://doi.org/10.15414/jmbfs.2015.4.5.383-386

15. Mitrović BM, Vitorović G, Vićentijević M et al (2012) Comparative study of (137)Cs distribution in broilers and pheasants and possibilities for protection. Radiat Environ Biophys 5:79–84. https://doi.org/10.1007/s00411-011-0391-8

16. Hove K (1993) Chemical methods for reduction of the transfer of radionuclides to farm animals in semi-natural environments. Sci Total Environ 137:235–248. https://doi.org/10.1016/0048-9697(93)90391-i

17. Voigt G (1993) Chemical methods to reduce the radioactive contamination of animals and their products in agricultural ecosystems. Sci Total Environ 137:205–225. https://doi.org/10.1016/0048-9697(93)90389-n

18. Voigt G, Müller H, Paretzke HG et al (1993) ^{137}Cs transfer after Chernobyl from fodder into chicken meat and eggs. Health Phys 65:141–146. https://doi.org/10.1097/00004032-199308000-00002

19. Arnaud MJ, Clement C, Getaz F et al (1988) Synthesis, effectiveness and metabolic fate in cows of the caesium complexing compound ammonium ferric hexacyanoferrate labelled with ^{14}C. J Dairy Res 55:1–13. https://doi.org/10.1017/S0022029900025796

20. Unsworth EF, Pearce J, McMurray CH et al (1989) Investigations of the use of clay minerals and prussian blue in reducing the transfer of dietary radiocaesium to milk. Sci Total Environ 85:339–347. https://doi.org/10.1016/0048-9697(89)90333-1

21. Peluffo RD, Hernández JA (2023) The Na^+, K^+-ATPase and its stoichiometric ratio: some thermodynamics speculations. Biophys Rev 15:539–552. https://doi.org/10.1007/s12551-023-01082-5

22. Zhang P, Idota Y, Yano K et al (2014) Characterization of cesium uptake mediated by a potassium transport system of bacteria in a soil conditioner. Biol Pharm Bull 37:604–607. https://doi.org/10.1248/bpb.b13-00871
23. Mills S, Yang B, Smith GJ et al (2023) Efficacy of Bifidobacterium longum alone or in-multi strain probiotic formulation during early life and beyond. Gut Microbes 15:2186098. https://doi.org/10.1080/19490976.2023.2186098
24. FAO/WHO. Food and Agriculture Organization and World Health Organization Expert Consultation. Evaluation of health and nutritional properties of powder milk and live lactic acid bacteria. [Internet]. Available from: http://www.fao.org/tempref/docrep/fao/meeting/009/y6398e.pdf
25. Gundlach J, Herzberg C, Hertel D et al (2017) Adaptation of *Bacillus subtilis* to life at extreme potassium limitation. MBio 8:e00861–17. https://doi.org/10.1128/mBio.00861-17

GPSR Compliance
The European Union's (EU) General Product Safety Regulation (GPSR) is a set
of rules that requires consumer products to be safe and our obligations to
ensure this.

If you have any concerns about our products, you can contact us on

ProductSafety@springernature.com

In case Publisher is established outside the EU, the EU authorized
representative is:

Springer Nature Customer Service Center GmbH
Europaplatz 3
69115 Heidelberg, Germany

www.ingramcontent.com/pod-product-compliance
Ingram Content Group UK Ltd.
Pitfield, Milton Keynes, MK11 3LW, UK
UKHW021012080726
473054UK00003B/76